Public Health Branding
Applying Marketing for Social Change

Edited by

W. Douglas Evans
Professor and Director of Public Health Communication and
Marketing, The George Washington University,
Washington, DC, USA

Gerard Hastings
Professor and Director of the Institute for Social Marketing and
the Centre for Tobacco Control Research,
University of Stirling and
The Open University, Stirling, UK

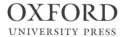

OXFORD
UNIVERSITY PRESS

OXFORD
UNIVERSITY PRESS

Great Clarendon Street, Oxford OX2 6DP

Oxford University Press is a department of the University of Oxford.
It furthers the University's objective of excellence in research, scholarship,
and education by publishing worldwide in

Oxford New York

Auckland Cape Town Dar es Salaam Hong Kong Karachi
Kuala Lumpur Madrid Melbourne Mexico City Nairobi
New Delhi Shanghai Taipei Toronto

With offices in

Argentina Austria Brazil Chile Czech Republic France Greece
Guatemala Hungary Italy Japan Poland Portugal Singapore
South Korea Switzerland Thailand Turkey Ukraine Vietnam

Oxford is a registered trade mark of Oxford University Press
in the UK and in certain other countries

Published in the United States
by Oxford University Press Inc., New York

A catalogue record for this title is available from the British Library

Data available

Library of Congress Cataloging-in-Publication Data

Public health branding: applying marketing for social change / edited by
W. Douglas Evans, Gerard Hastings.
    P. ; cm.
  Includes bibliograhical references and index.
  ISBN 978-0-19-923713-5 (alk. paper)
1. Public health—Marketing. I. Evans, W. Douglas. II. Hastings, Gerard.
  [DNLM: 1. Marketing of Health Services. 2. Public Health. 3. Advertising as
Topic. 4. Health Promotion. 5. Persuasive Communication. WA 100 P97683 2008]
  RA427.P82 2008
  362.1068'8—dc22
2008027677

Typeset by Cepha Imaging Private Ltd., Bangalore, India
Printed in Great Britain
on acid-free paper by
Biddles Ltd., King's Lynn, Norfolk

ISBN 978-0-19-923713-5

10 9 8 7 6 5 4 3 2 1

Foreword

Although branding has become a management priority for many top organizations, some people still wonder about the scope of branding. In what areas does branding apply? Just how pervasive is it? In my opinion, whenever and wherever people have choices, branding can matter. In choice settings, brands offer clarity and meaning to different alternatives under consideration. As it turns out, perhaps no choices are more important than those involved with public health. Choices in this domain are literally life or death.

Despite that sobering reality, there has been surprisingly little academic research that formally addresses public health branding. Although branding notions would seem to clearly apply, the recognition and adoption of branding principles is just now emerging in the public health arena. Scholars and managers have begun to delve into how to best design and implement marketing and branding concepts to improve public health. The good news is that – as is the case with virtually any branding application – basic branding principles apply to public health too.

Branding is all about creating awareness and image for an entity. In a fundamental sense, branding involves attaching a 'label' (for identification) and 'meaning' (for understanding) to a product, service, person, idea, etc. An individual must know what a brand is, what it is about and, most importantly, why that brand is or could be relevant for him or her. The brand itself is made up of different elements – a name, logo, slogan, or any other trademarkable information that can be used to facilitate identification and differentiation.

Positioning the brand is crucial in terms of ensuring that people understand the similarities and differences between the brand and related, possibly competing brands. What associations to the brand are or should be unique and which ones are or should be shared with other brands? Establishing that positioning depends on a host of different types of marketing activities. For example, brand-building communications may involve paid print or broadcast media, on-line or off-line social networks and word-of-mouth, PR and public relations, among other communication options.

Public health marketers have begun to use all these strategies and tactics in their attempts to influence socially desirable behaviors. They have labeled behaviors, crafted messages, and offered slogans to help people comprehend the medical and health consequences of what they should or should not do. They have done so by assuming, at least implicitly, that the most compelling competitive brand is the direct alternative to the proposed behavioral action in terms of inaction or existing behaviors, or vice-versa as the case may be.

At the same time – as is also the case with virtually any branding application – there are unique aspects of the public health setting that require some special consideration and thought. With public health, the brand is really about a health-related behavioral change, e.g., 'stopping smoking,' 'getting exercise,' or 'eating right.' A key challenge in public health branding is thus creating clearly defined brands for potentially fairly broad and complicated concepts. Public health marketers must decide what labels and meaning should be connected to desired, or even undesired behaviors, as well as to the personal or social costs and benefits that result from those behaviors.

For example, 'staying sober' may be used to brand a series of behaviors, and meaning may be attached to it by identifying relevant benefits. This brand may be reinforced by a symbol (e.g., a cocktail glass and/or needle within a circle and diagonal line to suggest 'no'), a slogan (e.g., 'Stay Smart. Stay Sober.' Or 'Live for Tomorrow.'), or other brand elements. The desired behavior of 'staying sober' may involve a number of more specific actions or behaviors such as: 1) avoiding potentially tempting people or situations or 2) engaging in rewarding, healthy behaviors through diet, exercise, and so on. These more specific behaviors could be branded in a way to identify and link them together, e.g., 'Act Right,' 'Eat Right,' and 'Exercise Right.' By branding these specific behaviors, they may become more salient and meaningful, making it easier for individuals to achieve the overall behavioral objectives.

Creating brand equity for a set of positive behaviors thus involves defining the desired behaviors in terms of carefully selected words, phrases, or images and then making sure that individuals can 'feel good' about doing the 'right thing' by understanding and appreciating the benefits they accrue from behavioral changes. The challenge is that the benefits individuals receive in return for these behavioral changes may be fairly intangible and seemingly removed, especially with respect to the more immediate benefits they might receive in exchange for engaging in undesirable behaviors.

One function that branding may be able to provide in public health marketing programs is to help individuals to communicate and signal to themselves, as well as to others, that they are engaging in desirable behaviors so that they are better able to realize more immediate benefits and receive positive reinforcement. For example, by displaying visible symbols or by describing themselves with a categorical label that, in either case, contains specific meaning with respect to a public health issue, individuals may be better able to achieve greater immediate satisfaction if they feel they have been 'credited' or acknowledged as having avoided undesirable behaviors or having embraced desirable behaviors.

The clear goal of public health branding is ultimately to change behavior and produce a more favorable human and financial cost-benefit. Behavioral change, however, is often preceded by perceptual and attitudinal shifts. In particular, to initiate behavioral change, public health branding may need to tap into powerful emotions as people see the positive consequences of behavioral change for self-esteem, social approval, and other behavior inducing feelings.

There are so many fascinating aspects to public health branding. The exciting part is that it is blossoming just as a new era in branding has emerged in the 21st century. Technological advances now allow for interactive and individualized messages of all forms.

More attention is being paid than ever before to corporate social responsibility and the role of the firm in improving the natural environment, local communities and social welfare as a whole. While corporate motivations vary from true interest in public health and welfare to mere public relations, these efforts can contribute to the success of public health brands. For example, via the internet, individuals can learn from and teach others and express their commitment to enact behavioral change and observe the successful changes of others. Corporate social responsibility can reinforce public health brands and help to create a social environment conducive to health behavior change.

The timing of this set of readings could not be better. The diverse chapters in this compilation are noteworthy in that they provide important insight and advances into both the theory and practice of public health branding. Public health branding will undoubtedly make tremendous strides in the coming years, and these readings can help to serve as an impetus for that progress.

Kevin Lane Keller
E.B. Osborn Professor of Marketing
Tuck School of Business at Dartmouth
March 2008

Preface

Introduction

Over a decade ago, an editorial in the journal *Tobacco Control* posed the question: 'What is the best known word in the world: Sex? Life? Death? Jesus?' 'No', came the answer, 'it's Coca-Cola'. This, the authors argued, was an impressive tribute to the power of branding, and that any attempts to tackle youth smoking would need to take on the tobacco brands.

This book picks up the baton, arguing that not only should public health challenge unhealthy brands, it should also develop its own healthy ones. It argues that by learning about concepts such as brand development, identity and equity we can do for public health what Philip Morris has done for teen smoking. This book brings together both theoretical learning and practical experience of public health branding from around the world, and demonstrates how one of the most powerful tools of marketing is being successfully adopted and deployed. It also looks towards the future, highlighting key challenges and mapping out the research agenda.

With luck, in future years Philip Morris will look enviously at public health, seeking to learn how it has developed such successful brands. And the best known word in the world will be 'health'.

Purpose and objectives of this book

Brands build relationships between consumers and products, services or lifestyles by providing beneficial exchanges and adding value to their objects. Brands can be measured through associations that consumers hold for products and services. Through brand promotion, these associations can become established and lead to a long-term relationship between the product or service and consumer. Similarly, public health brands are the associations that individuals hold for health behaviors or lifestyles that embody multiple health behaviors. Brands in both sectors can also apply to organizations, and upstream factors that promote organizational impact and wellbeing. Public health branding – building positive associations with healthy behaviors and lifestyle choices – is the primary strategy by which commercial marketing is applied in health communication and social marketing.

In the context of branding health behaviors, the purpose of this book is to examine the specific tactics and evidence of effectiveness of commercial marketing applied in public health programs. Through a series of evidence and practice reviews and case studies, the book argues that branding is a relatively new public health strategy that needs significant investment of resources and continued development of innovative methodologies to effect lasting population-level change. In recent years, public health branding has been successfully applied across a wide range of chronic and infectious disease issues and behaviors – from tobacco control to HIV/AIDS – and globally across the developed and developing world. Branding is critically important in public health because, very often, multiple behaviors need to be changed and maintained in order to have lasting health outcome benefits. Such behavior change can be more difficult than in product marketing and consumer choice, thus making the development of improved branding strategies a critical objective for public health.

Rationale for the book: why it is needed?

The translation and application of commercial marketing strategies into public health is the most important overall trend in social marketing. As discussed in the introductory chapter, recent writings on social marketing document the process of adapting commercial marketing approaches in social marketing, and the central role that such approaches now play. In public health, branding is one of the primary mechanisms for this translation and application. At the time of this writing, there is no book in print on the subject. Thus the time is right to examine how this field has adapted, changed, and in some ways expanded beyond the methods and purposes of commercial branding.

Audience

The primary audience for the book will be public health professionals, health communicators and social marketers, and researchers working in these fields. The intended audience is professionals who design, implement and study programs in health communication and social marketing. It will also be a useful book for advanced (postgraduate level) courses in public health, social marketing and related social science disciplines such as social psychology.

Additionally, the book will be of interest to business professionals and commercial marketers interested in 'cause marketing' (i.e. marketing to promote socially beneficial causes), corporate responsibility, and business philanthropy. If the reader already has commercial marketing knowledge, then the book will help in understanding marketing for social and health promotion purposes. It will demonstrate how knowledge about branding products like cigarettes, automobiles or shoes can be applied to branding health behaviors like responsible driving, avoiding tobacco use, or safer sex – and the ways in which branding strategies can be adapted to these ends. It will also address challenging questions about marketing and corporate responsibility. Should marketers promote products that kill one in two of their most loyal customers? Should McDonald's bear any responsibility for the obesity epidemic? This book can both help find the answers and provide solutions.

Scope

The book will review and clarify the concepts of branding, brand development and identification, and the higher-order concept of brand equity from the commercial marketing literature. It will then define public health branding and how this concept has been translated to date from the commercial world. The book will then address how commercial marketing has been translated and applied in public health communication and social marketing under the overarching strategy of branding. It will unpack specific commercial marketing tactics using case studies of public health programs. Case studies will cover a wide range of topics in public health – such as tobacco, drug and alcohol use, obesity, HIV/ADS, and reproductive health – to demonstrate the wide application of branding and related commercial marketing strategies. They will also include examples worldwide, including social marketing activities in Europe, the USA, and other parts of the developed world, as well as South Asia, Africa and other parts of the developing world. This will demonstrate the many and varied social, economic and cultural contexts in which marketing principles based on branding can be applied.

Major themes

Several major themes emerge from reflections on commercial and public health branding. The remainder of this volume addresses these themes in the context of underlying theory and case studies of specific branded health campaigns. Many of these themes converge and overlap, and each of the specific chapters attempts to identify these convergences and their potential significance for future public health brands and research on their effectiveness.

   The book is organized into three parts, reflecting the current state of research and marketing practice on public health branding. Part I focuses on theoretical foundations, including the basic concepts of branding, similarities and differences between commercial and public health branding, and theories of exposure, messaging, marketing, and behavior change that are typically used to develop and promote brands. Part II presents a series of case studies of major public health brands from across the world. This section describes the strategies underlying major brands in tobacco control, nutrition and physical activity, HIV/AIDS, and other topics. Part III focuses on the basic principles and practice of public health branding. Here we address a number of practical considerations in how public health brands can and have been developed and promoted, in addition to issues and challenges facing the field in various public health topics and global settings.

Part I

Part I focuses on theory and conceptual foundations, identifying the major themes described below.

Defining terms: what is public health branding? In Chapter 1, by Douglas Evans and Gerard Hastings, the authors describe basic concepts from commercial branding, and how those concepts have been translated into public health. The chapter compares commercial and public health branding approaches, and makes a broad distinction between the two domains of branding based on different purposes (selling products and services versus social benefit) and outcomes (purchasing versus improved health outcomes). However, through a series of examples, the chapter argues that while there are differences between the two sectors in terms of the value exchange between brand and consumer, the intervening marketing approaches to branding are quite similar.

Chapter 2, by Jonathan L. Blitstein, Douglas Evans, and David L. Driscoll picks up on the preliminary discussion in Chapter 1 on branding principles, theory, and strategies used to build commercial and public health brands, and how public health branding borrows from and is distinct from commercial strategies. For example, Chapter 2 asks the key question for public health campaigns: when is a public health message branded? Many social marketing campaigns seek to change behavior without branding their messages. What are the distinctive characteristics of branded health messages?

Psychological, communication and marketing theory and the research methods underlying branding Chapter 3, by Douglas Evans, Jonathan L. Blitstein, and James C. Hersey on the evaluation of brands, explores major behavioral precursors, such as attitudes and beliefs (e.g. perceived attributes) that are associated with brand exposure, as well as behavioral reactions (e.g. loyalty). This chapter examines major theoretical perspectives, such as social cognitive theory and the theory of planned behavior, that suggest mechanisms by which brand equity may influence health behavior. Chapter 3 also reviews methods to evaluate public health brands and theoretical and conceptual foundations for evaluating a brand's impact, such as message reaction and exposure theory, which explain immediate reactions to branded messages, and are associated with subsequent cognitive and emotional reactions and ultimately behavior.

Competition between commercial and public health brands Chapter 4, by Ross Gordon, Gerard Hastings, Laura McDermott and Douglas Evans, builds on the discussion in the preceding chapter and explores the purposes and methods of commercial and public health brands, and where they are in competition. Commercial brands can, and in many stark examples such as the tobacco industry, do have clear-cut profit motives that are contrary to public health. How are we to reconcile these tensions? How can public health brands learn from but also remain socially responsible in their competition with commercial brands?

Part II

Part II focuses on case studies and application of branding in public health. The chapters build upon the theory and conceptual foundations laid in Part I, and illustrate how major campaigns in the USA, Europe and Australia have conceptualized behavior change branding, implemented brand promotion efforts, and evaluated outcomes.

Countermarketing (oppositional) brands Chapter 5, by Gerard Hastings, Jo Freeman Renata Spackova, and Pierre Siquier, describes the European Commission's *Help* anti-smoking campaign, and how it is gradually developing into a multinational public health brand to rival those of the hazard merchants. Chapter 6, by Marian Huhman, Simani Price, and Lance D. Potter describes the *VERB, It's What You Do* physical activity brand. While not an oppositional brand, *VERB* has worked to counter media messages promoting sedentary behavior by branding sports and physical activity as cool, fun and exhilarating. Chapter 7, by Matthew C. Farrelly and Kevin C. Davis, discusses tobacco countermarketing campaigns, and their use of oppositional marketing strategies to go head-to-head with tobacco industry brands. Chapter 8, by Lela Jacobsohn and Robert Hornik, discusses the US Office of National Drug Control Policy anti-drug brand, the largest ever anti-drug marketing campaign, with a budget of over US$1 billion from 1998 to 2003. Jacobsohn and Hornik describe how it successfully built brand awareness, yet failed to achieve behavior change, meaning that it effectively promised without delivering. Chapter 8 also describes lessons for future public health brands.

Cultural, community, and individual differences in brand reactions Chapter 9, by Michael L. Hecht and Jeong Kyu Lee, explores community and cultural factors in creating public health brands, specifically in substance abuse. This chapter also contrasts the social elements of branding with the individual psychological elements discussed in Chapters 1 and 3.

Use of multiple brand promotion strategies In Chapter 10, on branding Down Under, Robert J. Donovan and Tom E. Carroll describe two major Australian public health brands: the *Freedom From Fear* campaign, which encourages men who use violence against their partners to voluntarily seek help to cease their violence; and the *Act-Belong-Commit* mental health promotion campaign, which aims to inform people of what they can and should do to maintain and strengthen their mental health. This chapter describes the brands underlying these campaigns and their promotion through multiple channels including mass media and community-based partnerships.

Part III

In Part III, which focuses on principles and practice of public health branding, the chapters focus on message strategies, global contexts, and limitations and future applications of public health branding.

Branding in global contexts In Chapter 11, Douglas Evans and Muhiuddin Haider describe a number public health brands from the developing world, including the *loveLife*, *Salama* and *Trust* HIV/AIDS prevention campaigns in Africa. They discuss specific strategies, challenges and evaluation findings, as well as distinctions between public health brands in developed and developing world contexts, such as social influences/context, media use/sources, and competition between public health brands and negative health influences, including commercial brands.

In Chapter 12, Muhiuddin Haider and Michelle J. Lee discuss branding of international public health organizations. They describe the organizational structures, processes and cultures to allocate brand-building resources globally, to create global synergies, and to develop a brand strategy that coordinates and leverages country brand strategies.

Message strategies Chapter 13, by Megan A. Lewis and Lauren A. McCormack, describes how tailored messaging strategies fit with branding strategies by helping to build brand equity. The authors describe the evidence for tailoring, providing examples of tailoring for specific cultural and individual differences. They go on to present the potential advantages over broader population-based communication strategies, discussing how tailoring and branding strategies can potentially work together and reinforce each other.

Social and ethical implications, limits, and appropriateness of branding In many cases, public health evidence is uncertain. In these situations, how should we proceed? In Chapter 14, Lauren A. McCormack, Megan A. Lewis and David Driscoll discuss the social and ethical implications, and potential limitations of branding in public health. They argue that branding, as a marketing technique, may not work as well when the clinical or public health evidence about the health topic is inconclusive and the message is complex (which is a growing phenomenon). They suggest some behavior change communication strategies that can serve as alternatives and complements to branding.

In Chapter 15, Douglas Evans and Gerard Hastings conclude the book with a discussion of where public health branding can go in the future, the impact of new media and technologies, including stealth and viral marketing strategies, and future research opportunities. They also build on the discussion of social and ethical issues, and potential limitations raised in Chapters 1 and 14. Overall, they conclude that public health branding is in its infancy but, with opportunities afforded by new media and increased public focus on health messages in the media, has tremendous potential to change public health practice for the better.

W. Douglas Evans

Contents

Contributors

Jonathan L. Blitstein
Research Psychologist, RTI International,
North Carolina, USA

Tom E. Carroll
Director, Carroll Communications,
Social Marketing and Research
Consultants, Adjunct Professor,
School of Public Health,
The University of Sydney,
Australia

Kevin C. Davis
Senior Research Analyst
RTI International, North Carolina, USA

Robert J. Donovan
Professor of Behavioural Research and
Director, Social Marketing Research Unit,
Curtin University, Perth,
Western Australia

David L. Driscoll
Professor and Director, Institute for
Circumpolar Health Studies, The
University of Alaska, Anchorage, AC, USA

W. Douglas Evans
Professor and Director of Public Health
Communication and Marketing,
The George Washington University,
Washington, DC, USA

Matthew C. Farrelly
Chief Scientist, Public Health Policy
Research Program, RTI International,
North Carolina, USA

Jo Freeman
Research Assistant,
Institute for Social Marketing,
University of Stirling, UK

Ross Gordon
Research Officer,
Institute for Social Marketing,
University of Stirling and The Open
University, Stirling, UK

Muhiuddin Haider
Associate Professor, School of Public
Health, University of Maryland, USA

Gerard Hastings
Professor and Director, Institute for Social
Marketing and the Centre for Tobacco
Control Research, University of Stirling
and The Open University, UK

Michael L. Hecht
Distinguished Professor, Communication
Arts and Sciences, The Pennsylvania State
University, Pennsylvania, USA

James C. Hersey
Principle Research Psychologist,
RTI International,
Washington, DC, USA

Robert C. Hornik
Wilbur Schramm Professor of
Communication and Health Policy,
Annenberg School for Communication,
University of Pennsylvania, Philadelphia,
PA, USA

Marian Huhman
Health Scientist,
Division of Adolescent and
School Health, Centers for Disease
Control and Prevention, Atlanta,
Georgia, USA

Lela Jacobsohn
Health Communication and Behavioral Scientist, Center for Injury Research and Prevention, Children's Hospital of Philadelphia, Philadelphia, PA, USA

Jeong Kyu Lee
Doctoral Student, Communication Arts and Sciences, Pennsylvania State University, Pennsylvania, USA

Michelle J. Lee
Strategic Information Assistant, Office of the US Global AIDS Coordinator, US Department of State, Washington, DC, USA

Megan A. Lewis
Senior Research Scientist, RTI International, North Carolina, USA

Lauren A. McCormack
Director, Health Communication Program, RTI International, North Carolina, USA

Laura McDermott
Research Officer, Institute for Social Marketing, University of Stirling and The Open University, Scotland, UK

Lance D. Potter
Senoir Study Director, Westat, Rockville, Maryland, USA

Simani M. Price
Senior Study Director, Westat, Rockville, Maryland, USA

Pierre Siquier
President, Ligaris, Paris, France

Renata Spackova
Account Director, Ligaris, Paris, France

Part I

Theory and conceptual foundations

1

Public health branding
Recognition, promise, and delivery of healthy lifestyles

W. Douglas Evans and Gerard Hastings

Summary

+ Brands in the commercial and public health sectors add value to the relationships between products or services and consumers.

+ Public health brands can be differentiated from commercial brands by their purposes (changing health behavior), nature of the exchange of value between brand and consumer, and outcomes (health behavior change).

+ Brands can apply 'upstream' – such as to organizations and government policies – as well as 'downstream' – to individual-level attitudes, beliefs and behavioral outcomes.

+ Branding is a global social marketing strategy that has demonstrated evidence of effectiveness across cultures, country settings and subject matter.

Introduction: what is a public health brand?

Basic notions from commercial branding

Commercial brands, and branding as a strategy to market products and services, are central to the global economy. Brands, recognition of brands, and the relationship between brand and consumer are essential to marketing and largely explain the tremendous success of product advertising and the growth of the global consumer economy since the early 20th Century. Brands have been defined as 'a set of associations linked to a name, mark, or symbol associated with a product or service' (Calkins 2005: 1). As this definition implies, the significance of brands is in the *associations* they represent, and the resulting behavior they can engender (e.g. buying a product, maintaining a relationship with the brand). In this respect, brands are very much like reputations – they precede the individual or organization and shape how the world responds.

Consider the example of Marlboro, one of the most successful brands of all time, and the leading brand of cigarettes worldwide. A report to Philip Morris (which subsequently became Altria) from marketing consultants Bruce Eckman, Inc. (1992) characterized the Marlboro brand as follows: 'All-American; hardworking/trustworthy; rugged individual, man's man (experienced, sure of self, confident, in charge, self-sufficient, down to earth, cool/calm, get the job done); admire his strength'. This reads very much like a desirable, masculine reputation – a kind of portrait or biographical sketch of a character – that many of us will likely admire and find socially desirable. That reputation is the basis for the associations Marlboro consumers may form with the brand, which in turn are the building blocks for the relationship between Marlboro and its consumers.

Given the proven harm caused by cigarette smoking, Marlboro's brand reputation may be entirely undeserved, but one has to admit it is a marvel of successful marketing. It is noteworthy that the Marlboro brand characteristics are quite separate from the physical product itself: they are marketing creations aimed at forming associations in the minds of consumers to build a relationship.

The associations consumers form with a brand – in the case of Marlboro mainly with notions of independence, strength and confidence – have both social and individual dimensions. Note that the social characteristic of being 'All-American' stands alongside 'rugged individual'. Brand associations are about both how we see ourselves, and about how we want to be seen by society and interact with others.

Commercial branding and brands represent complex concepts that have been defined based on several underlying constructs. Three main concepts help to illustrate the basic ideas:

◆ relationship between consumer and product or service (marketing focused on the consumer and building the brand–consumer relationship);

◆ value (customer and otherwise defined) added to a product or service;

◆ exchange (cost and benefit) between product or service and consumer.

At the outset, the basic notions of relationship, value and exchange highlight the fact that branding is more than simply a matter of *communicating* with consumers and persuading them to purchase a product, or take some desired action. Branding certainly utilizes communication strategies, but it is much more than that. Brands position products, services, behaviors and organizations by creating associations that can transcend any one advertisement or other promotional activity. Brands position their objects in the lives of consumers in the larger social and (through placement and promotion) physical environments in which we live.

Consider the Marlboro example again. The Marlboro Man created a social norm of smoking as a way to express independence, confidence and strength. These norms contributed to creating a social environment in which smoking was a socially desirable behavior. This was in part accomplished through specific product marketing efforts (e.g. television ads before the Fairness Doctrine took effect in 1971, billboards, event sponsorship and so on), but the brand itself was embedded in and helped to shape the social environment that reinforced and built the reputation of Marlboro as the cigarette brand of choice.

So if brands shape the social environments in which people live, what factors in the environment do they influence? In commercial branding, the effect of brands on individual consumers (what are the impacts of brand marketing activities on individual consumers and their relationship to the brand?) are of central importance. But, as Schultz and Schultz (2005) point out, brands influence and are influenced by broader, upstream environmental factors such as the constituencies (e.g. shareholders, boards of directors) surrounding the brand and its sponsor organization, in addition to the organization's larger reputation (corporate image) and its financial and general wellbeing. In other words, what financial value does brand marketing have for constituencies (e.g. higher share price) or the organization's bottom line, and how can the brand be valued as an overall organizational asset?

The notion of influencing upstream environmental factors as well as individual behavior is now prominent in public health as well. Historically, social marketing efforts to change modifiable health behaviors, such as preventing HIV/AIDS, have focused primarily on downstream, individual behaviors such as promoting condom use. Until recently, upstream efforts to change policies and larger environmental factors were given little attention. But in the 1980s and early 1990s, the exclusive focus on downstream behaviors was criticized and there was a call for more attention on social environmental conditions that could promote behavior change over the longer term (Wallack *et al.* 1993; Dearing and Rogers 1996). Social marketers responded by recognizing the upstream agenda (Hastings *et al.* 2000).

Consider the National Cancer Institute's American Stop Smoking Intervention Study (Project ASSIST). The purpose of ASSIST was to influence health policy by changing public acceptability of tobacco use and social norms in order to influence public policy (NCI 2005). ASSIST used media advocacy – 'the strategic use of mass media as a resource for advancing a social or public policy initiative' – to stimulate policy initiatives to restrict youth access to tobacco, promote clean indoor air laws, increase excise taxes, and restrict or ban advertising and promotion of tobacco (Evans *et al.* 2006). ASSIST branded tobacco control policies as the pro-social choice, and created a social movement to control and prevent tobacco use.

But whether the aim of a brand is to change individual behavior directly, or through changes in an organization or the social environment, brands are ultimately marketing tools, and branding is a marketing strategy. The key branding constructs cited earlier can be viewed in terms of the persuasive mechanisms that make the brand appealing and therefore an effective marketing tool:

- aspiration to an appealing external ideal;
- modeling of a socially desirable good;
- association with idealized imagery.

The concept of aspiration is central to a brand's marketing value, to its ability to influence consumers and create value – whether for the consumer, the sponsor or sponsor constituencies. Successful brands provide an external ideal to which consumers can aspire, and then deliver on the promise embodied in the ideal (as Wally Olins, one of the founding fathers of corporate affairs, reputedly expressed it: 'promise without delivery is like painting the toilet door when the cistern is broken'). Brands succeed by providing benefits to consumers, and distinguishing those benefits from the competition (Tybout and Sternthal 2005). Benefits are first promised through brand marketing that makes an external ideal salient – say, the power or sex appeal of driving a BMW – to which the consumer then aspires. Brands ultimately succeed to the extent consumers realize those promised benefits.

The concept of social modeling has long been understood by psychologists and certainly by commercial marketers. This concept is examined and thoroughly developed in the work of Albert Bandura (1986), in which social modeling plays a central role in social learning and the formation of knowledge, attitudes and beliefs (social cognition). In the context of branding, social models are figures that embody the ideals promised by the brand. For example, the Marlboro Man provided an appealing social model for the Marlboro cigarette's target audience. Social models have been applied in social marketing as well, such as the independent, rebellious youth featured in the American Legacy Foundation's *truth* campaign (Evans *et al.* 2002).

Imagery can be a powerful tool to build brand recognition, and can be a central component in creating intended (and unintended) associations. One of the main uses of imagery in brand marketing is to create the external ideal – the Marlboro Man riding out on the range, the BMW driver cornering nimbly on a windy road, or a *truth* campaign kid confronting the tobacco industry. Research on social imagery – on the process and effects of image formation due to social stimuli such as media and peer influences – shows that formation of social imagery can promote aspiration (Evans *et al.* 2004). The individual aspires to close the gap between his or her own self-image, and the external idealized image. Research suggests that social imagery formation plays an important role in determining adolescent health behaviors, such as smoking. For example, tobacco brand marketing portrays smokers as cool, popular, and having more friends (Aloise-Young and Hennigan 1996). Moreover, because adolescents typically value these traits, those who agree with these images are more likely to at least experiment with smoking (Barton *et al.* 1982; Burton *et al.* 1989).

From commercial to public health branding

The premise of this book is that there is much to be learned from commercial branding by public health practitioners and researchers who seek to change health behaviors – preventing smoking, encouraging condom use, or promoting nutritious eating and physical activity – and study the effects of such changes on population health. We argue that public health brands have been created in many contexts, that there is evidence they have a positive effect in changing health behavior, that more branded public health messages are needed, and that more research is needed on how they work and what health benefits accrue to audiences exposed to them. Branding is increasingly a central strategy in social marketing aimed at improving population health, and a promising public health strategy overall.

For example, in *Social marketing: why should the Devil have all the best tunes?* Hastings (2007) highlights the promise of branding. He notes a recent study conducted on behalf of the UK's National Institute for Health and Clinical Excellence and suggests that brands can be an effective way of reaching information-deprived communities. In the case of the

Scottish Health Education Group's efforts to reduce smoking and drinking and increase use of contraception, Hastings highlights the use of branding to communicate a lifestyle message of empowerment as the basis of an umbrella campaign addressing multiple behaviors with common elements and bases for prevention and control (Hastings 2007: 97).

Public health brands have the potential to embody multiple behaviors and behavior change messages. In so doing, they can help public health address significant challenges in terms of gaining and maintaining audience exposure and awareness of health messages due to funding limitations, difficulties competing with unhealthy product marketers with much larger budgets (consider that McDonald's – just one source of fast food in a huge industry – had an annual advertising budget of US$1.21 billion in 2003, compared with an average annual expenditure of US$68 million from 2001 to 2006 for the Centers for Disease Control and Prevention VERB campaign), and realize synergy based on underlying behavior change and persuasive mechanisms. This is because, as discussed earlier, brands are more than simply communication or any one health communication campaign of limited budget, scope and duration. Like commercial brands, brands can position health behaviors and the lifestyles they embody with the public, and thereby establish a long-term relationship that can be maintained beyond any individual campaign effort.

Public health brands are the associations that individuals hold for health behaviors, or lifestyles that embody multiple health behaviors (Evans *et al.* 2007a). In this chapter, we describe public health brands and their recent evolution as one of the primary strategies in social marketing and public health promotion. Public health branding is growing rapidly across topic areas from nutrition to HIV/AIDS, and is being used worldwide (Hastings 2007). The development of public health branding is illustrated by a recent systematic review by Evans *et al.* (forthcoming). Their work identifies some 37 studies that met search criteria for public health branding, all of which were published since 1990. Virtually all major topic areas in public health were represented by at least one branded health campaign, and in many cases evaluation findings demonstrated significant effects of the branded messages on health behavior (e.g. condom use or prevention of smoking initiation) and behavioral precursors (e.g. belief in effectiveness of condoms for HIV/AIDS prevention and self-efficacy to use them).

We argue that branding is critically important to future social marketing and public health promotion because, very often, multiple behaviors need to be changed and maintained in order to have lasting health outcome benefits. At the same time, social marketers typically have much smaller budgets and are 'on air' for a shorter time than their commercial counterparts. Recent research suggests that behaviors requiring one-time or limited changes may be more susceptible to the effects of health mass media campaigns than those requiring multiple changes and long-term maintenance (Snyder and Hamilton 2002; Evans 2006). As many health behaviors are complex and public health budgets are not large, health behavior change and maintenance can in some cases be more difficult than affecting consumer choice. This makes the development of improved branding strategies a critical objective for public health in order to prevent and control morbidity and mortality.

Complex, interrelated behaviors such as nutrition or unprotected sexual behavior are difficult to change through simple communication of health risks and benefits – the social context in which they occur needs to be recognized, and associations and relationships between behavior and desired goods for the consumer can be an effective strategy to promote health behavior. We argue that public health brands can serve these needs, and there is promising evidence that they can change and lead to maintenance of complex health behaviors.

For example, consider the example of smoking prevention behavior and the Legacy *truth* campaign. Smoking prevention behavior presents a complex health communication challenge in many respects. First, it represents in one sense the absence of behavior (i.e. not smoking), replacement of that behavior with something else (e.g. nonsmoking lifestyle choices, such as sports or participation in anti-tobacco program activities), and maintenance of the absent behavior (i.e. continued nonsmoker status). All of these factors are at play while, in the case of youth, the individual lives in a complex world of social and media influences and maintains nonsmoking status on a smoking uptake continuum (Pierce *et al.* 1996), represented by a set of knowledge, attitudes, and behaviors (no intention to smoke, haven't experimented with smoking). In the case of *truth*, a mass media campaign spoke to adolescent aspirations to become independent adults and to rebel against authority by channeling these needs against the tobacco industry and use of tobacco (Evans *et al.* 2005). At the same time *truth* was more than communication as it engaged numerous stakeholders and partners (e.g. the Ad Council, US state tobacco control programs, federal government agencies, schools of public health, and so on) and promoted community-based youth empowerment programs for community outreach and grassroots mobilization (Holden *et al.* 2005).

Thus the *truth* brand competed directly with tobacco industry brands by promising the benefits of a nonsmoking lifestyle to adolescents. More than just a communication campaign, *truth* competed not for a share of the smoking consumer market, but for the adolescent's choice between smoking and nonsmoking by providing a more beneficial lifestyle alternative. This kind of competition is at the heart of public health branding strategy.

In fact, it has been argued that branding of healthy lifestyles is in a sense part and parcel of public health – there is no getting away from it. Thus, branding as a strategy in social marketing and public health promotion is inevitable. Everything we do and say in public health has an image a tonality, the only question is whether we recognize and manage it, or ignore and fall victim to it (Lefevbre *et al.* 1995)

Distinguishing public health and commercial branding

We have introduced the idea of public health brands and given some examples, but what exactly do we mean by *branding healthy lifestyles*? Broadly speaking, public health brands are a complex set of associations between an individual and a health behavior or set of behaviors that embody a lifestyle. In one sense, they are quite like commercial brands in that they are made up of the relationship between the individual and the health behavior(s), the value that the behavior(s) provides to the individual, and the perceived benefit (or cost) of the behavior(s) by the individual.

Similarly, commercial and public health organizations can also brand themselves. For example, Richard Branson's Virgin brands offer an example of organizational branding that transcends any one product or service line, and positions the organization as modern, funny, hip, cool and, with recent efforts to 'green' its operations, as a friend of the environment and socially responsible (Specter 2007). A visit to the Virgin website (http://www.virgin.com/) confirms that Virgin is an organizational 'brand of brands' with taglines appearing prominently below the Virgin logo such as: 'This isn't a Website. It's our front door. Open it', and 'One little Website, a whole lotta Virgin'. The visitor is then offered a wide range of product and service offerings – from air travel to music – and reminded of Virgin's standing as the UK's leading brand (HPI Research 2007).

Compare Virgin with the Health Sponsorship Council (HSC) in New Zealand, the country's government agency that promotes health and healthy lifestyles. A visit to the HSC website (http://www.hsc.org.nz/) shows a clear-cut organizational brand focus in that HSC is positioned to 'market social change' by 'developing and delivering health promotion and marketing programmes' on spanning public health. HSC has developed specific branded programs (i.e. services) in tobacco control, sun safety, problem gambling and healthy eating, each with distinctive mission and objectives along with distinctive logo treatment, branded promise and benefits.

But there is a clear difference between commercial and public health brands that deserves examination. Public health does not brand products or services that can be directly purchased for a monetary price, but rather the benefit of engaging in or refraining from behavior(s) with health consequences.

This distinction between the purpose, nature of the exchange and outcomes of public health brands as compared with commercial brands has important implications. There may be differences in the relationship between consumer and brand. In the commercial world, relationships can be through product consumption, where the benefit typically accrues to the consumer by exchanging money for a product or service. But in public health, there is no comparable sense of consumption to speak of, but rather engagement in alternative behaviors (e.g. use of a condom to reduce risk of HIV infection). The value the public health brand provides to the consumer may come (in the case of tobacco or drugs) in avoiding consumption of an unhealthy product. Additionally, public health brands may be perceived differently, elicit differing reactions, and may be conceived differently by their developers on a number of dimensions.

For example, in conducting a systematic online search for published literature on public health branding, Evans *et al.* (forthcoming) operationalized 'public health branding' as any manuscripts in the published health, social science and business literature on branding or specific brands in health promotion marketing. The intent of the search was to identify articles reporting on the development, delivery or evaluation of branded messages through communication campaigns focused on health behavior and behavior change, as opposed to branding of products, services or other non-health outcomes.

Based on the use of certain key words, the authors found that some brands appeared to be aimed at public health promotion but were in fact exclusively aimed at selling products; meanwhile some other brands had both public health promotion and commercial components (e.g. promoting use of a particular brand of condoms for health and product sales purposes). One lesson of this research is that public health brands should be thought of as having promotion of health behavior and long-term public health benefit as their *sole* objective. This concept is important when we consider the efforts of many corporations, such as Altria and McDonald's, to implement marketing campaigns with an avowed health promotion and an underlying corporate promotion purpose, such as Altria's *Think Don't Smoke* campaign and a recent physical activity promotion campaign depicting Ronald McDonald riding a bicycle to the McDonald's restaurant (Wakefield *et al.* 2006).

At the same time, corporate social responsibility is a real phenomenon with potential health and other social benefits for the public. Multinational corporations such as British Petroleum (BP – 'Beyond Petroleum'), General Electric (GE – 'We bring good things to life') and Virgin (in its recent 'green' efforts) have branded themselves as seeking public good through improving the environment, health and overall human wellbeing in a variety of ways. These efforts indeed appear genuine, and a recent interview with Richard Branson (*The New Yorker*, 7 May 2007) demonstrates the commitment of some executives and corporate boards to social benefit through their corporate operations. But it is also clear from the Branson interview, and from the larger operations of such socially responsible corporations, that their purpose remains the service to shareholders not public health as an end in itself. After all, these organizations exist for the purpose of shareholder benefit.

So, while the motives (e.g. health vs. profit as a benefit) and outcomes (e.g. lifestyle adoption vs. product or service consumption) of commercial and public health branding differ, the principles and methods underlying branding in the two sectors are essentially the same. Both use characters (e.g. Smokey the Bear and the Marlboro Man), both can promote products (e.g. nicotine replacement therapy or clean needles) or services, and both can brand the organization as well as the offering. It is where public health and commercial brands start and end that they differ – in between they look very much alike. This distinction is important not only for understanding how these sectors are similar and different, but also the social and ethical implications of branding as a social marketing and public health practice, which is discussed later in this volume.

Brand equity

In this book, we follow recent research suggesting that brand equity is the overarching construct that characterizes brands and brand identification among target audiences. According to Aaker:

> Brand equity is a set of assets (and liabilities) linked to a brand's name and symbol that adds to (or subtracts from) the value provided by a product or service to a firm and/or that firm's customers. The major asset categories are: 1) Brand name awareness; 2) brand loyalty; 3) perceived quality; 4) brand associations.
>
> Aaker (1996)

Other authors in the marketing literature have elaborated the notion of brand equity, such as Kevin Lane Keller's focus on the relationship of the brand to the consumer. Keller defines what he calls *customer-based brand equity*:

> Customer-based brand equity is the differential effect brand knowledge has on the customer response to the marketing of that brand. Equity occurs when the consumer has a high level of awareness and familiarity with the brand and holds some strong, favorable, and unique brand associations in memory.

Keller (1999)

Keller argues that brand equity, and the power of brands to drive consumer behavior, lies in the experiences consumers have when they encounter the brand, and what they learn from those experiences (Keller 1999). One could view this as 'social learning' in Bandura's sense, and Keller argues that it is at the heart of brand equity. This in turn has consequences for the brand and its management, as the brand's development will be decided by consumers (e.g. recall the 'New Coke' fiasco in the 1980s), and managers must understand what their learned attitudes and beliefs are before deciding on new placement, price, product or promotional efforts.

The example of New Coke, a failed effort in brand transformation if there ever was one, demonstrates the importance of delivering on a brand's promise. Coca-Cola was invented in 1885 and first sold in 1894. Coke dominated much of the 20th-Century soft drink market, and was promoted as a refreshing soft drink with a secret formula and distinctive taste. It was the number one selling soda for most of the 20th Century. Between the 1940s and 1983, however, its market share declined from over 60 per cent to just 24 per cent. Pepsi, with its distinctive, sweeter taste, had significantly eroded Coke's market share. The famous 'Pepsi Challenge' campaign of the 1970s, in which blind taste tests in public arenas showed an overwhelming preference for Pepsi, contributed to Pepsi's gain in market share (Hays 2004).

In response, Coca-Cola developed the sweeter New Coke with a more Pepsi-like taste. The old Coke formula was taken off the market, and New Coke was introduced on 23 April 1985. New Coke initially showed strong sales figures. But soon negative news media attention and response from loyal Classic Coke drinkers, which had been predicted by New Coke focus group research that had been largely ignored by the company, led to the product's swift downfall (Schindler 1992). It seems the company had forgotten what made Coca-Cola a great brand: delivering a distinctive taste that consumers loved, expected, and associated with refreshment. Three months after the release of New Coke, the original formulation was brought back as 'Classic Coke' (and later just Coke) to assuage loyal Coke consumers, signaling the company's admission of a colossal branding blunder. New Coke is a case of a company losing touch with its consumers, and a brand failing to deliver on its promise.

The case of New Coke shows how consumers determine and drive the value of a brand. On a personal level, the consumer forms a social image of the brand (Chassin *et al.* 1981; Evans *et al.* 2004), based on their reception of the message (Petty and Cacioppo 1986), forming associations between their self-image and the brand. As a result, the consumer exposed to marketing efforts in support of the brand develops a level of equity, or value in their relationship with the brand. They become co-owners of the brand.

Brand equity can be viewed as a higher-order construct that captures the associations underlying a brand. Figure 1.1 presents a conceptual model to illustrate the component association constructs and their relationship to brand equity. Statistically speaking, brand equity can be considered a higher-order factor (Comrey and Lee 1992), and the association constructs as second-order factors, which are in turn made up of individual variables that may be (and have been in Aaker's work, and in public health studies such as Evans *et al.* 2005) measured through self-reports about brand identification and reactions by respondents exposed to the brand.

In Chapter 3 of this volume, Evans *et al.* argue that brand equity is the primary outcome variable of interest as an immediate result of audience exposure to branded health messages. That chapter explores the operational definition of brand equity and its components in depth, and describes methods to measure and evaluate its value as a predictor of health behavioral outcomes.

Public health and commercial branding strategies

As noted earlier, there are several primary mechanisms underlying commercial brands, including the relationship, value added, and exchange between product or service and consumer. Each of these commercial constructs has an analog in public health. For example, commercial marketers seek to build strong relationships (positive associations, brand identification and loyalty) between customers and product and service brands such as BMW, Nike and Marlboro. They use varying combinations of persuasive mechanisms such as aspiration, social modeling, or imagery to build and maintain positive brand associations, and thereby the relationship between brand and consumer.

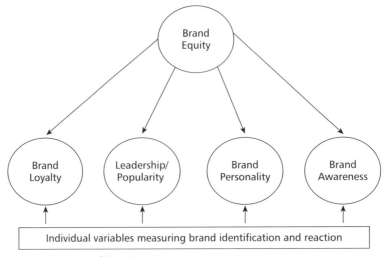

Fig. 1.1 Conceptual model of brand equity.

For example, in Fig. 1.2, BMW provides a social model by presenting a powerful vehicle that offers an adventurous, sexy lifestyle behind the wheel of a sports car.

Relational thinking and branding

The idea of relationship building as fundamental aspect of good business practice emerged during the 1980s. It flowed from research done in the service sector (e.g. banks) and business-to-business sector (e.g. marketing between component manufacturers and car producers) where the traditional marketing idea of focusing on ad hoc transactions was seen to be inadequate. In the case of services, the emphasis put on sales seemed to underplay the crucial construct of customer satisfaction. In business-to-business marketing, the mass, transactional assumptions in transactional marketing conflicted with the day-to-day reality of long-term, cooperative alliances between buyers. A more continuous and sophisticated model was needed.

The business sector as a whole also became increasingly conscious of the value of customer loyalty: it is much more expensive to acquire new customers than keep existing ones. The emphasis began to shift from one-off transactions to ongoing relationships (Grönroos 1997). Companies started to think not just about immediate, but long-term profitability. Indeed, it became apparent that individual transactions could lose money, provided the 'lifetime value' of the customer is positive. This has fundamental implications for the business function, greatly increasing the importance of customer service and satisfaction. An EIU survey conducted in 2002 suggests that this lesson has been well learnt. It showed that customer satisfaction is taking over from profitability as the prime determinant of performance-related pay (Richardson 2001).

Relationship building requires an ever-more intimate knowledge of the customer. Until recently, such insights were only possible on a small scale – a buyer dealing with a couple of dozen suppliers, or a local pub, for instance. But information technology has changed all that. Data mining, mobile communications, vastly enhanced computers, opportunistic and endemic data gathering all provide even the biggest operators with the

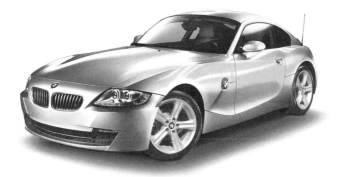

Fig. 1.2 BMW brands its Z4 roadster based on power, adventure and sex appeal. Reproduced with permission from BMW Corporation.

potential to understand and respond sensitively – and even individually – to their customers.

As with other human relationships, trust and commitment are crucial. Perhaps not surprisingly, this approach to marketing has been likened to marriage. Others have argued that this is taking the metaphor too far, reminding us that marketing is ultimately about profitability.

Nonetheless, there are many benefits to relationship marketing. If customers remain loyal then planning is much easier, pricing becomes less critical and the developing trust brings opportunities to sell new offerings. Relational thinking can also be applied to suppliers, retailers, competitors (through alliances), employees and other stakeholders.

Relationship building is epitomized in branding. It is the marketer's most powerful emotional tool, and therefore reinforces a key characteristic of any good relationship. In addition, brands can gradually become a fast and powerful way of confirming the synergy between marketer and customer. Indeed, as noted in the case of New Coke, it can be argued that successful brands are only part owned by the company – the customer also has a share. When Coca-Cola changed its formulation and ultimately went back to Coca-Cola Classic, this was partly put down to consumers' displeasure at *their* brand being adulterated.

For social marketers this suggests there are benefits to be gained if we move beyond what might be termed the 'intervention mentality', and instead think in terms of building long-term relationships with our customers. Experience, backed by well-established theory (e.g. the stages of change model), tells us that health behavior changes do not, for the most part, occur overnight. They involve a series of steps from initial contemplation through to reinforcement after the fact, a process that is both dynamic and precarious – the individual can regress or change heart at any point.

Furthermore, behavior change has both emotional and rational drivers. We know, for example, that despite their knowledge of the health consequences, young people smoke because it makes them feel adult and fashionable. It is this that explains the tobacco industry's huge – and extremely long-term – investment in evocative brands.

The move to relational thinking in marketing is acquiring its own momentum. As more companies move to this way of doing business – building trust and partnerships, emphasizing customer service and satisfaction and rewarding loyalty – those businesses that ignore it will become increasingly isolated and strident. If we in public health do not learn the lessons of relationship building and branding we will suffer a similar fate.

Finally, social marketing is founded on trust. It is not driven by profit but, at least ostensibly, a desire to benefit the target audience. It therefore has a very different, and perhaps morally higher, base than commercial marketing on which to build mutual respect with its customers. If commercial marketers can seriously argue that 'the presence of commitment and trust … is central to successful relationship marketing, not power and its ability to condition others' (Morgan and Hunt 1994), then social marketers have to listen. And public health brands have the potential to become a symbol of such trust.

Building relationships – how it works in public health

Public health brands can build relationships with audiences to encourage adoption and maintenance of preventive or health-promoting behaviors. Like commercial brands, they offer a brand promise, and typically ground their brand promotion in a 'call to action' that defines what the brand calls upon consumers to do. Figure 1.3 is a still from the Legacy Foundation *truth* campaign that captures the promotion of rebellion against the tobacco industry as a call to action to commit to a tobacco-free lifestyle.

In Chapter 5 of this volume, Hastings *et al.* discuss the European Commission's *Help* social marketing campaign which has also sought to develop and deliver on an attractive promise in the field of tobacco control.

Adding value – how it works in public health

Commercial marketers seek to add value to their products and services for consumers through the use of branding. A BMW *automobile* provides transportation, comforts and luxuries, and other practical benefits. However, the BMW *brand* conveys status, sense of power, sex appeal and other social goods that transcend the vehicle's practical utility.

Public health brands can also add value to the practical benefits of engaging in a preventive or health-promoting behavior beyond its immediate practical benefits (e.g. harm reduction or health enhancing). For example, the US Centers for Disease Control and Prevention (CDC) *VERB, It's What You Do* campaign to promote physical activity among tweens (pre-adolescent youth) sought to brand sports and exercise as cool, fun and exhilarating. It attempted to build a social norm of physical activity through a multi-component campaign that included mass media, community outreach and mobilization, and youth involvement and leadership (Huhman *et al.* 2005). The brand tagline 'It's

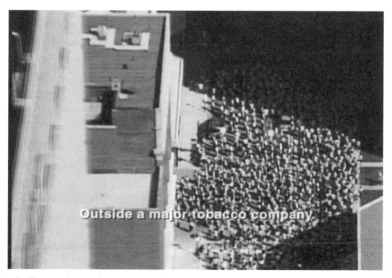

Fig. 1.3 Rebellion against tobacco. Reproduced with permission from the American Legacy Foundation.

What You Do' captures the essence of the brand promise: 'Nothing replaces the rush and exhilaration of physical activity. VERB ignites the desire for physical activity freeing kids to play out their dreams — I can't NOT play!' Be active, and you can live your dreams.

Beneficial exchange between producer and consumer – how it works in public health

Finally, commercial marketers seek to promote a sense of beneficial exchange between the producer and consumer in the brand. One might pay US$40,000 or more for a BMW, but in return receive a well-made, luxurious vehicle with the tremendous value-added features of the BMW brand such as sex appeal, a sense of power and status.

Public health brands can also promote a perceived beneficial exchange. In the *truth* campaign, the teen is offered independence, rebellion and 'coolness', which they obtain by refraining from smoking and maintaining a nonsmoking lifestyle.

An aspect of exchange in both the commercial and public health cases is *trust*. The value added by the BMW brand is due in large part to the fact that consumers trust BMW to deliver on its promised brand benefits. If BMW produced a minivan, it might very well dilute its brand and lose some of its perceived value of sex appeal or power, thus changing consumer associations for the worse. In effect, it would break faith by diluting consumer trust that the brand will consistently deliver on its promise. Don't look for a BMW competitor to the Honda Odyssey or Toyota Sienna anytime soon!

One way that public health brands have in the past diluted themselves and lost trust is by delivering negative messages or invoking fear appeals about risky health behaviors. Consider the US government's 'just say no' and 'this is your brain on drugs' anti-drug campaigns of the 1980s. Aimed at adolescents, these campaigns lost (or perhaps never established) trust with the target audience (primarily adolescents, and secondarily their parents) because they failed to appreciate the perceived benefits of the behavior they were competing against (e.g. marijuana use), were generally negative and lacked emotional or graphic appeal, and failed to offer a viable behavioral alternative. They offered nothing beneficial in return for giving up drug use. In brief, they violated most of the branding principles discussed in this chapter. In Chapter 8 of this volume, Jacobsohn and Hornik discuss how the well-funded US anti-drug campaign successfully built brand recognition while failing to change drug use behavior.

Compared with the commercial sector, branding is still in its infancy in public health. Campaigns such as *VERB*, *truth*, condom promotion efforts such as *loveLife* in Africa (Stadler and Hlongwa 2002), the work of HSC in New Zealand and many others that will be discussed in the rest of this volume, signify a new era in social marketing that has been growing since at least the 1990s. Branding is becoming more and more thoroughly established, and its principles are becoming widely adopted. Exit 'just say no', enter strategic branding as a cornerstone of public health practice.

Tactics underlying commercial brands and their analogs in public health

The overall marketing strategy of branding products and services is supported by a set of specific tactics that are used in varying combinations to build customer relationships, add value and create a beneficial exchange. There are four basic tactics: competition (value proposition), recognition, promise and delivery.

Technology, and integration of marketing tactics using multiple technology platforms, is increasingly a strategy of choice for commercial and social marketers alike. This has been driven largely by media saturation and advertising clutter, making it increasingly difficult for brand marketers to deliver their message and build recognition (Calvert 2008). For example, creating branded characters is a key to successful marketing aimed at children and youth (Institute of Medicine 2007). Popular television cartoon characters like Nickelodeon's SpongeBob SquarePants are used to sell products ranging from cereal to vacations, and animated characters such as Tony the Tiger serve solely as a spokesperson to sell a specific product, in this instance Kellogg's Frosted Flakes. Similarly, the Ronald McDonald character is used to sell the McDonald's brand, including the purchase of Happy Meals as well as his newer role as a physical fitness guru. By associating products and activities with fun, entertaining characters, interest in their products and brands is expected to increase (Kunkel *et al.* 2004). Premiums, such as a small toy in a McDonald's Happy Meal, are also used to increase product purchases by children (Calvert 1999).

Social marketers similarly compete by seeking to provide added value to their campaigns and broader lifestyle offerings. Under the *VERB* brand umbrella, for example, a series of products, activities and resources were developed for parents, schools, community-based organizations and other groups working with tweens (Huhman *et al.* 2005). These included 'Yellowball' (a promotional program for schools and community organizations that offered special rewards and recognition for being physically active), 'Make It Up' (a kit designed to help develop children's imagination as they participate in physical activities), and 'Crossover' (a kit to encourage participants to invent and play new games by combining existing games, like basketball and soccer).

As television advertisement clutter became an increasing problem for marketing products, advertising techniques began to include new approaches to supplement traditional ones. One such change is a shift from an 'in your face' to a more subtle 'hanging out with a brand' approach in which marketers attempt to disguise the intent of the ad. This approach to building audience recognition is known as stealth advertising (Gardner 2000). The theory behind stealth advertising is that advertising is most effective when consumers do not know it is advertising (Eisenberg *et al.* 2002). Brand recognition can best be achieved when the audience does not recognize the brand being consciously 'marketed'. In this way, the potential consumer's 'guard' will be down and they will be more open to persuasive arguments about the product. To implement this approach, marketers try to blur the line between the advertisement and the content where legally permissible (Eisenberg *et al.* 2002). One growing approach to stealth marketing is through online games and characters with which both youths and adults can interact and thereby learn about the brand without direct marketing (Gardner 2000).

The use of such techniques also presents an opportunity to build upon and deliver on a brand's promise. Offering value-added products, such as a toy in a Happy Meal or a *VERB* 'Make it Up' kit may build on the brand's promise of fun or involvement. The increasing prevalence of such approaches also tends to raise the stakes for brand marketers to come up with genuinely valued premiums for consumers deliver on the promise. The use of online interactive strategies, such as games, offers an opportunity to deliver added consumer value at little or no incremental cost. Other growing strategies to increase brand promise and delivery include product placement in other media venues (such as the classic example of Spielberg's ET character eating Reese's Pieces, which resulted in a 66 per cent spike in national sales, according to Mazur 1996), viral marketing, online personal information collection at interactive websites, and video news releases (Mazur 1996; Gardner 2000).

Design and evaluation of public health brands

What do we know about public health brands?

There is a growing number of public health brands, offering a body of material for review and examination of design elements, implementation strategies and evidence of effectiveness. These brands span the full range of major topics of chronic and infectious disease, and address most modifiable risk behaviors for morbidity/mortality, including HIV, tobacco, nutrition, physical activity, and so on (Evans *et al.* forthcoming). They also reflect the global scope of public health brands, with examples coming from Africa (e.g. *LoveLife*), Australia and New Zealand (e.g. *SunSmart*), Europe (e.g. the UK's *Fighting Fit*), Asia (*EXAMPLE*) and North America (e.g. *truth* and *VERB*).

As reported in Evans *et al.* (forthcoming), the published literature on public health brands provides us with some insight into how such campaigns have been designed, their promotional strategies, their effectiveness, and perhaps some insight and direction into future social marketing efforts. First, public health brands have been developed through all the overarching forms of marketing and promotion strategies, such as branded mass media campaigns, community outreach and community mobilization strategies. These latter efforts typically differ in many respects from mass media, often using messages and channels tailored to local community and cultural norms, and using local staff and community members to build source and message credibility (Evans *et al.* 2007b). Thus public health branding appears to be a versatile strategy that can and has been utilized in a broad range of campaigns.

Public health brands span most of the major fields of prevention and health promotion, including chronic and infectious disease prevention and promotion of protective behaviors. Not surprisingly, well-funded areas such as tobacco control and HIV/AIDS have contributed a large number of the existing public health brands, especially in the UK, USA and Africa. Lessons learned from these well-developed domains of public health branding are in turn spreading into new areas of public health over time. For example, the *Fag Ends* smoking cessation brand sponsored by the UK government is growing, and is expanding its efforts into nutrition and physical activity (Hastings 2007).

One area in which it branding appears to be growing is nutrition and communication of nutrition behavior. In July 2005, the National Cancer Institute (NCI) and the Division of Nutrition Research Coordination, both of the National Institutes of Health, held a state-of-the-science workshop entitled, 'Diet and Communication: What can communication science tell us about promoting optimal dietary behavior?' (Johnson-Taylor *et al.* 2007). A special issue of the *Journal of Nutrition Education* (March/April 2007), addresses the major themes of the workshop, including synthesizing ideas and future directions in the area. Health communication campaigns and branding are among the topic areas addressed.

Fitzgibbon *et al.* (2007) synthesize major themes and future directions. They make a case for applying successful marketing strategies used by the private sector and applying them to public health. Specifically, their paper describes branding as a potentially effective approach that has been used by the food industry and has been applied on a more limited basis, but successfully, in public health. As examples, they cite major US campaigns such as the NCI *5-A-Day For Better Health*, which promotes consumption of at least five servings of fruit or vegetables a day.

Both Fitzgibbon *et al.* (2007) and Evans *et al.* (forthcoming) have identified and described the marketing, psychological and other theories used to develop branded health messages. Not surprisingly, they find marketing theory to be the predominant theoretical basis for branded messages. Marketing theories cited in the literature typically deal with promotional or placement strategies (the '4 Ps' of marketing) used to deliver the brand to target audiences. Psychological theory appears less often, but does appear more frequently in reports on large, well-funded campaigns with more fully articulated behavior change objectives, such as *truth*, *VERB*, the UK's *Fighting Fat, Fighting Fit*, and the African *LoveLife* HIV prevention campaign (Wardle *et al.* 2001; Stadler and Hlongwa 2002; Evans *et al.* 2005; Huhman *et al.* 2005). Psychological theories are typically behavior change theories about the causal sequence from message exposure to behavior (through mediating variables) such as the theory of planned behavior and social cognitive theory (Bandura 1986; Ajzen 1991).

Techniques adapted from commercial marketing, such as audience segmentation, have been prominent in public health brands. Targeting technique is most frequently used to identify specific sociodemographic groups for branded messaging such as by age (e.g. youth for smoking prevention), gender, race or sexual orientation (e.g. young gay men for safe sex and HIV prevention). Relatively few brands have utilized tailored messaging, perhaps reflecting the newness of tailoring in public health and the difficulties of developing cost-effective brands using this technique. In Chapter 13 of this volume, Megan Lewis and Lauren McCormack discuss the potential of tailoring as a branding strategy, and its challenges.

As the field develops, it will be increasingly important to gauge the overall state of research and evidence base regarding public health brands. In the study by Evans *et al.* (forthcoming), nearly all the brands surveyed reported some evaluation effort, and qualified as 'good' on a quality scale based on 11 design, data collection and analysis elements (e.g. use of experimental design or measures of brand exposure).

The study did not however find many randomized experimental studies, or studies that used sophisticated measures and analyses of the effects of branding attributes on behavior, such as have been used in advertising research (e.g. multi-dimensional scales of brand equity). Increasingly, brand marketers in the commercial sector argue for the importance of rigorous brand evaluation using experimental designs in order to determine brand impact on consumer behavior and on upstream outcomes such as the brand as an organizational asset (Almquist and Wyner 1999). In public health branding, there is a need to develop more rigorous study designs and build upon existing work in public health brand measurement to increase precision and identify the potential mediating effects of brand uptake on the relationship between message exposure and health behavior change.

Conclusion

Commercial branding is among the most successful activities in the modern economy. In this chapter, we have examined the basic precepts of branding and related them to relatively new and emerging efforts to brand public health behaviors, policies and organizations. Commercial brands seek to sell products and services, while public health brands seek to change health knowledge, attitudes and behaviors. Commercial brands measure success in terms of sales and repeat business, while public health brands measure success in terms of changed behavioral mediators and health behaviors that prevent and control morbidity and mortality. The exchange of value between brand and consumer in the two sectors also differs, and this is due in part to differences in purposes and outcomes.

Firstly, most public health products do not have a monetary price, and, given the widespread correlation between greatest public need and disadvantage, this is often a desirable state of affairs. If the poor are in most need of our products, it seems to be completely unacceptable to charge for them; this would surely be regressive. However, experience in the commercial sector shows that price and value are closely interrelated: the value of a BMW is reinforced by its exclusive price tag and, at the other extreme, give-aways are often – figuratively as well as literally – taken for granted. Social marketing of condoms in developing countries provides instructive lessons here. Initial efforts to encourage contraception in India involved shipping out large quantities of free condoms. However, because they were free neither the distributors or the would-be users treated them with much respect. Product ended up moldering in warehouses, sell-by and storage instructions were not respected, and the product acquired a poor public reputation (Dahl *et al.* 1997; Harvey 1997).

For reputation read brand. Persistent poor value will accrete into a poor brand; conversely, BMW, for example, has been offering good value for decades and has thereby developed a very strong brand. Expensiveness is a key dimension of this brand, not just because it generates funds for the manufacturer to reinvest in high-quality production, but because it affects our perceptions of the offering. If a BMW cost the same as a Lada we would think less of them.

This phenomenon was thrown into relief by a brand we discuss often in this book. In the early 1990s, Philip Morris made a rare marketing mistake by dramatically cutting the price of Marlboro. It was seen as undermining not just its brand, but the very idea of branding. For a short while, the argument gained currency that the brand was finished and business in future would be simply about price. But Philip Morris reversed their decision, Marlboro regained its ascendancy, and the uncharacteristic aberration has become a classic business school case study to illustrate the importance of a consistent and coherent branding strategy, of which pricing is a key strand.

If we return to social marketing of condoms, the same lessons emerge. While the condoms were moldering in the warehouses, it was all too apparent that commercial products such as soft drinks were doing much better. They were well distributed (even the poorest village seemed to have a Coke machine), properly stored and readily consumed. Brand value was also very much in evidence. Success was due to commercialization: everyone in the supply chain stood to make money out of effective distribution. Even the final customer gained because the offering had added brand value, to which price contributed. Those marketing the condoms decided to follow suit and charge (a very modest) amount for their products. The result has been vastly increased condom usage and much wider availability (Dahl *et al.* 1997; Harvey 1997), along with some of the most sophisticated public health branding ever seen.

This does not suggest that we should rush to commercialize all social marketing efforts. But it does warn us to think carefully about what 'free' actually means. Health behaviors may not have a monetary cost, but they are nonetheless exchanged and have a value to the consumer. Social marketing that recognizes this value proposition succeeds in capturing the best lessons offered by commercial brands. In this chapter, we have argued that such efforts have an important ingredient for success against the competition.

References

Aaker, D. (1996). *Building strong brands.* New York: Simon and Schuster Inc.

Ajzen I. (1991). The theory of planned behaviour. *Organisational Behaviour and Human Decision Processes* **50**:179–211.

Almquist, E. and Wyner, G. (2001) Boost your marketing ROI with experimental design. *Harvard Business Review* **79**:135–41.

Aloise-Young, P. A. and Hennigan, K. M. (1996). Self-image, the smoker stereotype and cigarette smoking: Developmental patterns from fifth through eighth grade. *Journal of Adolescence* **19**:163–77.

Bandura, A. (1986). Social foundations of thought and action: a social cognitive theory. Englewood Cliffs, NJ: Prentice Hall.

Barton, J., Chassin, L., Presson, C. C., and Sherman, S. J. (1982). Social image factors as motivators of smoking initiation in early and middle adolescence. *Child Development* **53**:1499–511.

Borden, N. (1964). The concept of the marketing mix. *Journal of Advertising Research* **4**:2–7.

Bruce Eckman, Inc. Tobacco Document # 2045060177. Cited in: Ling, P. and Glantz, S. A. (2002). Why and how the tobacco industry sells cigarettes to young adults: evidence from industry documents. *American Journal of Public Health* **92**:908–16

Burton, D., Sussman, S., Hansen, W. B., Johnson, C. A., and Flay, B. R. (1989). Image attributions and smoking intentions among seventh grade students. *Journal of Applied Social Psychology* **19**:656–64.

Calvert, S. L. (1999). *Children's journeys through the information age*. Boston, MA: McGraw Hill.

Calvert, S. L. (2008). Using media to sell: marketing to children and media campaigns. *Future of Children* **18**(1):205–34.

Chassin, L., Presson, C. C., Sherman, S. J., Corty, E., and Olshavsky, R. W. (1981). Self-images and cigarette smoking in adolescence. *Personality and Social Psychology Bulletin* **7**:670–6.

Comrey, A. L. and Lee, H. B. (1992). *A first course in factor analysis* (2nd edn). Hillsdale, NJ: Lawrence Erlbaum.

Dahl, D. W., Gorn, G. J., and Weinberg, C. B. (1997). Marketing, safer sex, and condom acquisition. In M. E. Goldberg, M. Fishbein, and S. E. Middlestadt (eds.) *Social marketing: theoretical and practical perspectives*. Mahwah, NJ: Lawrence Erlbaum Associates.

Eisenberg, D., McDowell, J., Berestein, L., Tsiantar, D., and Finan, E. (2002). It's an ad, ad, ad, ad world. *Time* **160**(10).

Evans, D. (2006). How social marketing works in health care. *British Medical Journal* **322**:1207–10.

Evans, D., Wasserman, J. Bertolotti, E., and Martino, S. (2002). Branding behavior: the strategy behind the truth® campaign. *Social Marketing Quarterly* **8**:17–29.

Evans, D., Price, S., Blahut, S., Hersey, J., Niederdeppe, J., and Ray, S. (2004). Social imagery, tobacco independence, and the truth® campaign. *Journal of Health Communication* **9**:425–41.

Evans D., Price S., and Blahut, S. (2005). Evaluating the truth® brand. *Journal of Health Communication* **10**:181–92.

Evans, D., Ulasevich, A., Stillman, F., and Viswanathan, V. (2006). Tracking and evaluation of trends in print media. In F. Stillman and W. Trochim (eds.) *Evaluation of Project ASSIST: a blueprint for state-level tobacco control*. Bethesda, MD: National Cancer Institute Press.

Evans, D., Renaud, J., Blitstein, J., Hersey, J., Connors, S., Schieber, B., and Willett, J. (2007a). Prevention effects of an anti-tobacco brand on adolescent smoking initiation. *Social Marketing Quarterly* **13**:19–38.

Evans, D., Necheles, J., Longjohn, M., and Kristoffel, K. (2007b). The 5-4-3-2-1 Go! Intervention: social marketing for nutrition. *Journal of Nutrition Education and Behavior* **39**(S1):S55–S59.

Evans, D., Blitstein J., Hersey, J. Renaud, J., and Yaroch, A. (Forthcoming). Systematic review of public health branding research. *Journal of Health Communication*.

Farrelly M. C., Davis K. C., Haviland, M. L., Messeri P., and Healton, C. G. (2005). Evidence of a dose-response relationship between 'truth' antismoking ads and youth smoking. *American Journal of Public Health* **95**:425–31.

Fitzgibbon, M., Gans, K., Evans, D., Viswanath, V., Johnson-Taylor, W., Krebs-Smith, S., Rodgers, A., and Yaroch, A. (2007). Communicating healthy eating: lessons learned and future directions. *Journal of Nutrition Education and Behavior* **39**(S1):S63–S71.

Gardner, E. (2000). Understanding the net's toughest customer, *Internet World* **6**(3).

Grönroos, C. (1997). Value-driven relational marketing: from products to resources and competencies. *Journal of Marketing Management* **13**:407–19.

Harvey, P. D. (1997). Advertising affordable contraceptives: the social marketing experience. In M. E.Goldberg, M. Fishbein, and S. E. Middlestadt (eds.) *Social marketing: theoretical and practical perspectives*. Mahwah, NJ: Lawrence Erlbaum Associates.

Hastings, G. (2007). Social marketing: or, why should the devil have all the best tunes. London: Butterworth-Heineman.

Hastings, G., MacFadyen, L., and Anderson, S. (2000). Whose behaviour is it anyway? The broader potential of social marketing. *Social Marketing Quarterly* **6**:46–58.

Hays, C. (2004). The real thing: truth and power at the Coca-Cola Company. New York: Random House.

Holden, D., Evans, D., Hinnant, L., and Messeri, P. (2005). Modeling psychological empowerment among youth involved in local tobacco control efforts. *Health Education and Behavior* **32**:264–78.

Hornik, R. (2002). Public health communication: evidence for behavior change. Mahwah, NJ: Lawrence Erlbaum.

HPI Research (2007) http://www.hpiresearch.com/ped_caseStudies.php?case_study=5 (accessed 21 July 2007).

Huhman, M., Potter, L., Wong, F., Banspach, S., Duke, J., and Heitzler, C. (2005). Effects of a mass media campaign to increase physical activity among children: year-1 results of the VERB campaign. *Pediatrics* **116**:e247–e254.

Institute of Medicine (2007). *Food marketing to children and youth: threat or opportunity?* Edited by J. M. McGinnis, J. A. Gootman, and V. I. Kraak. Washington, DC: The National Academies Press.

Johnson-Taylor, W. L., Yaroch, A. L., Krebs-Smith, S. M., and Rodgers, A. B. (2007). What can communication science tell us about promoting optimal dietary behavior? *Journal of Nutrition Education and Behavior* **39**(S1):S1–S4.

Keller, K. L. (1999). *The Brand Report Card.* Cambridge, MA: Harvard Business School Press.

Kunkel, D., Wilcox, B., Cantor, J., Palmer, E., Linn, S., and Dowrick, P. (2004). *Report of the APA Task Force on Advertising and Children: psychological issues in the increasing commercialization of childhood.* Washington, DC: American Psychological Association.

Lefebvre, R. C., Doner, L., Johnston, C., Loughrey, K., Balch, G. I., Sutton, S. M. (1995). Use of database marketing and consumer-based health communication in message design: An example from the Office of Cancer Communications' '5 A Day for Better Health' program. In E. Maibach and R. L. Parrott (eds.) *Designing health messages. approaches from communication theory and public health practice.* California: Sage Publications, pp. 217–46.

Mazur, L. (1996). Marketing madness. *E Magazine: The Environmental Magazine* **7**(3).

McDermott, L., Stead, M., and Hastings, G. (2005). What is and what is not social marketing. *Journal of Marketing Management* **21**:545–53.

Morgan, R. and Hunt, S. (1994). The commitment-trust theory of relationship marketing. *Journal of Marketing* **58**:20–38.

Motsinger, B. and Vollinger, B. (eds.) (2005). *ASSIST: Shaping the Future of Tobacco Prevention and Control.* Bethesda, MD: National Cancer Institute Press.

Pierce, J. P., Choi, W. S., Gilpin, E. A., Farkas, A. J., and Merritt, R. K. (1996). Validation of susceptibility as a predictor of which adolescents take up smoking in the United States. *Health Psychology* **15**:355–61.

Schindler, R. M. (1992). The real lesson of New Coke: the value of focus groups for predicting the effects of social influence. *Marketing Research* **27**.

Snyder, L. B. and Hamilton, M. A. (2002). Meta-analysis of US health campaign effects on behavior: Emphasize enforcement, exposure, and new information, and beware the secular trend. In R. Hornik (ed.) *Public health communication: evidence for behavior change.* Hillsdale, NJ: Lawrence Erlbaum Associates, pp. 357–83.

Specter, M. (2007). Branson's luck. *The New Yorker*, 14 May.

Stadler, J. and Hlongwa, L. (2002). Monitoring and evaluation of loveLife's AIDS prevention and advocacy activities in South Africa, 1999–2001. *Evaluation and Program Planning* **25**:365–76.

Tybout, A. and Sternthal, B. (2005). Brand positioning. In Tybout and Calkins (eds.) *Kellogg on branding.* New York: John Wiley and Sons.

Wakefield, M., Terry-McElrath, Y., Emery, S., Saffer, H., Chaloupka, F., Szczypka, G., *et al.* (2006). Effect of televised, tobacco company-funded smoking prevention advertising on youth smoking-related beliefs, intentions, and behavior. *American Journal of Public Health* **95**:2154–60.

Wardle, J., Rapoport, L., Miles, A., Afuape, T., and Duman, M. (2001). Mass education for obesity prevention: the penetration of the BBC's 'Fighting Fat, Fighting Fit' campaign. *Health Education Research* **16**:343–55.

2

What is a public health brand?

Jonathan L. Blitstein, W. Douglas Evans, and David L. Driscoll

Summary

- Branding can be viewed by public health practitioners as a tool that will allow them to influence the perceived costs of engaging in health-promoting behaviors.
- Not all social marketing campaigns included branded messages, but all branded campaigns fall within the domain of social marketing activity.
- Branded campaigns promote a consumer orientation that emphasizes the nature of the exchange by appealing to the individual's self-interest. This approach will become increasingly important to the field of public health as individuals are required to take a more active role in managing their health.
- We can differentiate commercial brands from public health brands by recognizing that the brand object of a public health brand is the voluntary health-promoting behavior the individual is being asked to take up or maintain.
- To be successful, public health practitioners need to carefully consider factors such as demand, competition and timing in order that consumers perceive the brand as delivering its promised benefits.

When is a public health message branded?

Over the past 30 years, social marketing (Andreasen 2003; Grier and Bryant 2005; Evans 2006; Hastings 2007) or health marketing (Bernhardt 2006; Maibach *et al.* 2007), has expanded to become one of the predominant forms of communication in the field of public health and health promotion. Social marketers adapt marketing theories and concepts to design and implement communication strategies that promote socially beneficial change (Hastings and McDermott 2006). Social marketing campaigns in the realm of public health rely on theories of behavior change and marketing theories to promote changes in voluntary health behaviors such as smoking, diet and exercise, and sun-protective behavior.

One of the more recent tactics to gain attention in the realm of public health social marketing is the use of branding strategies (Evans *et al.* 2002; Wong *et al.* 2004). Branding has been embedded in the fabric of social marketing from its early days. Icons such as Smokey the Bear and McGruff the Crime Dog represent early efforts to incorporate Madison Avenue style tactics to promote social goods. But the strategic use of branding in public health, with an emphasis on value promotion based on aspiration and social modeling, is a relatively recent development. Terms like 'brand identity', 'brand equity', and 'value proposition' have only recently entered the public health lexicon.

Despite the growth of branding strategies, there is still a tendency to apply the term 'brand' to any communication campaign that has a logo or tagline attached, regardless of whether or not the communication represents a true branding effort. Additionally, there is a tendency to identify communications that promote branded health products that may serve public health goals (e.g. condoms for safe sex, water purification tablets to reduce water-borne bacteria) as representing *public health* brands. These campaigns are primarily aimed at inducing consumer purchase behavior, with positive health consequences as a secondary benefit of product use.

Aims of this chapter

Our goal in this chapter is to identify some of the key characteristics of branded communications and discuss the potential that branded messages offer the field of public health. Our main goal will be to show how branded public health campaigns can be differentiated from other public health campaigns. We will do this by reviewing the ways that branded communications provide a distinctive strategy to alter the perceived costs and benefits associated with a health behavior in a manner that makes the behavior more appealing to the message's audience. To support this position, we will first offer some insight into what it means for a product, service or health behavior to be branded. In the second section, we identify the characteristics that differentiate non-branded, or traditional, health communications campaigns from branded public health campaigns. Because branding is a marketing strategy, many readers will notice the overlap between the characteristics of branded campaigns and those of social marketing campaigns. In fact, we review some of these characteristics with the aim of emphasizing how using branding approaches and thinking like a brand strategist can provide additional insight into the development of social marketing campaigns. In the third section, we outline the characteristics that differentiate commercial sector health marketing from branded public health campaigns. Here, we focus on the specific strategies and approaches that differentiate product and service marketing from the marketing of health behaviors. Finally, we offer concluding remarks and discuss the use of branding as a potential strategy in the promotion of informed decision making.

Social marketing and branding

Social marketing employs commercial marketing principles and tactics to influence voluntary human behavior for societal benefit rather than commercial profit (Maibach and

Holtgrave 1995; Hastings and McDermott 2006). Social marketing can be distinguished from alternative approaches in public health promotion in part by its emphasis on the '4 Ps' of marketing – price, promotion, product and place – to influence voluntary behaviors (Grier and Bryant 2005; McDermott *et al.* 2005). Branding, a ubiquitous element of commercial marketing campaigns, has only recently gained traction among those employing social marketing in the field of public health. The increasing use of branding strategies in the development of public health social marketing campaigns offers an excellent opportunity to briefly revisit one of the basic concepts of social marketing – the principle of exchange – and discuss how *price* can be conceptualized in this domain and manipulated to increase the effectiveness of public health campaigns.

The exchange principle is an important, and often problematic, component of the social marketing process. Price, one of the '4 Ps' of social marketing, refers to the amount of money, time or energy that a consumer is willing to forfeit for the product or service being offered (Joyce and Morris 1992); price highlights the importance of recognizing the perceived costs and benefits of the campaign's product relative to the costs and benefits offered by the competitor(s) in understanding consumer behavior. Because social marketing is typically employed by public health and social scientists who believe the benefits of behavior change are self-evident, there is a tendency for the price and the exchange principle to be forgotten (Hastings and Saren 2003). This robs public health promoters of an influential lever for shifting behavior. When scientists fail to consider the perceived costs and benefits of alternative behaviors, and instead seek to alter modifiable health behaviors through information dissemination, the resulting campaign relies on the power of knowledge acquisition alone to promote behavioral change among message recipients. Branding brings the principles of exchange to the fore in public health campaigns. It reminds us that social marketing in public health, like any marketing activity, must consider the wants and needs of the target audience.

Why brand health behaviors?

The rise of social marketing in public health and the use of branding in the promotion of voluntary health behavior are tied to sweeping changes in healthcare and in our social construction of what it means to be healthy and well. The recognition that we are living in an era in which chronic disease and lifestyle factors are the leading causes of morbidity and premature loss of life has paralleled a growing emphasis on the individual's need to manage their own health. This shift has led to a new orientation in the field of public health that places greater emphasis on personal responsibility and individual choice in the prevention of disabling injuries and illness and the premature loss of life (Breslow 1999; Awofeso 2004). In tandem with this shift came a social movement that called for greater and greater levels of autonomy and individual responsibility in the field of healthcare. This can be seen in the rising call for health literacy (Ratzan 2001; Carmona 2005). Accordingly, educating the public to enable them to take personal responsibility for their health has become a leading objective of public health in the USA (Holman and Lorig 2004; Osborne *et al.* 2007; Redman 2007). Achieving this goal will require a greater understanding of the individual's perception of the target behavior – both in terms of the total burden (i.e. cost) associated with engaging in health-promoting behaviors and in terms of the cultural means and social aspirations tied to the behavior. Branding provides a mechanism to increase the salience and perceived value of the target behavior in the mind of the consumer. It reminds us that our target audience is comprised of agentic choice makers who have to balance numerous competing priorities in a world of limited time and resources. It also reminds us that if we expect our target audience to 'buy in' to our product, we not only have to effectively promote a desirable package through carefully selected outlets, we also have to provide it at a recognizable and realistic cost that offers a solution to our audience's needs.

What is a brand?

We begin by describing what we mean by a *branded message*. First and foremost, a branded message is a strategic communication designed to elicit a particular set of beneficial associations in the mind of the consumer which become linked to the brand's identity, providing equity or a sense of value (Aaker 1996; Ligas and Cotte 1999; Calder 2005). By a *strategic communication*, we mean that the brand's developers have engaged potential audience members in focus groups and other forms of consumer research to determine their needs relative to the product or idea being promoted. From this understanding of consumer needs, marketers develop a set of associations they wish to elicit, and use concept mapping or similar experimental techniques to help ensure that the aspirations and images evoked by the brand are actually received by the consumer as intended. The brand becomes a mental construct that provides the consumer with a sense of the value that is inherent in the brand concept above and beyond the values that may be recognized from the brand object (Keller 2003).

As Evans and Hastings discussed in the previous chapter, brand equity is a multi-dimensional construct that embodies each type of association between consumer and branded product, service, or behavior. *But, how does a brand develop equity?* Simply put, a brand acquires equity when the consumer recognizes that it provides him or her with a solution to a problem. More specifically, this involves the consumer becoming familiar with the brand, recognizing its perceived value, and forming positive associations that promote the intended exchange as a potential gain that provides the perceived benefit(s). As we will discuss, marketing solutions are predicated on the notion that individuals are goal-directed and self-interested problem solvers. Accordingly, brand equity offers a reason to view one product or service (or behavior) as the most effective solution to a particular problem. In general, there are three types of problems we seek to resolve and these problem sources correspond to the three types of attributes that are used to distinguish and provide equity in a brand. First, we use objects functionally to help us resolve problems in the world. Second, we use objects emotionally to help us resolve problems within ourselves. Third, we use objects expressively to help us resolve problems interacting with society. For example, you may enjoy a Pepsi-Cola because it is refreshing and thirst-quenching (a functional benefit), but you may also enjoy a Pepsi-Cola because of its association with a youthful and carefree lifestyle (a social identification benefit) or because you feel that it is a justified reward after a long afternoon of yard work (emotional benefit). As we will discuss later, these benefits reflect the set of associations the brand strategists hope to impart to the consumer to promote the value of the product and promote the desired behavior.

A brand is also a marker and a source of recognition. Commercial marketers go to great lengths to develop and protect the visible apparition of their brands – and for good reason. As Aaker (1996) points out, the brand is a 'mental box' where we store our beliefs, experiences and expectations. The brand image – the visible, iconic representation of the brand – becomes the 'thing-in-the-world' to which we attach our mental construals. But a brand is also a marker in the sense that we use brands to define and express aspects of ourselves. Brands are a salient component of contemporary culture that we use as markers of success and status, group membership, and self-description (Sherry Jr. 2005). In this way brands serve a totemic purpose. Ownership and display of the brand reflects the attributes of the brand upon the owner. For example, owing a Harley Davidson not only provides access to a select social circle, but marks you as an outlaw (Shouten and McAlexander 1995).

Perhaps most importantly, a brand is a promise. It is a social and implicit contract between the promoting agent (i.e. the seller) and the consumer audience. To buy the brand is more than an act of consumerism – it is an act of good faith wherein consumers place their trust in the promoting agent by believing that the brand will meet their expectations by providing the full range anticipated benefits. Accordingly, brand equity is not determined by the promoting agent or the brand strategist. Only when the promise made by the brand has been recognized by the consumer, is the brand's equity truly established.

Branding social marketing messages

In this section we identify a set of criteria that differentiate branded from non-branded public health messages, and in so doing, emphasize how branding can focus attention on the exchange principle and the price associated with the brand and the brand object. Of course, no single criterion is sufficient to determine whether or not a message is branded. Some non-branded messages have elements that make them look like branded messages. Furthermore, the processes of developing and maintaining a brand rely on both the actions of the brand promoter and the expectations and experiences of the target audience. Because audience reactions are often difficult to predict, branding cannot be reduced to a formulaic enterprise. It is only through consideration of a number of factors, such as the development of a brand identity and brand position, the value proposition (promise) of the brand, the aim of the communications activities, intention of the promoter, the development and management of the message, and the response of the target audience, that one can determine whether or not a public health message is indeed branded. With this caveat in mind, the following concepts can be viewed as a sort of 'Branding 101', an introduction to the basic concepts driving branded campaigns in public health.

Brand identity

Establishing a brand identity is the central task in the development of the brand. It encapsulates all the elements of the brand and becomes the central organizing fixture of all the associations that go into the creation of brand equity. Hence, development of a brand identity may be the most singularly important feature separating branded from non-branded communications efforts.

Aaker (1996: 68) defines brand identity as, 'a unique set of brand associations that the brand strategist aspires to create and maintain. These associations represent what the brand stands for and imply a promise to customers from the organization members.' The brand identity is the magnetic north of the brand. It is the singular and consistent anchoring point of all subsequent branding activities. It summarizes the anticipated associations the consumer will hold; it imparts to the consumer an expectation of what will be gained by taking part in the brand; it establishes a basis for the dyadic trust between the promoter and the consumer; and – perhaps most importantly – it provides a long-term organizing principle around which tactical application of the brand can be developed.

This long-term, strategic conceptualization separates branded from non-branded messages. The latter tend to be developed for a specific and tactical communication campaign. Campaigns that typically use traditional, or non-branded, messaging proceed with the belief that if the campaign is properly implemented, the target audience will be exposed to the message, and that sufficient exposure should lead to the desired behavior change (Randolph and Viswanath 2004). In contrast, successful execution of branded messages acknowledges the role of the consumer and requires a management orientation. Indeed, successful brand management is a product of continuous examination and reinvention of the 'story' of the brand to ensure that is it timely, relevant, and a facet of contemporary culture (Sherry Jr. 2005).

This notion of the brand identity as the result of a dyadic interaction between the consumer and the brand focuses attention on the exchange principle that underlies consumer decision making. Development and execution of a brand have been likened to an organic process in which the creation of the brand identity is a necessary first step – like planting a seed – the value of which is only realized once the consumer takes up the brand and evaluates the intended promise relative to the alternatives. Fruition occurs when the consumer's experience with the brand leads him or her to the recognition that it is the most appropriate solution or the best fit for the problem at hand. At this point, brand equity is harvested, the brand's yield is evaluated, and the brand manager must be ready to alter the brand identity should the consumer find that the brand does not live up to its promise.

Value proposition

Earlier we mentioned that a brand provides a solution to a problem and that the solution can be construed in terms of a functional, emotional or self-expressive benefit (Aaker 1996). These benefits are offered to the consumer as a yet-to-be-fulfilled promise that promotes the consumer–brand relationship. The key branding constructs noted by Evans and Hastings in Chapter 1 of this volume – aspiration to an ideal, social modeling and positive imagery – are the mechanisms by which the promise is delivered to, and realized by, the consumer. This complex sequence, beginning with the intentions of the brand strategist, encapsulates the functional, emotional and self-expressive benefits of the brand that drive the brand–consumer relationship which is summarized in the brand's value proposition (Aaker 1996).

The value proposition represents a simple and succinct answer to the basic question of the principle of exchange, *why should the consumer choose this product or service compared with the alternatives?* The value proposition should convey the brand's benefits to the consumer in terms that are direct and easy to grasp. It should also be specific enough to be directed to a particular consumer segment. A value proposition with these characteristics provides a natural bridge between the brand identity and the brand position, providing an organizing principle for the development of a communication strategy (Aaker 1996; Carpenter and Nakamoto 2005).

In the branding of public health messages, there are other considerations that strategists should consider in the development of the value proposition. For example, as we will discuss later on, factors such as competition and demand, which help to define the product category and competition for commercial brands, take on very different dimensions in a public health brand. The public health brand strategist should consider giving extra attention to these factors in the value proposition. This will help the audience members recognize the larger set of alternatives into which the target behavior falls, and will help establish the frame of reference for the consumer–brand relationship.

Consumer orientation

Branded communications are rooted in a consumer-based approach that acknowledges the need to develop messages that are relevant to the target audience, that align with the individual's self-interest, and that provide a reasonable expectation of value in exchange for engaging in the behavior being promoted (Houston and Gassenheimer 1987; Rothschild 1999; Chernev 2004). Understanding consumer's self-interest directs the brand strategist's choices with regard to the brand identity and its attributes.

Brands capitalize on consumer self-interest by targeting the wants and needs of the target audience. The brand does this by offering the consumer a solution to some real or perceived problem. This gives branded messages their market-driven orientation; they attempt to manage behavior by offering reinforcing incentives and/or consequences in a context that induces the individual to engage in voluntary exchange (Rothschild 1999).

The consumer orientation helps to ensure branded communications go beyond the simple information model of public health communication, which merely emphasizes the dissemination of empirically valid information (Maibach *et al.* 2006). The aim of dissemination approaches is to inform and educate the public, with the expectation that exposure to valid information will support the desired behavior change (Sutton *et al.* 1995;

Rothschild 1999). The problem with this expectation is that many people will decide that the empirically valid behavior is not aligned with their self-interests. Many people choose to engage in behaviors that offer short-term, tangible benefits at the expense of long-term consequences. These individuals are said to be acting myopically, referring to their short-sightedness. Others may evaluate the pros and cons and conclude that the potential gains from engaging in the desired behavior are not strong enough to warrant change. Rose (1992), for example, discusses the public health paradox. The paradox occurs because the behavior change aims of many public health campaigns are to reduce undesirable outcomes at the population level while the benefit to the average person is negligible compared with the sacrifice he or she is asked to make. Simply put, the changes that the average person is asked to make, though often small, are still more costly than the returns they are likely to realize.

Self-interest is manifest in the decisional processes consumers use to assess whether or not the exchange required to engage the branded object will benefit their long-term goals and aspirations. Exchange is the fundamental characteristic of any marketing activity. Houston and Gassenheimer (1987) emphasize the value transfer as the utility-maximizing functions of exchange behavior. In other words, people make exchanges to enhance their self-interests. An exchange occurs when two or more parties enter into an agreement through which each party seeks to gain benefits that will lead to the satisfaction of needs (Houston and Gassenheimer 1987). The recognition of exchange and its strategic use differentiates branded from non-branded messages.

In commercial sector marketing, most exchanges are characterized as restricted exchanges (Bagozzi 1975). These exchanges are dyadic, time-bound and involve costs that are easily determined and agreed to by both parties. They are dyadic in that they involve two agents, one the seller and the other buyer. The exchange is time-bound in that the buyer can anticipate that they will receive the value of the product immediately or shortly after purchase. The transfer of value (i.e. the purchase price) is a known quantity, as is the anticipated benefit of the product or service to be purchased. This last criterion is a key factor that promotes future exchange. So long as the agents involved in the exchange view their actions as increasing their utility (helping them to achieve some desired goal), they will continue to engage in marketing activities. In contrast, social marketing approaches are more complicated.

Exchanges promoted through social marketing and public health campaigns lack the typical quid pro quo structure of commercial marketing. According to Bagozzi (1975), social marketing is primarily concerned with the questions of why and how exchanges occur in relationships that promote social goods. These exchanges are characteristically complex and often involve symbolic exchange. In general, the consumer is asked to make a sacrifice or alter their current behavior in a way that can be viewed as evoking costs, in the sense that these changes reduce the individual's current subjective utility. These costs can be construed in terms of time as well as social and psychological expenses that are difficult to estimate. In return, the consumer is promised a future value that may be intangible, may require a number of intermediate steps to be realized, or may be realized by the prevention of a negative consequence. Accordingly, this promised value may be difficult to calculate, which means that exchanges involved in public health branding will require the consumer to accept risks. The lack of an easily accountable system of valuation, both in term of expenditure and gain, is a source of risk and a potential barrier that should be foremost in the minds of social marketers. Steps to simplify the calculus of the exchange and minimize the perceived risks associated with taking part in the branded behavior should be considered and incorporated into every step of the brand's development.

Brand position

So far we have discussed the development of the brand identity and the value proposition as two fundamental activities in the development of a branded public health message. While the brand identity provides a unifying structure and the value proposition summarizes the multidimensional facets of the brand's equity, the brand's position provides a roadmap that will direct the communications efforts designed to promote the brand and ensure that the brand concept will be received by the target consumer as intended. That is to say, the position imparts the promise.

Tybout and Sternthal (2005) identify four critical components of brand position. First, the brand position is aimed at a targeted consumer group. This targeting allows the brand promoter to create communications that emphasize the greatest advantages of the brand and tie equity to the need of the potential consumer. As this suggests, for any one brand, many potential positions can be developed. Indeed, it is the central, unifying brand identity that allows the brand promoter the flexibility to define greatest advantage in different ways for different segments without deviating form the core value propositions of the brand.

The second and third components of brand position are the frame of reference and the point of difference. The brand position is cast in a *frame of reference* that guides the consumer's understanding of the brand's benefits and situates the brand within a particular product category. The *point of difference* offers the advantage of the promoted brand over other members within the frame of reference. For example, BMW's brand position establishes its product's frame of reference as 'the luxury automobile category' and defines its point of difference as a high-performance car for the driving enthusiast, providing a better driving experience than any of its competitors; BMW's tagline, 'the ultimate driving machine' supports this image.

As these components demonstrate, one of the key functions of the brand position is to guide the targeted consumer toward an understanding of the value they will receive from the brand. Establishing a frame of reference and point of difference may be particularly challenging for promoters of public health brands. The intangibility of the brand combined with the lack of directly exchangeable competitors may provide limited comparatives. This point is elaborated later when we discuss competition.

The fourth and final component of brand position is the evidence that supports the claims made and provides consumers with a reason to believe that the promise will be delivered. Evidence is more important for branding efforts aimed at new products or when claims are more abstract. Established brands such as BMW or Levi's have less need to provide evidence of their products' ability to deliver due to the high levels of value these products have developed over the years. Developing sufficient and reasonable claims for public health brands is critical. Unlike commercial products and services which provide relatively immediate return on investment (you pay for and can assess the value of a BMW or a pair of Levi's almost immediately), the benefits of 'purchasing' a public health brand, such as increased physical activity or a smoke-free lifestyle, may take months or longer to accrue. In terms of creating powerful positions for public health brands, this suggests that providing claims that offer incremental evidence of the long-term changes likely to accrue from health-positive behaviors may be an effective strategy.

Verbal/visual cues

Commercial brand strategists expend a great deal of time and effort in developing language and visual elements that support the brand identity and value proposition in the mind of the consumer. These cues are then used repeatedly in communications activities to reinforce the brand in the mind of the consumer, to characterize the brand's product category, and to promote top-of-mind recognition. Verbal cues can include a product name, a slogan or tagline that will often also serve as a call to action, or the brand lexicon – a set of key words selected to highlight attributes of the brand concept in the mind of the consumer and consistently woven into branded messages (Calder 2005). Visual cues can include a logo, illustration, typography and color (Calder 2005).

The development of visual and verbal cues may be even more important to social marketers than to commercial marketers. First, public health brands are highly intangible. The behavioral targets of public health branding efforts are not packaged, not palpable, and not displayed on shelves. This lack of a percept (i.e. thing in the real world with which the brand is associated) adds to the difficulty of creating and maintaining brand equity. Second, public health brands are abstract. The concepts of 'a smoke-free lifestyle' or 'an active health information seeker' lack the kind of concrete, vivid, experiential detail that leads to the kind of mental representation that would promote specification and differentiation. This further complicates the development of brand equity.

Verbal and visual cues provide social marketers with an avenue to overcome these potential obstacles to effective brand development. In the development of the Centers for Disease Control's *VERB, It's What You Do Campaign* (Wong *et al.* 2004), the name 'VERB' was specifically chosen to convey a sense of activity. Public health brands that can successfully leverage verbal and visual cues to augment the salient and objective characteristics of the target behavior stand a far better chance of developing brand equity. We would argue that this is a necessary component of a well-developed public health brand, but not a sufficient component of branding. In fact, too often we see those with an incomplete understanding of brand development and management affix a logo or tagline to a communication effort and call it a branded campaign (see for example, Evans *et al.*, forthcoming).

Differentiating between commercial brands and public health brands

In this section we highlight and expand on the key factors that differentiate commercial sector branding from public health branding. Our principal aim is to highlight some of considerations unique to branding voluntary health-related behaviors. It is worth emphasizing that the primary distinction of public health brands is that they are the actual health behaviors that we wish to promote or prevent.

Brand object

We use the term 'brand object' to refer to the object of the branding effort; the thing to which the brand identity is attached. In using this term, we stress the fact that the product being branded is not always an object in the traditional sense. In fact, in the realm of public health branding, the thing to which the brand identity and brand equity are associated will never be an object in the traditional sense (Keller 1998). The brand object of a public health brand is the voluntary health-promoting behavior the individual is being asked to take up or maintain. This is one of the key distinctions between commercial sector branding and public health branding.

Behavioral goal

From our discussion of branding thus far, it should be obvious that commercial sector branding and public health branding have very different goals. In terms of the intended behavioral adaptation, the goal of commercial branding is to motivate an individual to purchase the branded product or service. This is a purchase that entails costs in the strict sense of a quid pro quo exchange, as previously discussed. In contrast, public health branding aims to induce behavior change so that the individual is motivated to engage in beneficial health-related behavior (Hastings and McDermott 2006). Certainly, this too has associated costs. The key distinction here is that the aim of a commercial sector branding effort is to induce commercial behavior – product consumption. The individual comes to acknowledge the brand's equity through acquisition of the product. Aside from those brands whose equity is deeply and singularly entrenched in functional benefits, use of the product may be a secondary issue in terms of deriving brand equity. For brands whose equity is derived primarily or exclusively from self-expressive or emotional benefits, product use may be a small component of the equation.

In contrast, the branded public health message is designed to promote engagement in a particular health-related behavior. While it may be necessary to purchase some consumer product to engage in the behavior (e.g. one should have appropriate running shoes before one begins jogging), the development of the consumer–brand relationship and the development of equity is derived directly from the engagement in the target behavior.

This is a crucial point in discriminating between two types of social marketing campaigns that include branding: campaigns that brand health products tied to health behaviors, and campaigns that solely brand health behaviors. As discussed, we view only the former as true public health brands. Consider these two options in the case of a social marketing campaign to promote safe sexual behavior. In the first case, the brand identity would be focused on the condom and the campaign communications would promote positive social models and aspirational imagery tied to condom use. The aim of this campaign would be to increase condom sales in the expectation that increased sales will lead to the desired change in risky sexual practice. In the second case, the brand identity would be focused directly on safe sexual behavior practices. Here the brand identity would be focused on voluntary sexual behaviors that reduce the likelihood of contracting STDs or having unwanted pregnancies. Positive social models and aspirational imagery would be related to a range of behaviors from communicating about sexual history to negotiating condom use with a partner. Notice that in the second case, the aim of the campaign is tied directly to the desired behaviors that will reduce risky sexual practices.

Demand

Demand is a marketing concept related to the consumer's tendency to act with self-interest. Primary demand refers to the consumer's choice to engage in, or not engage in, a particular category of product. Selective demand refers to the consumer's expression of preference within a particular category of products. Commercial marketers focus on selective demand and attempt to create differentiation and advantage for their product within the product class under the assumption that the decision to engage in this product class has already occurred (Rothschild 1999). Accordingly, the beneficial associations of the brand are tied to the product class and highlight the brand's promise is that it will fulfill the needs of the consumer in some way that offers greater advantage than other potential options in the product class. In contrast, social marketers are most often in a position of persuading the consumer to make a primary demand shift, often in a direction that seems to be at odds with the consumer's self-interest (Keller 1993). Thus, an important question for public health brand strategists becomes which set of behaviors should be branded (Keller 1998). Should the focus be on the benefits that accrue from engaging in the desired behavior, the costs associated in engaging in the undesirable behavior, or some combination of the two? This is a complex decision. It should be based on a number of factors: the desired behavior, its salience and importance, and the characteristics of the target audience.

Competition

The issue of competition is closely related to the two categories of demand. As pointed out in the previous section, commercial sector branding efforts aim to establish a position of superiority for the brand entry by differentiating it from other similar products and services. Here, competition is seen as other commodities in the same product class. In one sense, this makes commercial branding more straightforward than public health branding – it is easier to understand the competition. In the development of a branded public health message, promoters must consider the alternative primary demands among which the target audience can choose as sources of competition (Hastings 2007).

It is important for social marketers and those engaged in the branding of public health messages to recognize that they are always facing competition (Keller 1998). The sources of competition may not always be obvious, as they are in the case of commercial branding efforts, but any attempt to promote a change in behavior comes at the expense of alternatives, each of which should be viewed as a potential competitor. The more thought and attention we give to the forces that compete with our brands, the greater our chances of successfully promoting behavior change.

At the most fundamental level, the branded public health message must first overcome the persistence of current behaviors (i.e. habit). Many of our most basic health-related behaviors are highly automatic and heuristically driven. This is especially true for behaviors that have high levels of repetition and low engagement costs. This automaticity is – for the most part – a beneficial adaptation that frees cognitive resources for more important purposes. To overcome habit, public health strategists need to consider how they can incorporate concepts that convey low engagement costs to target audience members while simultaneously conveying sufficient benefit from engaging in the target behavior.

At a more obvious level, the branded message may also have to compete directly with countervailing commercial products. Perhaps the best examples come from one of the most thoroughly studied set of branded messages – the countermarketing efforts to reduce tobacco smoking. In the development of the *truth* brand, for example, public health brand strategists tapped into the same construct used by tobacco marketers to connect with youth – their natural tendency to rebel against authority figures (Evans *et al.* 2002). The *truth* brand, however, turned the tables on 'big tobacco' by establishing them as the authority figure and promoting the idea that tobacco marketers are manipulating youth. This is discussed more thoroughly by Farrelly and Davis in Chapter 6 of this volume.

Timing

Perhaps one of the biggest challenges faced by branded public health messages lies in expressing the terms of the exchange in a way that fits into the expectations of the consumer audience. Ultimately, the success or failure of a brand is based on its capacity to delivery on the promise it makes to the consumer. This requires time. To understand how time factors into the development of brand equity, consider the stages and the key characteristics in the diffusion of innovations model. The model suggests that during the persuasion stage an individual needs to recognize relative advantage, be able to test out or try the new product or behavior, and observe its benefits (Dearing *et al.* 1996; Rogers 2002). This is one of the reasons that commercial sector brands tend to be effective – the brand provides a relative advantage over its competitors and this promise is understood by the consumer. The consumer has direct access to the brand object, so that the benefits that derive from the brand can be assessed in close succession to the time that the purchase occurs.

In the social marketing of public health, the promised benefits are likely to be vague (better health) and realized at a time in the future that is not well defined. This has potentially weighty ramifications for the accrual of brand equity, as the effectiveness of the exchange can be diminished by poorly defined parameters of value and ambiguities in the timing of the promised benefits (Rothschild 1999). This suggests that public health practitioners interested in branding voluntary, health-positive behaviors need to carefully consider adaptive and creative brand strategies that promote equity through the identification of proximal and attainable objectives that can be tested and assessed by potential consumers. Establishing realistic timeframes for observing change is another approach that can be used to heighten the value of a branded behavior change.

A future challenge for public health branding: informed decision making

Earlier in the chapter, we discussed the growing movement toward increasing levels of autonomy and individual responsibility for health decision making. We also emphasized the role that market-oriented solutions can play in the promotion of voluntary behaviors. In this final section, we provide an example of the potential benefits of branding in public health. For this example, we provide a brief introduction to informed decision making (IDM), a behavior involved in an array of preventive health behaviors. IDM makes an excellent case study for the future of branded public health messages because the underlying behavior is highly abstract, complex, and its potential benefits are difficult to convey to the target audience. As we will discuss, branding provides an avenue to overcome these obstacles.

Informed decision making requires the decision maker to understand a number of complex factors. They must consider: (a) the nature of the disease or condition being addressed; (b) the clinical services available; and (c) their likely consequences (Briss *et al.* 2004). Additionally, they have to consider their preferences from among the various options available to them, participate in decision making at a personally desirable level, and, ultimately, either make a decision that is consistent with their preferences and values, or elect to defer decision making to a later time (Briss *et al.* 2004).

To date, we know of no efforts to develop a branded public health campaign that addresses IDM, but the complexity and the importance of IDM suggests that it could be an important target for future branding activities. The development of IDM brands will be challenged by the nature of the objectives and process.

The challenge in crafting a brand that promotes IDM will lie in gaining a greater understanding of the potential barriers and costs, including the cognitive costs associated with decision making, and identifying effective messages to marginalize those costs in relation to the benefits of engaging in IDM. The actual health outcomes of the behavior are entirely dependent on the options selected by the decision maker, and the uncertainty surrounding the decision means the health consequences of the decision made employing the IDM process cannot be described as superior to the alternatives. Most consumers have a low tolerance for uncertainty, complexity and ambiguity in their product selections, and would thus be uncomfortable participating in an IDM process.

The complexity is highlighted when we consider that the key attribute being promoted by an IDM brand is not the final decision, but the process by which that decision was made (i.e. was it an informed process?). Let us consider, for example, the case of screening for prostate cancer using the prostate specific antigen (PSA) test. From the perspective of traditional health communications, a prospective IDM message regarding the PSA would encourage audience members to carefully consider the risks and benefits of the PSA test described in a communication, assess their own values and preferences, and make a screening decision that is right for them. This approach does not consider the costs and barriers associated with IDM. But, in accordance with social marketing theory and methods, the value of IDM can be increased relative to those costs. In other words, the costs in time and energy required to participate in IDM could be offset by the perceived quality and personality of the brand – the image is that of a thoughtful and more independent thinker. Additionally, as a way to increase the objectiveness and salience of IDM, the branded public health message might target the more proximal goal of information seeking by evoking an image of thoughtfulness or 'a person who is in control' by directing the audience members to a website or to their physicians to seek to information that would lead to IDM.

Summary

This chapter has provided an overview of some of the characteristics that should be considered by public health practitioners interested in employing branding strategies in health communications campaigns. Starting with an overview of what a brand represents, we described a number of the hallmark activities that differentiate branded from non-branded communications. Chief among these are the strategic and purposeful development of an identity, position and value proposition. The culmination of these activities leads to the delivery of a branded message that offers value to the consumer and promotes the establishment of brand equity. We also discussed a number of factors that differentiate branding in the commercial sector from branding in public health. This distinction helps provide a division (albeit fuzzy) between branding aimed at products that contribute to the development of health and health promotion (e.g. brands that promote condom sales) and branding aimed at the altering voluntary health behaviors related to safe sexual practices (e.g. promoting communication among couples to reduce STDs and HIV/AIDS).

Perhaps most importantly, we have tried to emphasize the importance of considering the exchange that takes place in the adoption of new health-positive behaviors. Recognizing the importance of self-interest, public health practitioners engaging a branding strategy should make every effort to understand the exchange process from the perspective of the target audience. Developing branding messages in social marketing campaigns is one important way that public health practitioners can alter the cost–benefit ratio. This strategy is, however, dependent on the delivery of the brand promise and the establishment of brand equity. While the objective of branding is to establish and maintain brand equity, the function of branding is to alter to cost–benefit ratio of the inherent exchange. So, where equity is positive, and the consumer perceives benefits, the costs of the branded object are marginalized. This can lower barriers to cooperation and increase the likelihood of inducing the desired behavioral outcome (Wiener and Doescher 1991). As public health practitioners considering the costs to the target audience and what they will receive in exchange, the brand promise should be structured so that it offer a realistic description and explanation of the exchange process.

Finally, we suggest that public health brand strategist consider the how issues of timing and the delivery of the brand promise can be developed for behaviors that may require significant delay of gratification, such as physical exercise to promote healthy weight, or entail avoidance behaviors for which the function of the behavior is continued good health, as in practice safe sex behaviors.

References

Aaker, D. A. (1996). *Building strong brands*. New York: The Free Press.

Andreasen, A. R. (2003). The life trajectory of social marketing. *Marketing Theory* **3**:293–303.

Awofeso, N. (2004). What's new about the 'new public health'? *American Journal of Public Health* **94**:705–9.

Bagozzi, R. P. (1975). Marketing as exchange. *Journal of Marketing* **39**:32–9.

Bernhardt, J. M. (2006). Improving health through health marketing. *Preventing Chronic Disease* **3**, 1–3.

Breslow, L. (1999). From disease prevention to health promotion. *Journal of the American Medical Association* **281**:1030–3.

Briss, P., Rimer, B., Reilley, B., Coates R. C., Lee N. C., Mullen P., *et al.* (2004). Promoting informed decisions about cancer screening in communities and healthcare systems. *American Journal of Preventive Medicine* **26**:67–80.

Calder, B. J. (2005). Designing brands. In A. M. Tybout and T. Calkins (eds.) *Kellogg on branding*. Hoboken, NJ: John Wiley and Sons, pp. 27–39.

Carmona, R. H. (2005). Improving America's health literacy. *Journal of the American Dietetic Association* **105**(9):1345.

Carpenter, G. S. and Nakamoto, K. (2005). Competitive strategies. In A. M. Tybout and T. Calkins (eds.) *Kellogg on branding*. Hoboken, NJ: John Wiley and Sons, pp. 73–90.

Chernev, A. (2004). Goal-attribute compatibility in consumer choice *Journal of Consumer Research* **14**:141–50.

Dearing, J. W., Rogers, E. M., Meyer, G., Casey, M. K., Rao, N., Campo, S., *et al.* (1996). Social marketing and diffusion-based strategies for communicating with unique populaitons: HIV prevention in San Francisco. *Journal of Health Communication* **1**:343–63.

Evans, W. D. (2006). How social marketing works in health care. *British Medical Journal* **332**:1207–10.

Evans, W. D., Wasserman, J., Bertolotti, E. and Martino, S. (2002). Branding behavior: the strategy behind the truth campaign. *Social Marketing Quarterly* **3**:17–29.

Evans, W. D., Blitstein, J. L., Hersey, J., Renaud, J. M. and Yaroch, A. L. (forthcoming). Systematic review of public health branding research. *Journal of Health Communication*.

Grier, S. and Bryant, C. A. (2005). Social marketing in public health. *Annual Review of Public Health* **26**:319–39.

Hastings, G. (2007). *Social marketing: or, why should the devil have all the best tunes*. London: Butterworth-Heinemann.

Hastings, G. and McDermott, L. (2006). Putting social marketing into practice. *British Medical Journal* **332**:1210–12.

Hastings, G. and Saren, M. (2003). The critical contribution of social marketing: theory and application. *Marketing Theory* **3**:305–322.

Holman, H. and K. Lorig (2004). Patient self-management: a key to effectiveness and efficiency in care of chronic disease. *Public Health Reports* **119**:239–243.

Houston, F. S. and Gassenheimer, J. B. (1987). Marketing and exchange. *Journal of Marketing* **51**:3–18.

Joyce, M. L. and Morris, M. H. (1992). Pricing considerations in social marketing. In S. H. Fine (ed.) *Marketing the public sector: promoting the causes of public and nonprofit agencies*. New Brunswick, NJ: Transaction Publishers, pp. 101–13.

Keller, K. L. (1993). Conceptualizing, measuring, and managing customer-based brand equity. *Journal of Marketing* **57**:1–22.

Keller, K. L. (1998). Branding perspectives on social marketing. *Advances in Consumer Research* **25**:299–302.

Keller, K. L. (2003). Brand synthesis: the multidimensionality of brand knowledge. *Journal of Consumer Research* **29**:595–600.

Ligas, M. and Cotte, J. (1999). The process of negotiating brand meaning: a symbolic interactionist perspective. *Advances in Consumer Research* **26**:609–14.

Maibach, E. W. and Holtgrave, D. R. (1995). Advances in public health communication. *Annual Review of Public Health* **16**:219–238.

Maibach, E. W., Abroms, L. C. and Marosits, M. (2007). Communication and marketing as tools to cultivate the public's health: a proposed 'people and places' framework. *BMC Public Health* **7**(88).

Maibach, E. W., Van Duyn, M. A. and Bloodgood, B. (2006). A marketing perspective on disseminating evidence-based approaches to disease prevention and health promotion. *Preventing Chronic Disease* **3**:A97.

McDermott, L., Stead, M. and Hastings, G. (2005). What is and what is not social marketing: the challenge of reviewing the evidence. *Journal of Marketing Management* **21**:545–53.

Osborne, R. H., Elsworth, G. R. *et al.* (2007). The Health Education Impact Questionnaire: an outcome and evaluation measure for patient education and self-management interventions for people with chronic conditions. *Patient Education and Counseling* **66**(2):192–201.

Randolph, W. and Viswanath, K. (2004). Lessons learned from public health mass media campaigns: marketing health in a crowded media world. *Annual Review of Public Health* **25**:419–37.

Ratzan, S. C. (2001). Health literacy: communication for the public good. *Journal of Health Communications* **16**:207–214.

Redman, B. K. (2007). Responsibility for control: ethics of patient preparation for self-management of chronic disease. *Bioethics* **21**:(5):243–50.

Rogers, E. M. (2002). *Diffusion of innovations* (5th edn). New York: Free Press.

Rose, G. (1992). *The strategy of preventive medicine*. Oxford: Oxford University Press.

Rothschild, M. L. (1999). Carrots, sticks, and promises: a conceptual framework for the management of public health and social issues behaviors. *Journal of Marketing* **63**:24–37.

Sherry Jr., J. F. (2005). Brand meaning. In A. M. Tybout and T. Calkins (eds.) *Kellogg on branding*. Hoboken, NJ: John Wiley and Sons, pp. 40–69.

Shouten, J. W. and McAlexander, J. H. (1995). Subcultures of consumption: an ethnography of the new bikers. *The Journal of Consumer Research* **22**:43–61.

Sutton, S. M., Balch, G. I. and Lefebvre, R. C. (1995). Strategic questions for consumer-based health communications. *Public Health Reports* **110**:725–33.

Tybout, A. M. and Sternthal, B. (2005). Brand positioning. In A. M. Tybout and T. Calkins (eds.) *Kellogg on Branding*. Hoboken, NJ: Wiley and Sons, pp. 27–39.

Wiener, J. L. and Doescher, T. A. (1991). A framework for promoting cooperation. *Journal of Marketing* **55**:38–47.

Wong, F. L., Huhman, M., Heitzler, C., Asbury, L., Bretthauer-Mueller, R., McCarthy, S., and Londe, P. (2004). VERB – A social marketing campaign to increase physical activity among youth. *Preventing Chronic Disease* **1**:A10.

3

Evaluation of public health brands
Design, measurement, and analysis

W. Douglas Evans, Jonathan Blitstein, and James C. Hersey

Summary

- Brand equity is the higher order construct that captures the effects of commercial and public health brands on outcomes.
- This chapter focuses on the effects of brand equity on individual health behavior, but effects on upstream outcomes are important topics for future research.
- Brand equity mediates the effects of message exposure on consumer choice and health behavior.

Introduction: objectives of branding research

Brands seek to build relationships that enhance the value of products and services for consumers. By providing additional value for consumers, brands can instill a sense of loyalty and identification in consumers that causes them to continue purchasing the branded products and services over competitors. Brands accomplish this through associations with characteristics of the branded products or services that appeal to consumers, provide socially desirable models, and project idealized imagery to which consumers aspire. In short, brands project a personality with which consumers identify and seek to associate themselves through owning and using the branded products and services (Aaker 1996).

Factors such as loyalty, identification, personality and brand awareness, among others, operate as mechanisms that brand marketers use to promote consumer behavior (Keller 1998). Loyalty, for example, is at the foundation of relational thinking in recent work on branding (Hastings 2007), and may multiply the value of the individual's brand experience through diffusion to others (Reichheld 2003). These factors also represent the measurable effects of brand exposure on consumers that form the basis for individual-level brand research and evaluation. In this chapter, we argue that such individual-level factors are the constructs underlying brand equity, the higher-order construct that captures the effects of commercial brands on consumers, and public health brands on individual health behaviors.

Compared with commercial branding, it is much more challenging to evaluate the effects of public health branding campaigns. For instance, commercial brand managers have access to weekly data on sales and monthly data on market share, and these data are available for all individuals who purchase a product, not just on the subsample of a target audience who agree to participate in an evaluation. In addition, purchase decisions can often be influenced fairly quickly; in contrast; social marketing to promote healthy lifestyles involves ongoing behaviors that are embedded in interconnected community, cultural and family influences. One particular challenge is to evaluate the early effects of public health branding efforts, before long-term changes in behavior and health outcomes have been effected. This way, early feedback on the effects of social marketing campaigns can be used to refine brand promotion efforts.

Schulz and Schulz (2005) summarize the research methodology most commonly used in commercial brand research. They identify three main methodologies for evaluating brands: (1) consumer-based brand metrics, (2) incremental brand sales, and (3) branded business value. They describe each of the methodologies as explicating a pathway from consumer brand exposure to individual, financial or organizational outcomes associated with the brand. They note that '[t]he most common approach is to measure current brand perceptions, knowledge, and understanding, then track changes over time. These changes are then related to the marketing communication programs conducted on behalf of the brand' (Schulz and Schulz 2005: 246). The other two pathways measure sales and organizational outcomes of brands, as opposed to the effects of brands on individuals and their behavior.

Measurement and evaluation of public health brands, as with most research in public health generally, focuses on downstream effects (typically individual-level, or family or community-level) as the measure of program success. Likewise, the current chapter focuses on the marketing and communications pathway of the above model. However, measuring the organizational features and outcomes of brands may indeed be an important future direction for the field, and its potential importance should be acknowledged. As noted by Evans and Hastings and Haider in this volume, organizational standing may be crucial to public health brand promotion, and this is not just with respect to the organization's standing with the consumer, but also partners and stakeholders. Given that most social marketing brands are not funded directly by their customers (but by government agencies and philanthropies), this may be especially true.

For example, one of the key factors undermining public health branding the UK over the last few decades has been the government's reorganizing and reorienting the missions of social marketing organizations in response-changing policy agendas. In Scotland, for example, there have been four complete changes of identity for the national health promotion agency in the last 25 years (Hastings 2007). Campaigns as a whole often change identity (e.g. message platform and behavior change objectives) and fall victim to the same phenomenon. Thus a lack of organizational identity and longevity may be one of the key reasons public health brands have struggled to achieve the success of Marlboro and Coke. Future evaluations of public health branding should examine the second and third pathways in the Schulz and Schulz framework.

For current purposes, the consumer-based brand metrics methodology provides an illustrative framework within which to consider the objectives of public health brand research. Schulz and Schulz (2005: 247) note that 'if the consumer or prospect holds certain marketer-generated *right* attitudes and beliefs about the brand, they will most likely behave in the *right way* toward the brand'. For public health brands, the right attitudes and beliefs can be found in the elements of the brand identity that relate to the health promotion or disease prevention behavior (e.g. attitude that tobacco companies are trying to persuade young people to smoke, or belief that regularly eating junk food promotes obesity). Behaving the right way can be understood as acting and maintaining a pattern of behavior consistent with, and *based upon*, these attitudes and beliefs (e.g. not smoking because a manipulative industry is trying to get me to start smoking, or eating less junk food in order to maintain a healthy weight). Public health brand identification serves as the behavior change mechanism in the sense that it motivates internal arguments for a given health behavior. For example, 'I am living a smoke-free lifestyle because I can express a non-conformist attitude, demonstrate my individuality, and rebel against an industry that is trying to manipulate me by identifying with the *truth* brand'.

Conceptual evaluation framework

Evaluation of public health branding campaigns can be conducted in order to: (1) assess that brand messages are understood and relevant to target audiences (formative evaluation), (2) determine whether the target audience was adequately exposed to brand messages (process evaluation), and (3) measure the effects of exposure to branded health messages on related attitudes, beliefs and behavior (outcome evaluation). Table 3.1 provides an overview of the evidence sought at each of the three stages of branding evaluation.

Although the divisions between these stages are somewhat arbitrary, for the purpose of this discussion we consider formative evaluation as the evaluation of brand messages and potential brand before a campaign is launched; process evaluation as efforts to assess exposure to and reactions of a target audience to a brand; and outcome evaluation as efforts to assess the relationship of brand to health behavior.

Formative evaluation

Formative evaluation is often a very important aspect of branding efforts. In the context of branding, formative evaluation can help to assess the needs and values of a target audience for which a campaign is being developed. This might include a sense of the benefit of health behavior. Formative evaluation can assess reactions to a brand and potential brand messages.

The following lists the types of questions that might be addressed in formative evaluation of public health branding efforts:

- Questions to understand the target audience's needs, aspirations, values, current practices and competing behaviors.
- What message channels are used by the target audience?
- Do the brand-related messages capture the attention of the target audience?

Table 3.1 Evidence requirements by stage of branding evaluation.

Formative evaluation:

The brand and brand-related messages use channels that effectively reach the attention of the target audience

The brand-related messages capture the attention of the target audience

The target audience comprehends the messages associated with the brand and finds them personally relevant.

The target audience can identify the brand associated with brand-related messages

The target reacts favorably to potential messages associated with the brand

Exposure to the brand can prompt the target audience to engage in health-promoting behaviors

The images and associations held by the target audience do not prompt unintended negative reactions or behaviors.

Process evaluation:

(1) Evidence of substantial exposure of the target audience to the campaign brand

(2) Evidence that the target audience reacted positively to the campaign brand

---

Outcome evaluation:

(1) Evidence that exposure to the campaign brand influenced targeted beliefs, attitudes, and intentions

   (a) Evidence that the effects of campaign brand exposure were more strongly associated with changes in targeted beliefs than changes in non-targeted beliefs

   (b) Evidence that changes in targeted beliefs were associated with behavior (e.g. health promoting or protecting behaviors)

   (c) Evidence that the brand equity intervenes between campaign exposure and behavior (e.g. the association between campaign exposure and behavior is shown to be reduced when the targeted belief is controlled for statistically)

(2) Evidence that brand equity was associated with behavior

(3) Evidence that changes in behavior were not attributable to some other factor (e.g. other interventions, changes in the price of products, secular trends, or selection bias)

Criteria adapted from Hornik (2002)

- Does the target audience understand the messages associated with the brand?
- What messages do the target audience find personally relevant?
- Does the target audience think of the brand when they are exposed to brand-related messages?
- Does the target audience react favorably to potential messages associated with the brand?
- Does exposure to the brand prompt the target audience to engage in health-promoting behaviors?
- Do the images and associations held by the target audience about the brand prompt unintended negative reactions or behaviors?

Methods of formative evaluation can include one-to-one discussions, dyad and triad interviews, focus groups, and market testing. Table 3.2 shows the potential advantages and disadvantages of various types of research activities.

Table 3.2 Potential methods for formative evaluation.

Method	Advantage	Disadvantage
In-depth interviews	Unmediated reactions	Limited number of respondents; limited group interaction
Dyad/triad interviews	Easier to assemble; more time for each interview; respondents can prompt each other	Limited number of respondents
Focus groups	Opportunity for wider group interaction	Careful moderation to assure all participants share ideas and feelings
Market tests	Assess reaction to draft material	Limitation of generalizability
Web-panels	Quick response across the country	Limited to populations with internet access

Process evaluation

Historically, one of the most common failures of social marketing efforts is the failure to achieve sufficient exposure of target audiences to sustain health changes. Public health branding is important in helping to assure that related campaign messages can resonate beyond the individual message. Process evaluation helps to assess that the target audience has been exposed to campaign messages, and that in real-world circumstances, the target audience reacts favorably to the brand and brand messages. The first part of the section discusses approaches to assess exposure; the second discusses ways to assess reactions to the brand.

Measuring brand exposure and recall

There are two basic types of brand exposure and recall measures: self-report and environmental measures. Self-report measures capture individuals' aided (with prompts, such as summary information about the brand) or unaided (without prompts) awareness. Environmental measures use extant data about the delivery of a branded message, typically through mass media, in a given geographic area (e.g. a metropolitan statistical area). These two types of brand exposure have been widely used in branded health campaign evaluation (e.g. Farrelly *et al.* 2005; Hersey *et al.* 2005), and have important strengths and weaknesses that should be considered when analyzing the effects of branding on health behavior.

It is important to distinguish between *recognition* and *recall* of messages and media. A myriad of studies provide evidence that social marketing campaigns can be effective in changing tobacco-related attitudes, intentions and behavior (Sly *et al.* 2002; Farrelly *et al.* 2005; Hersey *et al.* 2005a, 2005b) and other health or problem behaviors (Hornik 2002). However, much of this effectiveness research is valid only to the extent that measures of campaign exposure are valid. Studies have examined measures of exposure to and/or memory of televised health marketing advertisements. Measures of *recognition* typically used in laboratory forced exposure designs have participants view an ad and indicate whether they have seen the message before, whereas *recall* measures provide study partici-pants with only a minimal verbal cue (Singh and Rothschild 1983). These studies have shown that recognition and recall measures are strongly correlated, and researchers seem to agree that both measures require respondents to access their long-term memory for at least minimal remnants of ad exposure (Southwell *et al*. 2002).

Furthermore, modern persuasion theories such as the elaboration likelihood model (e.g. Petty and Cacioppo 1986) suggest that individuals must engage in message 'elabora-tion' or the development of favorable thoughts about a message's arguments in order for long-term persuasion to occur. Thus, recall and recognition measures should predict subsequent changes in attitudes, beliefs and intentions toward campaign-targeted behaviors. A recent assessment of the extent to which these measures predict changes in behavior-related attitudes and intentions offers further evidence of their validity (Niederdeppe *et al*. 2007). Recent studies, such as the aforementioned work in tobacco control, the Centers for Disease Control's *VERB* campaign (Huhman *et al*. 2005), and ONDCP's anti-drug campaign (Hornik *et al*. 2003) have employed telephone survey methodologies that measure ad recall via measures of either confirmed ad awareness or aided recall of campaign brands.

Self-reported brand recall data

Self-reported recall of other mass media, including health messaging, is typically obtained by asking survey respondents whether they can recall having seen or heard specific advertisements (e.g. public service announcements or paid advertising). Self-reported awareness of branded health messages involves respondents recalling specific advertisements that are part of a branded campaign, and can also involve recall of specific brand attributes in the advertising.

The simplest form of self-reported awareness is aided awareness, which involves the respondent being asked whether they recall seeing an advertisement that had XYZ features. In the case of the branded campaign advertisement, these features would be chosen to identify brand attributes theorized to promote positive brand associations. For example, for the 'Verbatim' series of advertisements used in the Ohio *stand* campaign, respondents were asked the following aided awareness question: 'Have you recently seen any anti-smoking or anti-tobacco ads on television that show various Ohio teenagers talking directly into the camera about what they don't like about tobacco?' In other words, they were provided specific prompts about ad content as would be the case in any aided awareness survey question, but they were also asked about specific features of the ad that signified youth 'taking a stand' against tobacco use, which is the call to action of the *stand* brand.

A second, and generally more reliable, measure of self-reported exposure is confirmed awareness. A respondent is generally considered to have confirmed awareness if, having been asked about a given ad in the manner described above, they are able to then confirm their recall by identifying one or more specific scenes, screen shots, actors, actions or specific related items from the ad. For example, using the same *stand* Verbatim example, a follow-up question asked respondents, 'What happens in this ad?' Without any further prompting, respondents were given the opportunity to identify one pre-coded specific feature of the ad. In the case of the *stand* Verbatim ad, these features picked out specific brand attributes embedded in the video or audio such as (among other response options):

- Teenagers are standing up/fighting back to tobacco;
- Teenagers voicing their opinions about tobacco/tobacco companies;
- (Sarcastic tone) Thanks to tobacco companies for working to kill my family
- (Screen shot): '52 Ohioans die from tobacco every day. I don't want my dad to be one of them'

Environmental brand exposure data

Environmental measures of brand exposure rely on media market data such as gross rating points (GRPs) to provide estimates of population exposure in media markets. For example, many branded mass media campaigns buy advertising based on media outlet availability (e.g. appropriate television stations widely viewed by target audience) and media market characteristics (e.g. size, demographics, pricing). GRPs represent an estimate of viewership of paid media based on data derived from sources such as AC Nielsen. These data can be used to estimate population exposure to advertising aired during a given time on a particular station.

Environmental exposure data represent both a means of estimating branded campaign reach, and also a tool in evaluation in that they may introduce natural variation in brand exposure that can be used as an analytical tool, a kind of natural experimental control (Rossi and Freeman 1993). Farrelly *et al.* (2005) have used GRP data to estimate the impact on adolescent smoking over the first three years of the *truth* campaign. In this study, natural variation in media buying among media markets in a national campaign was used as a variable to account for differences in smoking behavior and changes in smoking over time in a population as a result of level of exposure. Figure 3.1 summarizes the variation in the *truth* campaign's exposure across the USA, with darker areas having higher scores on an exposure index based on GRPs of the campaign delivered in those media markets.

While the methods to assess the exposure to campaign messages are similar to those used in other campaigns – assessing confirmed awareness, assessing GRPs of exposure, and assessing exposure through interpersonal channels – we suggest that interpersonal channels can become particularly important in the instance of public health branding. This is because of the ways brands cut through message clutter is by the types of events, such as a *loveLife* concert, that can generate lots of communication among friends, co-workers and family.

Message receptivity and reactions

Elaboration likelihood model and related theories of message reaction

The manner in which messages are received can have a powerful effect on subsequent behavioral mediating variables and behavioral outcomes in a causal pathway (Petty and

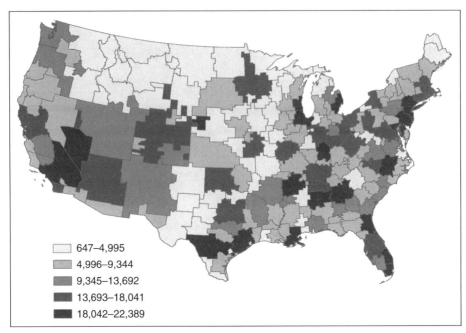

647–4,995
4,996–9,344
9,345–13,692
13,693–18,041
18,042–22,389

Fig. 3.1 Variation in *truth* campaign GRPs by media markets (2000–2002). Adapted from Farrelly *et al.* (2005).

Cacioppo 1986). One premise underlying branded health messages is that they provide a framework within which the audience can think about the proposed health behaviors, or lifestyle choices, and provide arguments or counterarguments that promote engaging and/or maintaining the behavior (Evans *et al.* 2005; Evans *et al.* forthcoming). The elaboration likelihood model (ELM) and related theories of message reaction and processing have been central in this conceptualization of how brands are related to message receptivity and reactions.

ELM distinguishes between two routes to persuasion: the central route and the peripheral route. Central route processes are those that require substantial thought, and are most likely to predominate under conditions that promote high elaboration. Central route processes involve careful scrutiny of a persuasive communication (e.g. a speech, an advertisement, etc.) to determine the merits of the arguments. Under these conditions, a person's unique cognitive responses to the message determine the persuasive outcome (i.e. the direction and magnitude of attitude change). So, if favorable thoughts are a result of the elaboration process, the message will most likely be accepted, and if unfavorable thoughts are generated while considering the merits of presented arguments, the message will most likely be rejected.

Peripheral route processes, on the other hand, do not involve elaboration of the message through extensive cognitive processing of the merits of the actual argument presented. These processes often rely on environmental characteristics of the message, like the perceived credibility of the source, quality of the way in which it is presented, the attractiveness of the source, or the catchy slogan that contains the message (Miller 2005: 129). Some research has considered emotional reactions (e.g. the likeability of the message or its environmental characteristics) to be a peripheral process that can affect reactions (Evans *et al.* 2005; Niederdeppe *et al.* 2007).

The two factors that most influence which route an individual will take in a persuasive situation are motivation (strong desire to process the message) and ability (actually being capable of critical evaluation). Which route is taken is determined by the extent of elaboration. Both motivational and ability factors determine elaboration. Motivational factors include (among others) the personal relevance of the message topic, accountability, and a person's 'thoughtfulness' (innate desire to think). Ability factors include the availability of cognitive resources (e.g. the presence or absence of time pressures or distractions) or relevant knowledge needed to scrutinize the arguments carefully. Under conditions of moderate elaboration, a mixture of central and peripheral route processes will guide information processing.

What role does message reaction play in brand equity?

Message reactions, both elaborated through central route and unelaborated through peripheral route processing, serve as mediators of the relationship between message exposure and brand equity. Positive associations can be built through both processes, but some form of positive initial message reaction is critical to brand identification and building equity in a public health brand.

Two widely used measures of message reactions based on ELM that have been associated with brand equity are message credibility and message likeability. Evans *et al.* (2005) have found that more positive reactions to individual *truth* campaign advertisements based on measures of credibility ('was this advertisement believable') and likeability ('was this advertisement likeable) were associated with more positive associations with the *truth* brand. The study considered the four latent constructs used to measure specific associations – loyalty, leadership, personality and awareness. Together, these four constructs form the higher-order *truth* brand equity construct.

The positive images of youth – as nonsmokers, rebels against the tobacco industry, and cool and edgy – depicted in *truth* message content have also been found to be correlated with decreased youth progression to established smoking (Evans *et al.* 2004). Positive social imagery depicting a social norm of not smoking, and of participation in a social movement against tobacco use, mediated the relationship between exposure to the *truth* campaign and decreased progression to established smoking. Given that such social imagery represents much of the message content underlying the *truth* brand, it is not surprising to find that *truth*'s brand equity mediates the relationship between the campaign and downstream outcomes.

Positive message reactions to the Ohio *stand* tobacco countermarketing brand have also been found to be associated with higher *stand* brand equity in a longitudinal cohort followed over a 20-month period during the campaign (Evans *et al.* 2007). Brand equity in *stand* was measured through a validated multidimensional scale adapted from the *truth* scale. The *stand* brand leadership/popularity subscale, which was based on descriptive social norms about the individual's social group (e.g. agreement with '*stand* is becoming more popular with kids like me') had the strongest prevention effect. This study concluded that social norms embodied in the individual items within this subscale appear to be the most important targets for social marketers employing a branding strategy, and may be applicable to health behavior change communications aimed at other risk behaviors.

Outcome evaluation

The third major type of public health brand evaluation is outcome evaluation – evaluations that assess the effects of brand equity and reaction to brand messages and health behavior. We recognize that effective evaluation is often able to combine process and outcome evaluation and at the same time offer immediate formative feedback to help enhance the campaign effort. At the same time, brand reactions and outcomes are correlated, and thus process and outcome evaluation efforts work hand in hand.

There are two main approaches to public health brand outcome evaluation. The first is to assess the correlation between brand equity and sustained behavior change. The second is to assess the role of brand equity in mediating the relationship between campaign exposure and sustained behavior change.

Evaluating the effects of brand equity on health behavior

Brand equity

In Chapter 1 of this volume, Evans and Hastings described the notion of brand equity as a set of associations between the consumer's self image and his or her social image of the brand. These individual associations, positive or negative, with specific attributes of the brand collectively determine an overall level of brand equity. In this chapter, we seek to operationalize the notion of brand equity by articulating the specific associations, brand attributes and collective characteristics of consumer perception and develop a system of measurement.

Brand equity is a measurable, higher-order construct or, in operational terms, a latent variable, that is in turn composed of multiple component constructs, as suggested by the earlier quote from Aaker (1996). In public health research, these constructs have been operationalized to reflect the asset categories of public health brands. For example, 'brand loyalty' can be translated as maintenance of a health behavior (e.g. avoiding smoking, or regular physical activity) once the behavior has been initially adopted in response to a branded health message (e.g. from anti-tobacco campaigns such as Legacy's *truth*® or physical activity promotion such as the Centers for Disease Control's *VERB*). Other asset categories are outlined in the next section.

Dimensions of brand equity relevant to public health

We propose that individuals form complex associations with public health brands, and thus value the relationship and make a commitment to living a certain lifestyle (e.g. not smoking, exercising regularly, or always using condoms). Product and service brands are based on the same underlying principles. Thus, the application of brand equity measures to health behavior-based lifestyles is in many ways similar to product and service brand equity. As discussed in Chapter 1, Aaker (1996) has developed a scale to measure brand equity along ten dimensions: the *Brand Equity Ten*. To examine the level of brand equity in the *truth* tobacco countermarketing campaign, Evans *et al.* (2002) developed a variant of Aaker's model. Their study analyzes the relevance of Aaker's dimensions as they relate to *truth* brand equity. Table 3.3 summarizes these dimensions and their relevance to *truth*.

In this analysis, monetary dimensions are considered irrelevant to *truth*. There are several reasons why monetary dimensions of commercial brand equity are not directly relevant to public health brand equity, and this distinction helps to illuminate the purposes and objectives of branding in the two contexts.

First, as noted in this chapter and elsewhere in this volume (see Chapters 1, 4 and 11), brands are about relationships between product and consumer, and about the underlying value or exchange of value added by the brand to a product or service for a consumer. In the commercial sector, value is a function of the cost of the item relative to the consumer wants and needs satisfied by purchasing the branded product or service (Calkins 2005). As described in Chapter 3, this reflects a restricted exchange, one in which value is recognized by both parties and the benefits derived from the exchange are obtained in close temporal proximity. It is primarily a trade-off of the monetary cost and benefits provided by the purchase. Non-monetary costs certainly can and do factor in consumer decision making, but monetary costs are typically primary in considering whether to engage in an exchange, such as purchasing a product.

In public health, however, the exchange is essentially non-monetary. It is true that engaging in a health behavior such as choosing not to smoke, or increasing physical activity, may have associated monetary costs, or have costs that could be calculated for some purposes in monetary terms (e.g. cost of personal time spent exercising instead of working). However, the primary costs associated with engaging in behaviors promoted by branded health messages are non-monetary. Adopting and maintaining such behaviors – whether using condoms to prevent HIV/STDs, or eating five servings of fruits and vegetables per day to promote good health and maintain a healthy weight – are not purchases. Money or its equivalent is not expended for the purpose of obtaining the object of the brand (i.e. product, service, behavior, etc.). The trade-off between cost and benefit is one of a behavior and an alternative (smoking vs. not smoking), and about the social and other lifestyle benefits realized by one behavior or another (e.g. being more socially accepted by engaging in one or another).

Many of these costs are based in the social, psychological or self-presentation consequences of engagement. For example, an individual who decides to quit smoking would forfeit the social contact opportunities associated with the 'smoke break' and may limit contact with smoking friends to achieve his or her goal. Similar, a teenager who decides to maintain a smoke-free lifestyle risks social marginalization if the prevailing attitude of their social milieu attaches positive personality value to 'being a smoker'. In this chapter, we argue that these costs are a substantial element of the non-monetary exchange of value underlying the relationship between public health brands and individuals adopting health behaviors.

Table 3.3 Aaker's brand-equity dimensions and *truth* dimensions.

Aaker's dimensions	Relevance to *truth*
Price premium	Participation in *truth* doesn't have a *monetary price*, so the dimensions are the individual's investment of time and effort (i.e. opportunity costs) associated with adopting the *truth* lifestyle.
Satisfaction/loyalty	*Satisfaction/loyalty* is a direct measure of how willing customers are to stick to a brand. One standard measure is whether the customer would recommend the product to a friend. This is highly relevant to the campaign's goal of teens' promoting a nonsmoking lifestyle among peers.
Perceived quality	*Perceived quality* is highly associated with other brand identify measures, including specific functional benefit variables (what does this product do for me?). Perceived quality measures typically ask the respondent to compare the product to competitors. *Truth* has two kinds of competitors (and measures): (1) tobacco industry-sponsored anti-smoking campaigns and (2) tobacco product ads.
Leadership/popularity	*Leadership/popularity* attempts to measure how the product rates as compared to others (is it the number one product?), how 'in' it is, and how innovative it is perceived to be. It is difficult to define a relative leadership position for *truth* (it could perhaps be compared to industry-sponsored anti-smoking campaigns, such as Philip Morris' *Think Don't Smoke*), but *truth* popularity can be measured and compared to tobacco industry ads.
Perceived (monetary) value	As *truth* is not purchased, *perceived value* is not applicable.
Brand personality	*Brand personality* is the Aaker measure most directly applicable to *truth*. These are the associations people make with the brand, and how customers differentiate it from other brands. *Truth* seeks to create a social image of an appealing lifestyle without smoking. Cigarette advertising attempts to create an idealized social image that includes smoking. This is the essence of the 'brand war' between *truth* and cigarette advertising. These questions measure how well *truth* is succeeding in getting teens to equate their self-image with the idealized *truth* social image.
Organizational associations	*Organizational associations* involve the customer's perception of the relationship between the producer with the product. People like to buy products from trusted organizations. The *truth* campaign explicitly avoids linkages with Legacy. But product characteristics are surrogates for the organization, so the proposed questions ask about the most important association – between the campaign and telling the truth.
Brand awareness	*Brand awareness* is a standard measure of the presence of the product in the mind of the customer. When they think of the product, they think of what? One question asks specifically about awareness of key campaign messages.
Market share	*Market share* can be captured by analysis of gross rating points data.
Market price	*Market price* is not applicable because *truth* is not purchased.

Identifying and compensating for these costs is essential in the development of effective brands, and accounting for them is essential in the measurement of brand effectiveness.

Measuring brand equity

Based on our reinterpretation of Aaker's brand equity dimensions, *truth* branding scales have been adapted from his *Brand Equity Ten* measures (Aaker 1996). The *Brand Equity Ten* is a set of standardized marketing and advertising research scales intended to be applicable across all products and market sectors. The scales were however developed with traditional products in mind, such as automobiles and toothpaste. We have designed a set of Aaker-type measures to fit the branding of *truth*, which is a set of attitudes, beliefs and behaviors about not smoking.

Evans *et al.* (2005) report on the development of a multidimensional brand equity scale designed to assess uptake of the *truth*® tobacco countermarketing brand. The scale was implemented in a series of nationally representative media tracking studies in US metropolitan areas targeted by *truth*. The scale was used as part of a larger telephone survey conducted with youth and young adults aged 12–24 as part of the national evaluation of the *truth* campaign from 2000 to 2002. Table 3.4 summarizes the *truth*® brand equity scale.

What are the hypothesized effects of brand equity on health behavior?

Brand equity occurs when individuals who are exposed to brands form associations with them. In turn, by forming the *right* kinds of associations, individuals will view the target behavior as more beneficial (or less costly) and will be led towards behaving in the *right way* – that is, in ways that promote health and prevent disease as a matter of self-interest. There is a causal hypothesis implicit in this view: exposure to a brand causes to associations, which in turn lead to some level of equity in the brand, and in turn lead to behavior. For example, exposure to the HIV/AIDS prevention brand, *loveLife*, which promotes responsible condom use as part of a young, hip lifestyle, leads to positive associations with *loveLife*, which in turns leads to regular use of condoms (Stadler and Hlongwa 2002).

In operational terms, public health brand equity functions as a mediating factor in the relationship between brand exposure and health behavior. In other words, the hypothesized behavioral mechanism through which public health brands are associated with prevention and health-promoting behavior is brand equity. Understanding brand equity in this way, important questions surround the evidence for the mediating effects of brand equity.

There is a large and growing conceptual and statistical literature on mediation as a tool for theory-based intervention design and for modeling and evaluating intervention effects. In general, a given variable may be said to function as a mediator to the extent that it accounts for the relation between the predictor and the criterion (Kenny 2007). Mediators are the intervening factors that tie elements of the communicated message to changes in the behavior of the communication receiver. Mediation analysis allows researchers to decompose associations between the independent and dependent variables in order to reveal the underlying causal mechanisms though which the intervention produces the desired behavior change. It allows researchers to assess whether program

Table 3.4 The *truth*® brand equity scale.

Construct	Measures
Price premium (willingness to invest time/effort)	I'd like to help *truth* get the word out. I'd defend *truth* if someone were putting it down. I'd wear a *truth* T-shirt.
Satisfaction/loyalty	If I had the chance, I would tell other kids my age to watch the *truth* ads.
Perceived quality	I pay more attention to *truth* ads than other anti-tobacco ads out there. *Truth* ads are better than other anti-tobacco ads out there. *Truth* ads are better than ads for cigarettes and other tobacco products.
Leadership/popularity	*Truth* ads are becoming more popular with kids like me. *Truth* ads are for people like me.
Brand personality	Would you say that the young people in truth ads generally Take control of their lives Take risks Rebel against authority Act independently The kids in *truth* ads are just like me. The kids in *truth* ads are like the kids I hang out with.
Organizational associations	When I see anti-smoking ads on TV, I can always tell which ones are *truth* ads. The *truth* ads are always honest. Other anti-smoking ads on TV are always honest.
Brand awareness	When you think of the *truth* ads, you think It's dumb to smoke cigarettes. Tobacco companies are trying to get young people to smoke. Smoking is not cool. Young people have better things to do than smoke. Not smoking is a way to express your independence. Young people can take action against tobacco companies.

impacts follow the prescribed theory of behavior change and provides practical information on how programs can be improved (MacKinnon *et al.* 2002).

The classical approach to mediation (see for example, Baron and Kenny 1986; Holmbeck 1997), assumes that the mediating variables account for an observed relationship between program inputs and measured outcomes. Accordingly, this approach requires the analyst to demonstrate a significant association between the intervention (molar) and the desired outcome as a necessary first step in the process of evaluating mediation. A mediated relationship is one in which the path relating A to C is mediated by a third variable (B). The mediated relationship would look like the following:

Tobacco prevention message (A) → belief that tobacco industry is manipulating me (B) → choice not to initiate smoking (C)

More recent theorists have taken a broader view of mediation, which has been described as an intervening variables approach. Under the intervening variables approach, program inputs, mediating processes and outcomes are all viewed as parts of a sequence of events (Collins *et al.* 1998; Shrout and Bolger 2002). While still similar in many ways to the classical approach, the intervening variables approach offers more freedom to program evaluators, allows the mediators to be conceived of in different ways, and extends applicability of mediation analysis.

Mediating variables are often contrasted with moderating variables, which pinpoint the conditions under which an independent variable exerts its effects on a dependent variable. Whereas moderator variables specify when certain effects will hold (external influences that may confound observed mediation and outcomes), mediators speak to how or why such effects occur. For example, choice may moderate the impact of incentive on attitude change induced by discrepant action, and this effect is in turn mediated by a dissonance arousal-reduction sequence (Baron and Kenny 1986). A moderating relationship can be thought of as an interaction. It occurs when the relationship between variables A and B depends on the level of C.

The best explanation of the above relationship is a combination of mediating and moderating variables. Tobacco prevention messages may promote a decision not to smoke, but making and maintaining that decision may also require reinforcement by peers. Thus, there is an interaction between messages and peer influences that serves as a moderating variable. Message exposure only reduces the propensity to initiate smoking, or progress from experimentation to established smoking, to the extent that peers agree with and reinforce anti-tobacco message content.

What is the evidence for these effects?

The case of *stand* provides a nice example of the evidence for prevention effects of brand equity on health behavior. In the *stand* evaluation, brand equity was conceptualized with respect to the campaign, its target audience (11–18-year-olds in Ohio) and call to action: 'Make a difference in the lives of important people around you by *Standing Up* against tobacco use.'

There were three main brand constructs for *stand*:

◆ Loyalty (will you continue with behavior?)
◆ Leadership (is the brand better than competitors?)
◆ Personality (do you perceive the brand characteristics as cool?)

In combination, these constructs comprise *stand* brand equity. The campaign's testable hypotheses were that youth with higher brand equity in *stand* would:

◆ be more likely to sustain nonsmoking lifestyle;
◆ perceive messages superior to tobacco industry; and
◆ perceive brand to have socially desirable personality.

Evans *et al.* (2007a) evaluated *stand* brand equity by examining maintenance of nonsmoking behavior and lack of intentions to initiate smoking (e.g. remaining a nonsmoker and indicating no intention to become a smoker, which defined a 'closed to smoking' youth category). Evidence consisted of associations between the above mentioned individual *stand* constructs and the overall brand equity construct, and future (absence of) smoking behavior and intentions to initiate smoking. Data were gathered from a longitudinal cohort of youth who were asked about their exposure to *stand*, brand associations (individual variables forming the *stand* brand equity constructs), and smoking intentions and behavior.

Figure 3.2 and Table 3.5 illustrate data from *stand* and evidence for prevention effects of brand equity on smoking initiation. Figure 3.2 illustrates a statistically significant reduction in the percentage of target audience youth who had never smoked in year 1 of the campaign among those who reported awareness of the *stand* brand, controlling for sociodemographic and other relevant confounding variables, compared with youth who reported no awareness of the brand. Table 3.5 illustrates results from multinomial logistic regressions that demonstrate the prevention effects of *stand* brand equity and identification with specific branding factors, on smoking initiation, controlling for relevant confounding variables. Respondents who had greater brand equity at baseline (BL) were less likely (i.e. had an odds ratio (OR) lower than 1.00) to ever be smokers at an eight-month follow-up (L1) and to a somewhat lesser extent at a 20-month follow-up (L2).

Brand equity as a mediator

The central tenet of public health branding evaluation is that message-specific branding measures and the higher-order construct of brand equity mediate the relationship between branded health message exposure and intended behavioral outcomes. For example, in the *truth* campaign, Evans *et al.* (2005) found that four second-order factors (constructs based on individual branding measures, that in turn form a higher-order brand equity scale) – brand loyalty, identity, personality and awareness – both individually and collectively mediated the relationship between *truth* advertising exposure and

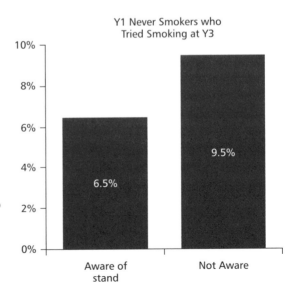

Fig. 3.2 Lower probability of initiating smoking after 20 months among youth who had never smoked at baseline and were aware of the *stand* brand compared with youth who were unaware of the brand.

Table 3.5 Odds ratios and confidence intervals (CIs) from the multinomial logistic regressions of smoking initiation on brand equity and control variables.

Construct	BL-L1 Respondents (CI)	BL-L2 Respondents (CI)
Brand equity scale	0.92*	0.91*
	(0.86, 0.98)	(0.86, 0.97)
Gender (male)	1.13	0.91
	(0.56, 2.29)	(0.37, 2.25)
Age (15–17)	1.23*	1.04
	(1.02, 1.48)	(0.83, 1.31)
Race/ethnicity (white)	0.76	0.68
	(0.43, 1.34)	(0.34, 1.38)
Friends smoke (one or more)	9.71***	8.56***
	(4.62, 20.41)	(3.40, 21.57)
Brand loyalty subscale	0.82*	0.79*
	(0.70, 0.96)	(0.66, 0.94)
Gender (male)	0.81	0.74
	(0.43, 1.53)	(0.33, 1.67)
Age (15–17)	1.21*	1.13
	(1.03, 1.43)	(0.91, 1.41)
Race/ethnicity (white)	0.83	0.74
	(0.50, 1.37)	(0.38, 1.44)
Friends smoke (one or more)	12.08***	11.48***
	(6.34, 23.00)	(5.00, 26.40)
Brand leadership/popularity subscale	0.53***	0.58**
	(0.41, 0.67)	(0.43, 0.79)
Gender (male)	1.09	1.15
	(0.61, 1.96)	(0.56, 2.34)
Age (15–17)	1.25*	1.07
	(1.03, 1.52)	(0.87, 1.32)
Race/ethnicity (white)	0.82	0.77
	(0.53, 1.28)	(0.45, 1.32)
Friends smoke (one or more)	10.67***	8.24***
	(5.94, 19.17)	(4.01, 16.90)
Brand personality subscale	0.77*	0.81†
	(0.64, 0.93)	(0.64, 1.03)
Gender (male)	1.07	1.07
	(0.57, 2.00)	(0.49, 2.31)
Age (15–17)	1.23*	1.07
	(1.01, 1.50)	(0.87, 1.32)
Race/ethnicity (white)	0.85	0.78
	(0.54, 1.35)	(0.43, 1.42)
Friends smoke (one or more)	8.33***	7.12***
	(4.31, 16.08)	(3.22, 15.75)
Brand awareness subscale	0.79**	0.82**
	(0.69, 0.91)	(0.72, 0.94)
Gender (male)	1.02	0.99
	(0.55, 1.89)	(0.46, 2.11)
Age (15–17)	1.17	0.99
	(0.96, 1.43)	(0.80, 1.23)
Race/ethnicity (white)	0.70	0.66
	(0.44, 1.13)	(0.37, 1.19)
Friends smoke (one or more)	9.05***	8.60***
	(4.72, 17.36)	(3.91, 18.96)

Reference value for control variables listed in parentheses.

*** $p < 0.001$, ** $p < 0.01$, * $p < 0.05$, † $p < 0.10$

smoking uptake. In other words, respondents (youth aged 12–18) with higher brand loyalty, identity, etc. were less likely to become smokers.

Figure 3.3 provides a simple illustration of the hypothesized role of brand equity as a mediating construct.

The *truth* campaign is a nice example of branding evaluation, but there have been many branded health campaigns across most of the major topics in public health. Infectious and chronic disease, one-time (or few-time) behaviors and behaviors requiring long-term maintenance have all been the subject of branded health campaigns (Snyder *et al.* 2002). Looking across these communication efforts, what is the evidence to suggest that brand equity functions as a mediator?

Mediation and moderation in targeted health message evaluation

As Evans and Hastings discuss in Chapter 1 of this volume, branded health messages are a species of targeted health messages – the most direct application of commercial targeting strategies in public health. Targeting strategies seek to aim specific messages at specific population groups to maximize message effects based on a theory of change. Public health brands operate on a theory of what associations specific population groups are likely to form with specific messages, or combinations of messages. Thus, public health brands inherently are concerned with audience characteristics and the social context (potential moderators) in which branded messages are delivered.

Mediating effects of public health brands should be considered in the context of hypothesized moderators – the theory of effects and behavior change underlying the brand should be considered in beginning any evaluation. For example, branded health campaigns consider cultural characteristics – cultural targeting or tailoring – to be essential to message strategy. Specific advertisements, or flights of ads, have been developed in campaigns such as *truth*, *VERB*, and the ONDCP anti-drug campaign specifically for African-American, Hispanic and other population groups in order to build brand equity with these specific audiences (Hornik and Yanovitsky 2003; Evans *et al.* 2005; Huhman *et al.* 2005). Evaluation of these campaigns must also consider different reactions to ads by cultural or racial/ethnic

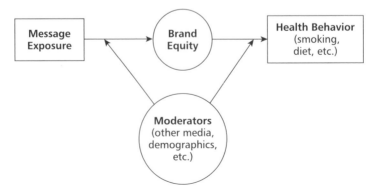

Fig. 3.3 Brand equity as a mediating construct.

groups, and build in measures of audience sociodemographic characteristics to multi-variate models used to analyze campaign effects on behavior and the role of brand equity as a mediator. Evans *et al.* (2005), for example, incorporated respondent race/ethnicity as a moderator in a two-step structural equation model (SEM) to test the role of *truth* brand equity as a mediator of campaign effects on smoking uptake.

Moderators can come in many forms, but there are several clear-cut categories that can affect reactions and outcomes of health communication messages. These include:

- personality and sociodemographic characteristics;
- other media effects (e.g. advertising for opposed products and services, such as from tobacco companies or junk and fast food producers);
- cultural characteristics and norms that are associated with behavioral outcomes of interest (e.g. food preferences or views on sexuality);
- community characteristics (e.g. availability of opposed products or physical features such as walkability that could promote or inhibit health behaviors);
- social influences or social environment (e.g. family or peer influences);
- environmental moderators of public health brand effects.

Public health branding research typically studies four major moderating influences on health behavior:

- competing brands and messages in the media;
- population and cultural characteristics (sociodemographics);
- social environmental influences;
- physical environmental influences;
- competing messages and media.

Marketing and advertising of commercial products is omnipresent in modern society. Having grown up in the early 20th Century as a means of building the consumer economy as a tool to sell the surplus fruits of mass production (Mazur 1996), marketing exploded with the advent of television advertising, and has grown exponentially again with the emergence of the world wide web and alternative media such as gaming plat-forms, cell phones and other handheld devices (Calvert *et al.* 2005). It has been estimated that the average American consumer is exposed to over 40 000 advertisements per year (Kunkel *et al.* 2004; Kunkel and McKinley 2007).

The omnipresence of media influences is especially pronounced for youth and young adults. As Roberts and Foehr (2008) have observed, 'young people surrounded by media in their homes and schools, but the portability that goes with increased miniaturization of digital media means that kids can remain connected almost anywhere they wish to go'. Moreover, these authors also note that media multitasking (i.e. using multiple media concurrently) has become increasingly prevalent, one result of which is that kids report exposure to substantially more hours of media content than they report hours using media.

All of this media exposure tends to crowd out and compete with social marketing messages aimed at changing health behavior. Food advertising promotes consumption of fast and junk foods, tobacco advertising promotes smoking. The appearance of attractive, socially desirable imagery and actors in movies, television or advertising smoking or eating high-fat foods and looking good normalizes unhealthy behaviors. Branded health campaigns seem like small fish swimming in a big pond.

Product marketing campaigns are on the air 24 hours a day, 7 days a week, with much larger advertising budgets. Branded health campaigns operate with much smaller budgets, have limited on-air duration, and generate less total exposure. Consider that the *truth* campaign had a total budget of approximately US$300 million from 2000 to 2002, the largest expenditure ever for an anti-smoking campaign, and yet the US tobacco industry spent approximately US$13 billion a year in advertising and promotion and generated far greater exposure. Their advertising continues at increased levels, while *truth*, like all other branded health campaigns, has decreased in spending and exposure generated over time.

A related challenge for social marketing is message competition with unhealthy product marketers, such as tobacco companies, which may use deceptive marketing practices. There has long been speculation in the tobacco control movement that the tobacco industry uses 'prevention' marketing as a way of obscuring branded anti-tobacco campaigns and creating message confusion, and even 'boomerang' (opposite of intended smoking prevention) effects (Henriksen *et al.* 2006). Wakefield *et al.* (2006) examined the question whether tobacco industry sponsored smoking prevention advertising aimed at parents (the industry's main target audience, rather than adolescents for whom prevention is the primary goal) had any beneficial effect on adolescent smoking behavior (the prevention target). They found little relation between exposure to tobacco company sponsored, youth-targeted advertising and youth smoking outcomes. Among adolescents in grades 10 and 12, greater viewing of tobacco company parent-targeted advertisements was, on average, associated with lower perceived harm of smoking, stronger approval of smoking, and stronger intentions to smoke in the future.

One could argue that the tobacco industry competes with branded anti-tobacco marketing by 'killing it softly' with confusing message targeting and messages intended to create a boomerang effect. Such effects are an important obstacle to public health branded messages, and should be the target of future studies on competing messaging and message effects.

The overall picture for branded health campaigns is that they operate in a crowded and highly competitive environment. Exposure and becoming salient and of interest to target audiences is a major challenge, and the effects of competing commercial messages must be accounted for both in message strategy and in evaluating branded campaign effects on behavioral mediators and health behavior.

Population and cultural characteristics

Social norms, such as descriptive norms about how people perceive normative behavior in their community and subjective norms about how people perceive others *should* act, can be a powerful influence on health behavior and decision making (Fekadu and Craft 2002; Eisenberg and Forster 2003). At the same time, public health social marketing campaigns pay careful attention to cultural, racial/ethnic, and other population-specific norms in developing and delivering behavior change messaging. For example, the *truth*,

VERB and anti-drug campaigns all had major ad flights directed at general, multicultural, mainstream audiences, and also specific flights directed at African-American, Hispanic, Asian and Native American populations (Farrelly *et al.* 2002; Hornik *et al.* 2003; Huhman *et al.* 2005).

Public health brand equity studies typically utilize sociodemographics as moderating variables to capture differences in the effects of targeted messages on distinct population groups. For example, Evans *et al.* (2007a) conducted multinomial logistic regressions to examine the effect of *stand* brand equity on adolescent smoking initiation, and controlled for the effects of race/ethnicity, gender and other sociodemographics. There were small, but statistically significant differences in reactions to *stand* between racial/ethnic groups, with white adolescents being less likely to initiate smoking than other groups. At the same time, a small but statistically greater number of non-white adolescents dropped out of this longitudinal study, raising the question of how non-responding African-American, Hispanic and other adolescents may have responded differently to the branded campaign. These are important questions for public health branding research to explore in the future.

Social environmental measures

The social environment, such as peers and family health behaviors, can have a powerful influence on adults and young people, and moderate the effects of branded health messages. Social cognitive theory (SCT) posits four sources of self-efficacy information, the most potent of which Bandura (1986) asserts is 'enactive mastery', or learning through trial and error. Another source is 'social modeling', or individual behavior formed by the attitudes and behaviors of people who serve as the adolescent's role models. For tobacco, SCT variables that support smoking include opportunities for observation and modeling of smoking, opportunities to use tobacco, social norms supportive of smoking (e.g. favorable image of smokers), and reinforcement for behavior.

In particular, advertising, television, movies and news media can provide role models that play an important role in the formation of attitudes about tobacco use, especially among young people (Pollay 1995). Cigarette advertisements, for example, provide image-based information to adolescents about smokers and may contribute to adolescent attitudes regarding smoking and smokers (Schooler *et al.* 1996). American youth are routinely and heavily exposed to some form of tobacco industry marketing, but the impact of this exposure on smoking behavior is not as well understood by researchers (Jacobson *et al.* 2001) and is likely to be complex. In future studies, appropriate measures will be crucial to evaluate how pro- and anti-tobacco images in the media translate into social images for adolescents.

Physical environmental measures

In addition to the social environment, physical characteristics of the individual's environment can moderate the effects of brand equity on health behavior. The 'built environment' can be a powerful influence on health-related decisions, and has been widely discussed and studied in recent years in connection with nutrition and physical activity in the context of the burgeoning global obesity epidemic (IOM 2005). For example, highly walkable, mixed-use neighborhoods have been associated with increased physical activity in the form of more walking for transportation (Frank *et al.* 2005).

The IOM (2006: 263–64) has developed a number of recommendations for communities that include expanding opportunities for physical activity in recreational facilities, parks and playgrounds; building sidewalks, bike paths and routes for walking or bicycling to school; and increasing street and neighborhood safety, especially in low-income, inner-city populations at high risk of childhood and adult obesity.

Recently, branded health campaigns have sought to encourage community utilization of physical activity resources and thus interaction with the built environment. The Consortium to Lower Obesity in Chicago Children has created the *5-4-3-2-1 Go!* initiative, which uses a healthy lifestyles branding strategy aimed at improving family food choices and increasing utilization of community physical activity resources (Evans *et al.* 2007). This initiative offers a model of how to change the social environment, and thereby increase healthy interaction with the built environment, through branding physical activity and increased consumption of healthy foods.

Future directions

Clearly there is a need for more research and testing of measures and instrumentation of branding and brand association. As noted in Evans *et al.* (forthcoming), most public health brand evaluations have focused on measuring brand exposure and awareness, and have had limited or no measures of brand associations. The role of public health brands as mediators of health behavior calls for valid and reliable measurement of such associations. It also calls for close attention by evaluators to the branding strategies used in campaigns, and development of highly-sensitive measures that capture brand imagery, cognitive and affective features intended by campaign developers to activate positive associations with brand characteristics and thereby motivate health behavior change and long-term maintenance.

Analyzing public health branding data

The main point of this chapter has been that public health brand equity operates as a mediator between branded message exposure and health behavior change. It operates through processes of message receptivity (credibility, likeability) and has effects on downstream attitudes, beliefs and related social cognitions that promote health behavior. Thus we are proposing a causal theory – or at least the beginnings of a theory – about how brand equity affects health behavior. What is the evidence for this view and how are these processes supposed to work?

Effects of brand equity on health behavior

Treating brand equity as a mediator, we hypothesize a causal pathway leading from message exposure, through brand equity and subsequent attitudinal mediators, to health behavior. In other words, we assume a set of independent, mediating and dependent variables will be estimated in a path model. Structural equation models are now widely used to estimate path models (Bentler 1995).

In an SEM to estimate the mediating effects of brand equity, we use either a self-report (e.g. confirmed awareness) or environmental (e.g. GRP) measure of branded campaign exposure as the independent variable. The mediating variable will be the higher-order brand equity factor, and/or its component factors such as brand awareness or personality. Dependent variables in our explanatory model will include health behaviors (observed or self-reported) such as smoking initiation or uptake (progression from nonsmoker to established smoker status), time spent in moderate or vigorous exercise, food choice and consumption (fruits and vegetables, low-fat dairy, junk or fast foods), or condom use. Moderating variables will be to account for all known or hypothesized sources of external influence, such as relevant other media effects (e.g. in an anti-smoking analysis, exposure to tobacco industry advertising), social environmental effects (e.g. peer influences), and sociodemographic characteristics. Once all the model variables are identified and a causal pathway hypothesized, an analytical model can be constructed.

Modeling effects of brand equity on behavioral precursors and health behavior

To illustrate the modeling of brand equity, consider the following model developed to test the *truth* brand equity scale using a two-stage SEM approach. This model was drawn from a study by Evans *et al.* (2005) that used a national cross-sectional survey of youth from the Legacy Media Tracking Survey that had been designed to help assess youth exposure and reactions to the *truth* campaign. The data selected for this analysis were based on the national sample of 12–17-year-olds collected in mid-2001, approximately 18 months after the launch of the *truth* campaign. The study assessed affinity to the *truth* brand using the measures adapted from Aaker (as shown in Table 3.2.).

For this analysis, the sample was split into two randomly selected subsamples ($n_1 =$ 1136 and $n_2 = 1170$) to allow for cross-validation of the findings (Cudek and Brown 1983; MacCallum *et al.* 1994). The first-order confirmatory factor model was comprised of four oblique (i.e. correlated) constructs representing different factors or dimensions of brand equity (loyalty, leadership, personality and awareness). Maximum likelihood CFA was performed to solve for parameter estimates in the calibration sample. The parameter estimates were then applied to the validation sample. That is, unstandardized factor loadings were constrained to be equal in both models, but error variances were re-estimated in the validation sample. This method, referred to as 'fixed-structure' cross-validation is the most stringent form that allows for sampling error (MacCallum *et al.* 1994). Data-model fit was then assessed by utilizing previously reported joint criteria (Hu and Bentler 1999). Additionally, coefficients were compared between subgroups by testing these parameter constraints in a multiple population analysis with a Lagrange multiplier test (Byrne 1994; Bentler 1995). Correlational techniques such as CFA and SEM have been reported previously in the study of anti-marijuana (Stephenson 2003), anti-heroin (Stephenson 2002), and anti-smoking advertising campaigns including the *truth* campaign (Evans *et al.* 2005).

The next step was to specify and test the theoretical second-order factor structure of brand equity. Again, maximum likelihood was used to estimate parameters on both the calibration and validation samples. Fit was assessed and the second-order loadings were cross-validated between the random subgroups in the manner described above. EQS 5.7 (Bentler 1995) was the software package used for analysis. After cross-validation, both the first and higher-order CFAs were performed on the combined dataset to estimate a factor model that would be applicable to other studies involving the *truth* brand equity construct (Evans *et al.* 2005).

Finally, several measures of 'factor quality' were calculated to ensure that the factors had acceptable reliability and that they accounted for the desired proportion of variance in the original, measured variables. The first of these measures, variance extracted, is a measure of the variability in the measured variables explained by the first-order factors, and the variability in the first-order factors explained by the higher-order construct. In the current investigation, the desired value of this index is equal to 0.5, indicating that at least one half of the total variance should be accounted for by the factor. In a factor with k indicators, variance extracted is of the form:

$$\text{Variance Extracted} = \Sigma \frac{(\text{standardized factor loading})^2}{k}$$

The next index is the reliability of the construct (RC) and has been previously reported (Fornell and Larker 1981: 45–6; Raykov 1997; Hancock and Mueller 2001: 198–9). RC is a ratio of variance explained by the construct in a standardized loading metric to the total standardized variance of that construct. The total variance is the sum of explained and unexplained (i.e. error) variance. Acceptable values of RC are equal to 0.7. RC is denoted as the following:

$$\text{RC} = \frac{\Sigma(\text{Standardized loading})^2}{\Sigma (\text{Standardized loading})^2 + \Sigma (\text{Error Variance})}$$

The final factor quality index, coefficient H, is similar to RC. Coefficient H is actually the squared multiple correlation between the construct and the optimum linear composite formed from the indicators (Hancock and Mueller 2001). Where RC can potentially yield reliability estimates that are less than that of the best indicator, coefficient H cannot. If all factor loadings are equal, coefficient H will be equal to RC, if not coefficient H will be larger. Additionally, coefficient H is unaffected by the sign of factor loadings, and cannot be reduced by the addition of indicators. The recommended value of coefficient H is 0.7. Coefficient H for a factor is represented as:

$$\text{Coefficient H} = \cfrac{1}{1 + \cfrac{1}{\dfrac{\Lambda_1^2}{(1-\Lambda_1^2)} + \dfrac{\Lambda_2^2}{(1-\Lambda_2^2)} + \dots + \dfrac{\Lambda_k^2}{(1-\Lambda_k^2)}}}$$

with 1,2, … k indicators, where Λ represents a standardized factor loading.

Figure 3.4 depicts the resulting SEM of *truth* campaign outcomes, and shows the mediating effect of *truth* brand equity on smoking uptake.

Future directions

There are many potential directions for future branding research, but one of the most important may be the development and evolution of public health brand equity. Commercial marketers and market researchers are keenly interested in changing perceptions of their brands, and the influence of new competing products and social changes on their brands. But little research has been done on changes in public health brands, and in the associations target audiences have for them, over time.

There are several hypotheses worth considering. Individuals with high brand equity communicate with their peers about the branded campaign, creating a diffusion effect. Social conditions may change due to moderating influences such as changing social norms (consider how the social acceptability of smoking has evolved since the 1970s) or changes in marketing and advertising (consider the promotion of organic food and glamorization of exercise such as running and working out at fitness clubs). Additionally, if branded campaigns such as *truth* persist over time, their aggregate reach and frequency will increase, which will tend to increase total brand equity. Over time, brand equity and its component constructs (e.g. brand awareness, or personality) may increase and have a stronger correlation with campaign exposure and a stronger mediation effect.

Analytical techniques such as longitudinal growth modeling (LGM) offer substantial opportunities to study the evolution of branded campaigns. LGM is a more recent and

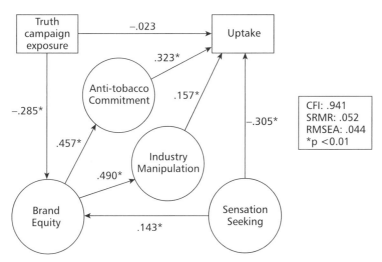

Fig. 3.4 Structural equation model demonstrating *truth* campaign brand equity mediating effects. Source: Evans *et al.* (2005). Reproduced with permission from *Journal of Health Communication*.

flexible alternative to classic methods for analyzing longitudinal data, such as repeated-measures ANOVA. It may be used for both descriptive and hypothesis testing purposes, both of which are important to this study. At its simplest, LGM estimates two important quantities of interest using a minimum of three time-ordered measurements. These quantities are used to describe the linear trend of a behavior or outcome over time. The first quantity is the intercept or initial status. This gives an overall estimate of the level of an outcome at the beginning of the time-span examined. The second quantity is the slope, representing the rate of change in the outcome. Together, these values form the longitudinal linear trend or trajectory of a behavior. One key feature of LGM is the estimation of variability in behavioral trajectories, such that each individual (or other micro-level unit) has a unique trajectory. This allows for (1) tests of the covariance between initial status and linear slope (e.g. do individuals who start lower at baseline have the greatest increases over time on the behavior of interest) and (2) incorporation of covariates as predictors of initial status and linear growth over time.

Using an LGM model, we can answer important questions longitudinal questions about public health brand equity, such as the following:

◆ What are the attitudes toward the brand prior to campaign exposure?

◆ What is the change in attitudes, intentions, and beliefs from one time point to another in the absence of brand exposure?

◆ Do those with lower intentions to engage in branded behaviors (e.g. remain tobacco-free, increase exercise, use a condom) at the beginning of the campaign tend to have greater increases in intentions over time compared with those who have greater intentions at the beginning?

Estimating the normative rate of change in a behavior such as smoking, or construct such as brand equity in *truth*, is important because effects of exposure to branded health messages should be estimated in relation to this overall trend. Other methods for longitudinal data that ignore this change over time that occurs in the absence of treatment may find no program effects or even conclude that the behavior has worsened despite exposure to the health messages.

Longitudinal studies of branded campaigns have been relatively rare (Evans *et al.* forthcoming), but new studies provide opportunities to examine changes in brand equity over time. For example, in the evaluation of the *5-4-3-2-1 Go!* obesity prevention campaign, researchers are collecting longitudinal data from a sample of community members in a randomized trial. The primary focus of analyses will be to determine the main effects attributable to *5-4-3-2-1 Go!* brand equity. Additive treatment growth models will be used to test these effects (Muthén and Curran 1997). Intervention effects – attitudes and beliefs about healthy foods and physical activity, reductions in sedentary behavior, increased utilization of community physical activity resources, improved healthy food choice – will be assessed as deviations from the normative trend in change over time in intentions, beliefs and attitudes that may be attributed to exposure to the branded *5-4-3-2-1 Go!* message. The difference in rates of change from the normative trend will be measured by estimating a third quantity in addition to the initial status and normative rate of change. This third value is a second slope factor and represents change over time due to *5-4-3-2-1 Go!* brand equity.

Studies such as this offer a model for future brand equity research that can test key outstanding questions about the efficacy and effectiveness of public health brands:

- To what extent, and under what conditions, do public health brand equity effects increase over time?

- How does the relationship between public health brands and audience change over time?

- What effects do changes in social norms and other moderators such as the media and marketing environment have on brand equity and its mediating effects?

- How can public health marketers improve the effectiveness of their brands in changing and maintaining health behaviors over time?

References

Aaker, D. (1996). *Building strong brands.* New York, NY: Simon and Schuster Inc.

Bandura, A. (1986). *Social foundations of thought and action: a social cognitive theory.* Englewood Cliffs, NJ: Prentice Hall.

Baron, R. M., and Kenny, D. A. (1986). The moderator-mediator variable distinction in social psychological research: conceptual, strategic and statistical considerations. *Journal of Personality and Social Psychology* **51**:1173–1182.

Bentler, P. M. (1995). *EQS structural equations program manual.* Encino, CA: Multivariate Software, Inc.

Bentler, P. M. and Chou, C. P. (1987). Practical issues in structural modeling. *Sociological Methods and Research* **16**:78–117.

Byrne, B. M. (1994). *Structural equation modeling with EQS and EQS windows: basic concepts, applications, and programming.* Thousand Oaks, CA: Sage.

Calvert, S. L., Rideout, V. J., Woolard, J. L., Barr, R. F., and Strouse, G. A. (2005). Age, ethnicity, and socioeconomic patterns in early computer use: A national survey. *American Behavioral Scientist* **48**:590–607.

Cudek, R. and Brown, M. W. (1983). Cross-validation of covariance structures. *Multivariate Behavioral Research* **18**:147–67.

Eagly, A. H. and Chaiken, S. (1993). *Psychology of attitudes.* Fort Worth, TX: Harcourt, Brace, Jovanovich.

Eisenberg M. E. and Forster J. L. (2003). Adolescent smoking behavior: measures of social norms. *American Journal of Preventive Medicine* **25**:122–28.

Evans, D., Wasserman, J., Bertolotti, E., and Martino, S. (2002). Branding behavior: The strategy behind the truth[sm] campaign. *Social Marketing Quarterly* **3**:17–29.

Evans, D., Price, S., and Blahut, S. (2005). Evaluating the truth[sm] Brand. *Journal of Health Communication* **10**:181–92.

Evans, D., Renaud, J., Blitstein, J., Hersey, J., Connors, S., Schieber, B., and Willett, J. (2007a). Prevention effects of an anti-tobacco brand on adolescent smoking initiation. *Social Marketing Quarterly* **13**:19–38.

Evans, D., Necheles, J., Longjohn, M., and Kristoffel, K. (2007b). The 5-4-3-2-1 Go! Intervention: social marketing for nutrition. *Journal of Nutrition Education and Behavior* **39**(S1): S55–S59.

Evans, D., Blitstein, J., Hersey, J., Renaud, J., and Yaroch, A. (Forthcoming). Systematic review of public health branding. *Journal of Health Communication.*

Farrelly, M. C., Healton, C. G., Davis, K. C., Messeri, P., Hersey, J. C., and Haviland, M. L. (2002). Getting to the truth®: Evaluating national tobacco countermarketing campaigns. *American Journal of Public Health* **92**:901–7.

Farrelly, M. C., Davis, K. C., Haviland, M. L., Messeri, P., and Healton, C. G. (2005). Evidence of a dose-response relationship between 'truth' antismoking ads and youth smoking. *American Journal of Public Health* **95**:425–31.

Fekadu, Z. and Kraft, P. (2002). Expanding the theory of planned behavior: the role of social norms and group identification. *Health Psychology* **7**:33–43.

Frank, L. D., Schmid, T. L., Sallis, J. F., Chapman, J., and Saelens, B. E. (2005). Linking objectively measured physical activity with objectively measured urban form: Finding from SMARTRAQ. *American Journal of Preventive Medicine* **28**(S2):117–25.

Hastings, G. (2007). *The potential of social marketing: or, why should the devil have all the best tunes.* London: Butterworth-Heinemann.

Henriksen, L., Dauphinee, A. L., Wang, Y., *et al.* (2006). Industry sponsored anti-smoking ads and adolescent reactance: test of a boomerang effect. *Tobacco Control* **15**:13–18.

Hersey, J., Niederdeppe, J. Evans, W. D., Nonnemaker, J., Blahut, S., Holden, D, Messeri, P., and Haviland, L. (2005a). The theory of truth®: how counterindustry campaigns affect smoking behavior among teens. *Health Psychology* **24**:22–31.

Hersey, J. C., Niederdeppe, J., Ng, S. W., Mowery, P., Farrelly, M. C., and Messeri, P. M. (2005b). How state counter-industry campaigns help prime perceptions of tobacco industry practices to promote reductions in youth smoking. *Tobacco Control* **14**:377–83.

Hornik, R., Maklan, D., Cadell, D., Barmada, C., Jacobsohn, L., Henderson, V., *et al.* (2003). *Evaluation of the National Youth Anti-Drug Media Campaigns: 2003 report of findings.* Report prepared for the National Institute on Drug Abuse (Contract No. N01DA-8-5063), Washington, DC: Westat.

Harnik, R. and Yanovitsky, I. (2003). Using theory to design evaluations of communication compaigns: the case of the national youth anti-drug media campaign. *Communication Theory* **13**: 204–24.

Hu, L. and Bentler, P. M. (1999). Cutoff criteria for fit indexes in covariance structure analysis: Conventional criteria versus new alternatives. *Structural Equation Modeling* **6**:1–55.

Jacobson, P., Warner, K., Lantz, P., Wasserman, J., Pollack, H., and Ahlstrom, A. (2001). *Combating teen smoking: research and policy strategies.* Ann Arbor, MI: The University of Michigan Press.

Keller, K. L. (1998). Branding perspectives on social marketing. *Advances in Consumer Research* **25**:299–302.

Kenny, D. (2007). Mediation and moderation. Available at: http://users.rcn.com/dakenny/mediate.htm (accessed 22 October 2007).

Kunkel, D. and McKinley, C. (2007). Developing ratings for food products: lessons learned from media rating systems. *Journal of Nutrition Education and Behavior* **39**(S1): S25–S31.

Kunkel, D., Wilcox, B., Cantor, J., Palmer, E., Linn, S., and Dowrick, P. (2004). *Report of the APA Task Force on Advertising and Children: psychological issues in the increasing commercialization of childhood.* Washington, DC: American Psychology Association.

Macallum, R. C., Roznowski, M., Mar, C. M., and Reith, J. V. (1994). Alternative strategies for cross-validation of covariance structure models. *Multivariate Behavioral Research* **21**:1–32.

MacKinnon, D. P., Lockwood, C. M., Hoffman, J. M., West, S. G., and Sheets, V. (2002). A comparison of methods to test the significance of the mediated effect. *Psychological Methods* **7**:83–104.

Mazur, L. (1996). Marketing madness. *E Magazine: The Environmental Magazine* **7**(3).

Muthén, B. and P. Curran. (1997). General longitudinal modeling of individual differences in experimental designs: a latent variable framework for analysis and power estimation. *Psychological Methods* **2**:371–402.

Niederdeppe, J., Farrelly, M. C., and Haviland, M. L. (2004). Confirming 'truth': more evidence of a successful tobacco countermarketing campaign in Florida. *American Journal of Public Health* **94**:255–7.

Niederdeppe, J., Davis, K. C., Farrelly, M. C., and Jarsevich, J. (2007). Stylistic features, need for sensation, and confirmed recall of national smoking prevention advertisements. *Journal of Communication* **57**:272–92.

Petty, R. E. and Cacioppo, J. T. (1981). *Attitudes and persuasion: classic and contemporary approaches.* Dubuque, IA: William. C. Brown.

Petty, R. E. and Cacioppo, J. T. (1986). *Communication and persuasion: central and peripheral routes to attitude change.* New York: Springer-Verlag.

Petty, R. E. and Wegener, D. T. (1999). The elaboration likelihood model: Current status and controversies. In S. Chaiken and Y. Trope (eds.) *Dual process theories in social psychology.* New York: Guilford Press, pp. 41–72.

Pollay, R. W. (1995). Targeting tactics in selling smoke: Youthful aspects of 20th century cigarette advertising. *Journal of Marketing Theory and Practice* **3**:1–22.

Reichheld, F. F. (2003). The one number you need to grow. *Harvard Business Review* **81**(12):46–54.

Roberts, D. and Foehr, U. (2008). Trends in Media use. *Future of Children: Children, Media, and Technology* **18**(1):11–39.

Rossi, P. and Freeman, R. (1993). *Evaluation: A Systematic Approach.* Thousand Oaks, CA: Sage Publications.

Schooler, C., Feighery, E., and Flora, J. A. (1996). Seventh graders' self-reported exposure to cigarette marketing and its relationship to their smoking behavior. *American Journal of Public Health* **86**:1216–21.

Schulz, D. and Schulz, H. (2005). Measuring brand value. In A. Tybout and T. Calkins (eds.) *Kellogg on branding.* Hoboken, NJ: John Wiley and Sons.

Shrout, P. E., and Bolger, N. (2002). Mediation in experimental and nonexperimental studies: New procedures and recommendations. *Psychological Methods* **7**:422–45.

Southwell, B. G., Barmada, C. H., Hornik, R. C., and Maklan, D. M. (2002). Can we measure exposure? Evidence from a national campaign. *Journal of Health Communication* **7**:445–53.

Stephenson, M. T. (2002). Sensation seeking as a moderator of the processing of anti-heroin PSAs. *Communication Studies* **53**:358–80.

Stephenson, M. T. (2003). Examining adolescents' responses to anti-marijuana PSAs. *Human Communication Research* **29**:343–69.

Wakefield, M., Flay, B., Nichter, M., and Giovino, G. (2003). Effects of anti-smoking advertising on youth smoking: a review. *Journal of Health Communication* **8**:229–247.

Wakefield, M., Terry-McElrath, Y., Emery, S., *et al.* (2006). Effect of televised, tobacco company-funded smoking prevention advertising on youth smoking-related beliefs, intentions, and behavior. *American Journal of Public Health* **96**:2154–60.

4

Building brands with competitive analysis

Ross Gordon, Gerard Hastings, Laura McDermott, and W. Douglas Evans

Summary

◆ This chapter demonstrates how competitive analysis can help build brands in public health by offering customer insight; help to develop strategic alliances; and help deal with the competition from the hazards merchants.

◆ Key lessons can be generated to help inform these outcomes by using the following forms of competitive analysis: case studies of commercial brands; internal document analysis; and studies of the deleterious effects of commercial brands.

Introduction

This book is about the public health sector emulating the huge success of commercial brands. This chapter focuses on a key dimension of this brand management success: competitive analysis. It begins by discussing why competitive analysis is helpful in brand management, not just in commerce, but also in public health. It then goes on to discuss three ways of analysing the competition: case studies, internal document analysis and studies of harmful marketing. Finally, key lessons are drawn.

Competing as well as copying

Competition is a crucial driver of the whole business process; it focuses minds and optimizes performance. It also provides a vital management tool. Analysing the competition helps a company to get its bearings, position itself in the market and adjust its course as circumstances change.

What is true for business in general is equally true for the more proscribed task of brand management. McDonald's examines competing brands like Burger King and KFC to help define and hone its brand positioning; likewise, the Adidas brand manager will plot the Adidas brand's trajectory against that of Nike and Converse. This cross-referencing also jumps sectors, as with the ad executive who described Marlboro Lights as the

'Diet Coke of cigarettes' (The heading Edge Consultancy 1997). In this guise competitive analysis provides an invaluable way of mapping consumer perceptions – we can all immediately understand what that ad executive meant. These consumer perceptions underpin brand strategy, and they are just as important in public health as in business.

Brand competition can also be more direct and aggressive, with little love being lost between the protagonists. The New Coke fiasco (see Chapter 1), for instance, was driven by the company's neurosis about Pepsi's success. Pepsi has responded by stoking the fire with its ongoing 'Pepsi Challenge' campaign, an overt attack on Coke's position as brand leader. This introduces a slightly uncomfortable notion for us in public health: are our brands really going to engage in this kind of combative competition with one another? One could speculate whether it is a matter of *truth* versus *VERB*. Let us hope not – it certainly need not be so. Even in the free market, competitors can become collaborators; for example, the Star Alliance brings together a clutch of airlines that might at first glance be thought to be fierce rivals. The alliance, however, is the product of intelligent competitive analysis, which has convinced each participant that cooperation is more rewarding than competition.

Similar alliances can be useful in public health; for instance, tobacco control is being advanced by a panoply of public health brands, from cancer charities to advocacy groups. To do this, groups need to understand each other, where they fit in the consumer's mind and that the whole can sometimes be greater than the sum of the parts.

A more combative form of competition emerges when we consider what World Health Organization (WHO) dubs the 'hazard merchants', in particular the big tobacco firms. Few in public health would advocate a strategic alliance with Philip Morris.

Commercial brand managers certainly pay close attention to competition from outside the market, and take muscular action when necessary. Branding can play a key part in the ensuing battle, but for commercial brand managers it brings no guarantee of success. A few years ago, Shell Oil got a severe mauling from Greenpeace when it tried to dispose of its Brent Spar oil rig by sinking it off the Scottish coast. Although the UK government supported the company's actions and subsequent analysis suggested that science was on its side, the oil company had to back down. It had become a battle for hearts as well as minds, and Greenpeace had a far more trusted and reliable reputation than Shell. Its brand won the day.

The fast food, alcohol and tobacco industries, among others, look on public health with the same caution and focus as the oil industry now looks on environmental pressure groups. If we are to meet their gaze with confidence, we need our own brands just like Greenpeace. This may lead to confrontation, but not necessarily. Philip Morris may be a partner too far, but competitive analysis might throw up opportunities for working with pharmaceutical companies or sections of the food industry.

In summary, while at first glance competition may seem a rather inappropriate construct for a discipline like public health, which is built on notions of consensus and caring, it can in reality bring four key strengths to our brand building efforts. First, it helps us to understand our customers better and thereby ensure an improved fit between our brands and their lives. Second it enables us to develop successful strategic alliances to give our brands better leverage. Finally it helps us deal with the competition from the hazard merchants by informing countermarketing campaigns that will undermine their brands and, where necessary, challenging them directly.

Competitive analysis in practice

This chapter will now examine three approaches to analysing the competition:

- case studies of commercial brands in the tobacco and alcohol markets – discussing their effects on health and society and showing how critical marketing can provide a tool for providing solutions;

- analysis of companies' internal documents – examining documents that have been used in fields such as tobacco control to inform research and decision making surrounding marketing;

- studies of the deleterious effects of commercial branding – primary research into the behavioural effects of commercial branding in areas such as tobacco, alcohol and food marketing.

In each case we summarize the key benefits and lessons these analyses can bring to public health branding.

Case studies

Case studies are useful because they allow us to examine who the competition is, what they are doing and what strategies and techniques they use that might be useful if transferred to public health branding. More fundamentally, the information case studies can help us to understand our customers better. Here we examine case studies of commercial brands in the tobacco and alcohol markets: Marlboro and Camel in the tobacco industry, and Budweiser and WKD in the alcohol industry. We will examine their brand strategies and key learning points for public health branding.

Tobacco

Marlboro Marlboro is a brand of cigarette made by Altria and is the world's best-selling international cigarette brand (Altria 2007).[1] Marlboro is named after Great Marlborough Street, the location of its original London factory. The brand dates back over 100 years to 1902 when Philip Morris, a London-based cigarette manufacturer, created a subsidiary to sell several of its brands including Marlboro. In the 1920s, Marlboro was advertised as a woman's cigarette using the slogan 'Mild as May'. However the brand faltered during and immediately after the Second World War and was temporarily removed from the market. In the 1950s Marlboro was reintroduced with marketing that tapped into the popularity of the romanticized cowboy and was able to increase sales by 5000 per cent.

This was the period in which the Marlboro Man was introduced, a brand image that is regarded as one of the biggest marketing icons. *USA Today* listed the Marlboro Man as

---

[1] Note that Altria divested Philip Morris, maker of Marlboro, on March 28, 2008.

number one on their list of imaginary luminaries, the 101 most influential people who never lived. Essentially, Marlboro was transformed from a feminine brand into a masculine one by the use of advertising featuring rugged cowboys at nature with only a cigarette. The success of the campaign and the use of the Marlboro Man helped Marlboro become one of the world's leading tobacco brands. Marlboro has also been very effective in delivering tangible benefits. It has been shown that Marlboro cigarettes have had ammonia compounds added to them to increase the potency of the nicotine in them without measurably increasing the quantity. Some pharmacologists have contended that the quicker the nicotine absorption, the more satisfying and reinforcing its psychological and addictive effect becomes (Kluger 1996).

The size and impact of the Marlboro brand was very clearly demonstrated by the events of Marlboro Friday on 2 April 1993. Philip Morris announced a 20 per cent price cut to their Marlboro cigarettes to fight back against the low-price competitors eating into their market share. As a result, shares in major household brands such as Heinz and Coca-Cola, along with the owner of Marlboro – Philip Morris – nosedived. The price cut was interpreted as an admission of defeat from the brand, that marketing and branding was ineffective, and that price promotion was the way forward. The events were subsequently described as signifying the death of the brand. This view proved wrong, however, as Marlboro and branding in general recovered to once again become dominant once Marlboro realized its mistake and reversed the decision to discount.

Marlboro has also had an enduring association with sport, especially motor racing. Until 1996 it had a long and successful sponsorship of the McLaren Formula 1 racing team which won many championships, offering a huge level of brand exposure around the world. Marlboro has also sponsored the Ferrari team, which was for a time known as Scuderia Ferrari Marlboro. The brand has also sponsored Indy Car racing in the USA, World Rally Championship teams and races and also motorcycling events. All these branding activities have provided Marlboro a high level of worldwide exposure and brand recognition.

Camel The Camel brand of cigarettes was introduced by US company R.J. Reynolds Tobacco (RJR), the world's second largest tobacco firm, in 1913. The Camel name and imagery were chosen as travels to faraway places were in vogue during the early 20th Century and viewed as exotic and desirable; the image of the camel was used to symbolize this effectively. Prior to launch, the brand was promoted in advance using teaser advertising campaigns stating that 'the Camels are coming', a play on a traditional Scottish folk song 'the Campbells are coming'. The promotion strategy, once the brand was on sale, included the use of a circus camel 'Old Joe', which would go through town distributing free cigarettes. The brand's tagline, which was used for several decades, was 'I'd walk a mile for a Camel'. The brand enjoyed strong sales throughout much of the 20th Century, and was supplied to soldiers during the Second World War, becoming one of the three dominating brands on the market after the war along with Lucky Strike and Chesterfield. Endorsement by personalities such as US newscaster Edward Murrow, who smoked up to four packs per day, contributed to the brand's popularity. Similar to Marlboro, Camel established itself as a masculine brand, using rugged, outdoor imagery with a distinct logo, packaging and style. The town of Winston-Salem where RJR was founded was nicknamed 'Camel City' at one time, a reflection of the brand's popularity.

Camel has also used brand stretching by launching Camel boots and Camel clothing. On occasions this has been used to circumvent tobacco ad bans. For example, in Norway in 1975 following a tobacco ad ban, adverts for Camel boots appeared in the print media.

Like Marlboro, the Camel brand has sponsored motor racing events in the form of the International Motor Sports Association Camel GT racing series, as well as sponsoring the Lotus Formula 1 team in the late 1980s. Camel also sponsored the Honda team in the AMA Superbike competition, and the Camel Trophy off-road race between 1980 and 2000.

The Joe Camel figure was created as a brand mascot in the 1950s, although it did not become widely used until the figure was rediscovered in the 1980s. Joe Camel was a cartoon-type character that featured in print media advertising and, prior to 1987, appeared in animated TV adverts – essentially cartoons.

The branding activity pursued by Camel has helped it maintain its position as one of the world's leading cigarette brands. Like Marlboro, the Camel brand has been carefully designed and maintained over the years using strong promotional campaigns with imagery and appeals to values that identify the product to consumers.

Key lessons

Longevity Marlboro and Camel have both been around for 100 years or more and have continuously maintained and developed brand image, allowing them to build up a relationship between the brand and its customers over a long period of time. This enables such brands to build up a degree of trust: they are well established, well known, familiar and have built up a relationship with their customers. Continuity is the key here; longstanding commercial brands have been doing it for years and will keep on doing it. Successful brands are the result of decades of careful effort and design. Contrast this with the situation in the public sector in which reorganization, retrenchment and political change often result in rebranding or brands appearing and disappearing with regularity. Take the UK approach to health promotion as an example: in Scotland the body responsible for health promotion has been rebranded four times in the last 25 years, preventing formation of an established brand to can help brand recognition and customer loyalty. In New Zealand, however, the Health Sponsorship Council was established in 1993 and has built brands and relationships with its audiences. What we can learn from commercial brands is that longevity is vital.

Subtlety The two tobacco brands are used with great subtlety. The link with masculinity, for instance, is achieved through imagery and association with appropriate sports. The issue is not forced nor is their image undermined. And yet their methods are very powerful. Marlboro was so successful in changing from a woman's cigarette in the 1920s that the brand's sales increased 5000 per cent in the 1950s as it pursued a masculine image. Importantly this use of subtlety is about respecting the customer and not patronizing them with paternalistic or unsophisticated branding. This is an important lesson that needs to be taken onboard in the field of public health.

Delivering tangible benefits. Strong brands deliver tangible benefits. As noted in Chapter 1, any good brand should facilitate recognition, make a promise and deliver satisfaction. The last point is vital, as promise without delivery is extremely damaging. The tobacco brands examined in our case studies have been successful in adhering to this process by ensuring that the product is always consistent and reliable. Marlboro has even used ammonia technology to increase the potency of the nicotine in its cigarettes, thereby delivering satisfaction to its customers. In the public health sphere this is an important lesson. One may establish a public health brand with a major promotional drive behind it, gaining recognition and making promises about the services it can offer, but if the framework is not in place to deliver the services or product effectively then customer satisfaction cannot be delivered and the brand will be badly damaged.

Alcohol

Budweiser Budweiser – often referred to as Bud – is a global beer brand owned by the US Anheusur-Busch Company based in St Louis. The brand was introduced in 1876 in the USA but has since expanded to many markets around the world, allowing Budweiser and Bud Light to become the number one and two beer brands in the world, generating $3.4 billion in profits for Anheusur-Busch in 2004 (Anheusur-Busch 2004). Major expansion markets for Budweiser include China, Mexico, Argentina, Finland and Russia, demonstrating that Budweiser is a truly global brand. The brand's tagline is currently 'Budweiser, King of Beers' and the brand name is one of the most recognized in the world.

Budweiser has been marketed strongly for over 100 years. In the early 1900s, the company commissioned early phonograph companies to record popular music tunes to promote the brand. Several advertising campaigns for the brand have entered the popular culture in the USA, the UK and other markets. One particularly memorable campaign was the 'Whassup' campaign, which made use of viral marketing. Prior to any ads appearing, mobile phone text messages were sent to a database of key customers giving them advance information about the campaign. Once these had appeared, the slogan was then sent out so that it could be passed on by the receivers to their friends. This was supported by a website offering interactive activities, including further opportunities to forward the slogan, messages and characters from the adverts to friends using both e-mail and text messaging. The campaign was very successful – 'Whassup?!' became a popular catchphrase in many languages and a musical version of the ad made it into the UK chart listings.

Another campaign featured three animated cartoon-like frogs named by their different croaks, 'Bud', 'Weis' and 'Er', which was also very successful in promoting the brand and strengthening its presence in popular culture.

Budweiser is heavily involved in sports sponsorship, being a major sponsor of the FIFA World Cup, the FA Premier League as well as being beer sponsor of a number of clubs in the English Football League. The brand was also headline sponsor of the British Basketball League in the 1990s and is official partner and sponsor of a number of sporting franchises in the USA. This has resulted in the Budweiser brand becoming synonymous with sports especially, association football.

WKD Launched in 1996, WKD is vodka-based drink operating in the flavoured alcoholic beverage (FAB) market, and is owned by Beverage Brands UK Ltd, a relatively small player compared with Diageo and Bacardi-Martini, who dominate the market. However, the WKD brand has been strongly marketed in the UK recently and the brand has used many new and innovative ways to market itself. WKD is one of the top five selling FABs, and in 2004 the brand's marketing budget was approximately £25m (*The Grocer* 2004).

The brand range includes WKD Original, available in three formats – Vodka Blue, Vodka Iron Brew and Vodka Silver, and WKD 40, a shot-based drink. WKD, which is positioned in the youth-targeted FAB market, has been marketed in such a way as to have particular resonance with young people. The brand name WKD, a play on the word 'wicked', is a commonly-used term among young people to express approval, and is a component of fashionable 'street' language.

WKD has been marketed using innovative advertising in the conventional media using language and situations identifiable to the young, new media and viral marketing, and sponsoring activities and events associated with young people. This activity has been backed by aggressive pricing – the product is cheaper than many of its competitors.

The WKD brand has been promoted in a major TV advertising campaign featuring adverts in which people play tricks on their friends, with the adverts encouraging consumers to get in touch with their WKD (wicked) side and ending with the caption, 'Have you got a WKD side?' The substitution of the word 'wicked' with the brand name 'WKD' is a marketing technique becoming increasingly common. Therefore, while the brand name itself identifies with the language of young people, the use of the word 'WKD' in the TV adverts utilizes another meaning of the word in such a way as to appeal to youth.

WKD has also been advertised in an extensive poster campaign using billboards across the UK, particularly in student towns and in premises such as student unions, complementing WKD-sponsored student tours. The brand has also used flyposting, in particular to advertise web microsites or competitions.

Beverage Brands has used sponsorship of events associated with its target consumer group as a way to market WKD. The brand sponsors scoreboards at a number of English Premiership football grounds and has previously sponsored diverse sports such as yachting and ice hockey. WKD was also one of the sponsors of the UK television channel ITV's coverage of the Euro 2004 football championships and has sponsored dance music events and a range of student events in pubs around the UK. Again, in sponsoring such events, WKD is associating with activities enjoyed by young people and is building a brand name that identifies with the fashionable and cool.

The WKD brand has a sophisticated website that includes a number of features such as video games, events advertising, competitions and a section for VIP members.

The WKD brand has also used viral marketing – the website offers an e-mail postcard service, and a 'windup service' allowing users to send bogus letters by e-mail to their friends. WKD has made use of mobile phone text messaging to run text-and-win competitions for the brand.

In the field of product development, WKD has endeavoured to keep things fresh by releasing new variations of the product. In 2002, WKD 40, a shot-based variant of WKD with a 40 per cent ABV, was launched in Iron Brew and Blue variants. In 2003, WKD Original Vodka Silver was launched to complement the two existing WKD Original drinks, giving a wider range of flavours. WKD Original was also launched in large 70 cl bottles in 2001 in an effort to boost sales in the off-licence trade (*The Grocer* 2001).

WKD has been marketed aggressively towards the 18–25-years age group and has been the subject of a large marketing budget for a number of years. Aggressive pricing and innovative marketing techniques such as extensive use of viral marketing, sponsorship of sport and student events, and clever media advertising have enable WKD to build a brand that appeals to young people and especially young males as well as the typical female drinkers of FABs. As a result, WKD has been able to increase market share at the expense of competitors despite an overall decline in sales of FABs.

Key lessons

Innovative use of new media Websites, mobile phone text messaging and viral marketing are channels of communication that can be harnessed and used in the public sector. The new media channels used by Budweiser and WKD tend to be used most widely by younger people who embrace such technologies willingly. Furthermore, new media are much more interactive and democratic than traditional marketing channels (consumers can actually influence and often control content). Clearly the lesson here is that in public health branding there is a requirement to embrace innovative new media channels to be able to reach audiences and be accessible.

Cultural relevance Budweiser and WKD have been very successful in developing their brands in such a way as to ingratiate the brand into popular culture through the use of marketing campaigns that resonate with young people. This involves taking the brand beyond a mere product but developing it as a feature of contemporary culture; this technique can also be used in the public sector. Alcohol brands in particular have been effective in appealing to a youth audience through involvement with youth culture such as sports, music and fashion. Alcohol sponsorship is a significant channel of marketing activity for the alcohol industry with music festivals and venues, sports teams and competitions, and a whole range of cultural events being sponsored by alcohol brands. This enables the brands to fit in with youth culture and reach young people. The use of new media channels complements this process and allows brands to become culturally relevant and accessible.

Co-ownership of the brand The third lesson we can extrapolate from examining the case studies of Budweiser and WKD is the importance of branding and how it instils a sense of co-ownership with consumers. Many of the popular commercial brands we see around us are such a part of life for consumers that many identify with their favourite brands as matching their self-image. At a societal level, brands are often used by people to tell other people about themselves, who they are, what they stand for and so on (Murphy 1987). Therefore branding is important in people's lives and the commercial sector has been very effective in creating this state of affairs by making its brands culturally relevant. For example, WKD has created an innovative and culturally relevant marketing campaign for its products using language, media and cultural references to which a young audience will relate. For some consumers, the WKD brand almost acts as a badge. Similarly, the Budweiser 'Whassup' campaign was so successful and far-reaching that it became a part of the cultural lexicon in several countries. Much of this branding activity is underpinned by extensive and ongoing consumer research which enables commercial brands to understand the lifestyles of their customers and enables them to construct the brand around their lives. In the field of public health, by recognizing that branding is important in people's lives we can better construct brands that will be relevant to the lives of our consumers, enabling them to better identify with them.

Internal document analysis

Another way in which we can conduct competitive analysis is by examining internal documents from the commercial sector. This helps us to scrutinize the marketing practices of products that may have a harmful effect on society and can illustrate malpractice. It can also help to inform countermarketing strategies. A wide range of documents can be analysed, such as contact reports between clients and marketing agencies, client briefs, media briefs, media schedules, marketing budgets and market research reports. Normally litigation or government intervention is required to obtain such documents; in the UK, for example, internal industry documents have been requested by the House of Commons Health Select Committee. In the case of tobacco industry documents, however, some material was initially leaked by whistleblowers. Qualitative analysis of these documents is normally conducted around key themes (Silverman 1995) and this process has been used to analyse industry documents in the areas of tobacco, food and pharmaceuticals (Hastings and MacFadyen 2000; McDermott and Angus 2003; Devlin *et al.* 2005).

Analysis of industry documents has perhaps been most widely used to examine tobacco marketing, and research reports have been used as a tool for tobacco control. Documentary analysis of the tobacco industry's actions has generated much controversy and interest. Blanke (2002) comments that, 'by exposing, in tobacco executives' own words, the dishonest and starkly cynical nature of their statements and actions, the documents deprive the industry of credibility, undercut its current arguments and focus the debate on its own behaviour'.

Documentation analysis has been used extensively in the field of tobacco control to inform research and decision making surrounding tobacco marketing by examining tobacco industry documents to assess how their products are marketed to consumers. For example, various studies have demonstrated that the tobacco industry has targeted young people with their marketing strategies (Pollay 2000; Cummings *et al.* 2002; Anderson *et al.* 2006). Several studies have shown that tobacco companies have sought to avoid regulation and undermine government policy or tobacco control efforts, treated voluntary regulation codes with cynicism, and established a clear link between branding and consumption; their use of all marketing channels and, in some cases, low regard for their customers (describing one segment as 'slobs') have also been described (Glantz *et al.* 1995; Hastings and MacFadyen 2000; Carter 2002).

In tobacco control, analysis of internal industry documents has been used in several ways, all of which address the competition. Findings have been used to inform media advocacy, litigation and public inquiries, international organizations' investigations (e.g. the World Health Organization, the Framework Convention on Tobacco Control) and regulation and legislation. The importance of tobacco industry documents for informing public health strategy is discussed elsewhere in the literature (Bero 2003).

Documentary analysis has also been used to examine internal communications in the food industry. Analysis conducted at the request of the House of Commons Health Select Committee examined internal documents from the UK food industry to determine whether marketing communications and strategies were adhering to regulation and codes of practice. The research found evidence that brands aimed to increase consumption of unhealthy foods, encouraged 'pester power' (where marketing strategies manipulate children to pester parents or their family members to purchase unrequired goods or services), and used sophisticated marketing strategies and techniques and a high level of understanding of children to target them with their marketing activity (McDermott and Angus 2003).

In recent years, the marketing practices of the pharmaceutical industry have also been subject to scrutiny and criticism. In the UK, the House of Commons Health Select Committee commissioned a study of internal marketing documents that it had obtained from five UK pharmaceutical companies (Devlin *et al.* 2005). A qualitative analysis was undertaken on the documents to examine whether the marketing of prescription-only medicines to health professionals contravened the specifications outlined in the Association of the British Pharmaceutical Industry's self-regulated Code of Practice.

The research highlighted considerable concerns about how the current Code of Practice was working. It showed that the marketing of prescription-only medicines had on occasions transgressed the Code. For example, the general public and patients *are* seen as deliberate targets for marketing (the UK code prohibits this), and campaigns targeting health professionals use emotional drivers, irrational constructs and branding strategies that are far removed from the Code's requirement for communications to be 'accurate, balanced, fair, objective and unambiguous'. The findings from this analysis can inform development of the regulatory codes surrounding pharmaceutical marketing.

Internal document analysis can tell us some interesting and important things about branding. First, it can help expose bad practice and the hypocrisy of anti-health brands like Marlboro. Second, as in the case with the pharma documents, it helps to illustrate how crucial branding can be even when rigorous, scientific decisions are being made by highly-trained professionals (ie doctors prescribing). This shows that emotional decision making matters; we all need to feel reassured and confident about our choices. Finally, the role of branding in pharma also provides an opportunity to highlight the contrast in research approaches involved in new drug production (randomized controlled trials and positivism) versus brand building (ethnography and exploration). This is particularly relevant to the public health field given its tendency for research approaches based on

randomized controlled trials and positivism. The lessons we can learn by using document analysis can also help us to inform countermarketing strategies and regulation.

Studies of the deleterious effects of commercial branding

The final strand to competitive analysis that we examine is the deleterious effects of
commercial branding. We have already demonstrated that branding is a major component of commercial marketing and is successful. However, there is also research evidence
that suggests that some of this activity can have a harmful effect on individuals and
society. Studies on the effects of commercial marketing belong to the critical marketing
paradigm. The impact of commercial branding and wider marketing on health and societal welfare has been well researched and documented by social marketers (Gordon *et al.*
2007). Critical studies of the effects of commercial marketing on behaviour have been
carried out in the areas of tobacco, food and alcohol marketing. This activity forms an
important strand of the critical marketing debate – and through this kind of critical
examination social marketing provides a tool for identifying solutions. Here we examine
how studies of tobacco and alcohol marketing have contributed to the critical marketing
debate by constructing an evidence base that can be used to inform decision making,
regulation and legislation.

Tobacco marketing

Branding is one of the key marketing strategies employed by the tobacco industry to
promote its product and has been since tobacco brands first appeared. There is a well-
established evidence base linking tobacco marketing to behaviour, including awareness
of and involvement with tobacco brands, brand choice and smoking behaviour (Smee
1992; MacFadyen *et al.* 2001; Lovato *et al.* 2003). Research has been widely published on
the behavioural effects of general tobacco marketing, including branding, but there is
also brand-specific evidence of an effect. Hafez and Ling (2005) conducted analysis of
tobacco industry documents to assess the impact of Marlboro's global branding strategy
on young people. It was found that Philip Morris conducted research on young people
throughout the world, focusing on lifestyles, brand studies and marketing effectiveness.
The research identified core similarities in the lifestyles and needs of young consumers
worldwide, including independence, hedonism, freedom and comfort. Philip Morris
adopted a global marketing strategy that branded Marlboro using this information to
position it as a product that would appeal to young adults. A standardized brand identity
was used along with advertising messages to target the shared values of and appeal to
young people around the world (Hafez and Ling 2005). Furthermore, tobacco industry
research documents have emerged which have gone some way to explain how Marlboro
changed their cigarettes to make them more addictive and help them dominate the
market (Kluger 1996).

There is also research that indicates the impact the branding activity of Camel
cigarettes has had. Research published in the *Journal of the American Medical Association*
in 1991 on brand logo recognition among children aged 3 to 6 years old found that Joe
Camel was more easily recognisable than Mickey Mouse, Bugs Bunny or Barbie.

Approximately 30 per cent of 3-year-old children correctly matched Joe Camel with a picture of a cigarette, with a figure of 91.3 per cent of 6-year-olds managing to make the match (Fischer *et al.* 1991). The American Medical Association requested that RJR withdraw the campaign but the request was initially refused. Due to further pressure, however, the Joe Camel campaign was eventually withdrawn in 1997 and replaced with a supposedly more adult campaign featuring beautiful and exotic women. Research carried out in Turkey on the recognition of cigarette brand names and logos among primary school children indicated that Camel was the most recognizable logo and Marlboro the most recognisable brand name (Emri *et al.* 1998).

The importance of branding the tobacco industry is now magnified given the introduction of wide restrictions on other forms of tobacco marketing. Rather than witness the death knell of tobacco marketing, many companies have used branding as a tool with which to continually market tobacco products. Indeed, many tobacco companies including Philip Morris and RJR have used 'brand stretching', the diversification of the brand to non-tobacco merchandise and services to circumvent restrictions on tobacco promotion. Examples include Camel boots and clothing, Marlboro cigarette lighters and the Marlboro Classics range of clothing. Brand stretching has been found to have an effect; research has shown that schoolchildren who are exposed to clothing resulting from brand stretching are four more times likely to smoke than other children, with 32 per cent of those surveyed owning at least one branded item (Bonn 1997). Recent research carried out in the UK has indicated that despite the ban on most forms of tobacco marketing, there is still a strong influence from branding on adolescent attitudes towards smoking and intention to smoke (Grant *et al.* 2007).

Alcohol marketing

Turning now to alcohol marketing we find that, as in the tobacco industry, branding is one of the key pillars of the marketing mix. In many markets, such as those comprising young people, it is a key dimension of the marketer's offering. As a result, brand names like Budweiser, Bacardi and Smirnoff have acquired enormous value. This is ever truer given changes in the alcohol industry itself over the last 20 years, which has witnessed mergers and consolidation of the market with a number of key global brands emerging. The focus on multinational brands supported by huge marketing budgets has resulted in changes in the way alcohol is marketed. In the UK alone, the alcohol industry spends over £800 million per year in marketing its products (Euromonitor 2004). Alcohol is now marketed using the full range of channels available in the marketing mix, and there is a growing trend for expenditure to shift away from the traditional channels of direct advertising in the print and broadcast media to 'below the line' activities such as sponsorship, special promotions, viral marketing, the use of new media such as websites and mobile phone communications, and experiential marketing (Hastings *et al.* 2005). This activity is so extensive that it is argued that alcohol brands have become a part of the entertainment, cultural and sporting milieu (Caswell 2004).

There is considerable debate over the effect of alcohol marketing including branding on drinking behaviour. The evidence on alcohol marketing and consumption comprises two types of evidence: (1) econometric studies that use time series data to examine the relationship between aggregated alcohol consumption and supply variables such as advertising expenditure (Duffy 1990; Lee and Tremblay 1992; Calfee and Scheraga 1994) and (2) consumer studies examining the relationship between drinking behaviour and psychological effects such as recognition, appreciation and rewards derived from alcohol advertisements (Aitken *et al.* 1988). Though both types of studies have demonstrated links between alcohol advertising and behaviour, doubt remains over the strength and comprehensiveness of the evidence base, certainly in the minds of policy makers. Consider, for example, this statement in the Alcohol Harm Reduction Strategy for England:

> There is no clear case on the effect of advertising on behaviour. One recent study suggests that such an effect may exist, but is contradicted by others which find no such case. So the evidence is not sufficiently strong to suggest that measures such as a ban on advertising or tightening existing restrictions about scheduling should be imposed by regulation.

> Prime Minister's Strategy Unit (2004: 32)

However, recent longitudinal research into the effects of alcohol marketing on youth drinking have established a causal link (Ellickson *et al.* 2004; Stacy *et al.* 2004; Snyder *et al.* 2006). Further research that will add to the evidence base is ongoing in the UK and New Zealand.

In terms of the effects of alcohol branding as a specific element of marketing, some research evidence has suggested it has an effect on attitudes and behaviour. Aitken *et al.* (1988) conducted a study on young people's perceptions of and responses to alcohol advertisements and found that respondents were aware of brand imagery and found it appealing. Another study found that levels of awareness of beer advertising are linked to greater knowledge of brands, increasingly positive beliefs about drinking and higher intentions to drink as an adult (Grube and Wallack 1994). Criticism has been levelled at Anheusur-Busch for the use of cartoon-like characters that generate the attention of children for deliberately targeting young people in an effort to develop brand loyalty at a young age. Research carried out in the USA in 1996 found that the Budweiser frogs were more recognizable to children aged 9–11 years than the Power Rangers, Tony the Tiger or Smokey the Bear (Lieber 1996). There are also concerns over alcohol brands and sports sponsorship, with research indicating that sports with large numbers of youth participation or spectators are often sponsored by alcohol brands, leading to calls for greater regulation (Maher *et al.* 2006).

Again the importance of critical social marketing research in informing regulation and decision making is demonstrated here, especially when considering the statement of the UK government above. By evaluating the impact of commercial alcohol marketing on drinking behaviour and also offering insights into how alcohol is marketed, such critical studies provide valuable information and findings that can assist in developing policy and regulation that could restrict alcohol's deleterious effects on society.

Many of these studies carried out by social marketers have moved beyond establishing effect on behaviour but have informed decision making and regulation. For example, much of the work published in the UK (see MacFadyen *et al.* 2001) informed the UK government's decision to implement an advertising ban on tobacco products. Critical marketing has therefore played an important part in addressing the effects of tobacco branding on behaviour by informing regulation and tobacco control policy. Studies examining the impact of tobacco marketing on behaviour have helped build a considerable evidence base that has been used to guide policy and regulation (Hastings and MacFadyen 2000; Pollay 2000; MacFadyen *et al.* 2001; Cummings *et al.* 2002; Lovato *et al.* 2003). Social marketing has an important part to play in the critical marketing paradigm as it offers an understanding of both the commercial and social sectors, and of the good and the bad that marketing can bring to society (Hastings and Saren 2003). By exposing the malevolent side of tobacco marketing, such as targeting youth, the findings of critical social marketing research have led to advertising or wider marketing bans being introduced in the UK, Finland, Brazil and New Zealand, among others. Furthermore, critical marketing has also influenced the first ever international agreement to limit marketing activity – the Framework Convention on Tobacco Control (WHO 2003). This demonstrates how critical marketing research can move towards solutions by creating an evidence base that informs regulation and decision making.

However, it is important that the correct regulatory solutions are found once an evidence base has been established. For example, many of the advertising bans that have been introduced, such as on tobacco marketing, focus on the paraphernalia of branding (advertising) rather than its essence (the brands themselves).

There is also a need to engage in media advocacy and debate around the implications from research findings and the subsequent regulatory or policy response to them. Achieving the desired outcomes for public health in this process, winning the debate and engendering policy change, can be made easier with the support of a strong and relevant brand. For example, it is easier to attack the big tobacco companies with the support of the Cancer Research UK brand; likewise, the support of the British Medical Association provides an immediate advantage because it is a well-established brand that people already trust.

Conclusion

This chapter demonstrates that competitive analysis is a valuable tool that can be used to inform public health branding strategies by offering customer insight, helping to develop strategic alliances and dealing with the competition from the hazard merchants. By using the analysis techniques described, key lessons can be extrapolated to help achieve these outcomes.

The case studies generate some key lessons for public health branding. The importance of longevity was illustrated. It helps us think beyond discrete, short-term changes in behaviour towards generational approaches that involve forming meaningful, trusting and lasting relationships with our target audience(s). Many successful commercial brands have been around for a long time – Lucky Strike for 136 years, Coca-Cola for 115 years, Smirnoff for 83 years and McDonald's for 67 years.

We have learned that subtlety is a useful lesson we can take from commercial branding. Commercial brands are very effective at creating a brand identity through subtle means using media such as advertising or sponsorship. In public health, we too must respect the customer, use subtlety and not insult the intelligence of our audience nor appear paternalistic.

The vital importance of delivering tangible benefits has been highlighted as one of the key lessons we can take from competitive analysis of commercial brands. Many commercial brands are very effective at delivering customer satisfaction, whether through consistency of product, great customer service, or like Marlboro, product development.

Furthermore, the value of the innovative use of new media has been discussed. Commercial brands such as Budweiser and WKD have reached consumers though the very effective use of innovative channels of communication such as viral marketing and websites. These channels are also more interactive and democratic and have great appeal for younger consumers. The innovative use of new media in public health branding offers a good way of reaching end users more effectively.

Commercial organizations are often very successful at making sure that their brands are culturally relevant. Using contemporary cultural references and associating with cultural events and activities such as music, sport and fashion are very effective branding techniques. This enables brands to fit in with culture and reach people, especially youth audiences, effectively.

Commercial brands are also successful at creating a sense of co-ownership of the brand for consumers. Values, lifestyle choices and cultural references identified and used in the branding strategies of Marlboro and WKD such as independence, freedom and irreverent humour have been used to model these brands around their customers' lives. This helps the brands build more effective and lasting relationships with their customers.

We can also see the value of creating strategic alliances from examining the commercial world, which can be very effective in progressing a public health agenda such as in tobacco control. Strategic alliances to share research and learning and create advocacy groups are often a very effective use of resources.

Internal document analysis helps to expose bad commercial branding practice and highlight hypocrisy of brands that are potentially damaging to public health. Furthermore, document analysis reinforces how crucial branding is in any corporate strategy. This form of analysis also illustrates the differences in approach towards research found in the commercial sector (ethnographic and exploratory) compared with that in public health (randomized controlled trials and positivism).

Finally, studies on the deleterious effects of commercial marketing help inform regulation, decision making and litigation by building up a scientific evidence base. It highlights where branding is having an adverse impact on health and society, thus informing regulation and similar efforts to offset these negative effects. The ability of such research to inform regulation and decision making has been established and demonstrated (Hastings and Saren 2003; Gordon *et al.* 2007).

These lessons generated by competitive analysis, using the techniques discussed in this chapter, can bring four key strengths to public health branding. First, competitive analysis offers customer insight and thereby ensures an improved fit between our brands and their lives. Second, it enables us to develop successful strategic alliances to give our brands better leverage. Finally, it helps us deal with the competition from the hazard merchants by informing countermarketing campaigns that will undermine their brands and, where necessary, challenge them directly. Competitive analysis is therefore a key tool for building competitive public health brands.

References

Aitken P. P., Leather D. S., and Scott A. C. (1988). Ten-to sixteen-year-olds' perceptions of advertisements for alcoholic drinks. *Alcohol and Alcoholism* **23**:491–500.

Altria (2007). Altria Group, Inc. 2007. Annual Report. Available at: http://www.altria.com/download/pdf/investors_AltriaGroupInc_2007_AnnualRpt.pdf (accessed 5 May 2008).

Anderson S. J., Dewhirst T., and Ling P. M. (2006). Every document and picture tells a story: using internal corporate document reviews, semiotics, and content analysis to assess tobacco advertising. *Tobacco Control* **15**:254–61.

Anheusur-Busch (2004). International beer operations. Available at: http://www.anheusur-busch.com/Stock/2004AR_InternationalBeerOperations.pdf (accessed 5 May 2008).

Bero, L. (2003). Implications of the tobacco industry documents for public health and policy. *Annual Review of Public Health* **24**:267–88.

Blanke, D. (2002). *Towards health with justice: litigation and public inquiries as tools for tobacco control*. Geneva: WHO Tobacco Free Initiative.

Bonn, D. (1997). Tobacco promotion bans will work. *Lancet* **350**: 1831.

Calfee, J. and Scheraga C. (1994). The influence of advertising on alcohol consumption: A literature review and an econometric analysis of four European nations. *International Journal of Advertising* **13**: 287–310.

Carter, S. M. (2002). Mongoven, Biscoe and Duchin: destroying tobacco control activism from the inside. *Tobacco Control* **11**:112–18.

Caswell, S. (2004). Alcohol brands in young peoples' everyday lives: new developments in marketing. *Alcohol and Alcoholism* **6**:471–6.

Cummings, K. M., Morley, C. P., Horan, J. K., Steger, C., and Leavell, N. R. (2002). Marketing to America's youth: evidence from corporate documents. *Tobacco Control* **11**:5–17.

Devlin, E., Hastings, G., and Anderson, S. (2005). Dealing in drugs: An analysis of the pharmaceutical industry's marketing documents. In *House of Commons Health Committee Report – The influence of the pharmaceutical industry – 4th report of session 2004–05 Volume 2, 22 March, Appendix 33 (PI125)*. London: Stationery Office.

Duffy, M. (1990). Advertising and alcoholic drink demand in the UK: some further Rotterdam model estimates. *International Journal of Advertising* **9**:247–57.

Ellickson, P. L., Collins, R. L., Hambarsoomians, K., and McCaffrey, D. F. (2004). Does alcohol advertising promote adolescent drinking? Results from a longitudinal assessment. *Addiction* **100**:235–46.

Emri, S., Bagci, T., Karakoca, Y., and Barisc, E. (1998). Recognition of cigarette brand names and logos by primary school children in Ankara, Turkey. *Tobacco Control* **7**:386–92.

Euromonitor (2004). Market Report: Alcoholic Drinks in the United Kingdom. London: Euromonitor.

Fischer, P. M., Schwartz, M. P., Richards, J. W. Jr, Goldstein, A. O., and Rojas, T. H. (1991). Brand logo recognition by children aged 3 to 6 years. Mickey Mouse and Old Joe the Camel. *Journal of the American Medical Association* **266**:3145–8.

Glantz, S. A., Barnes, D. E., Bero, L., Hanauer, P., and Slade, J. (1995). Looking through a keyhole at the tobacco industry: The Brown and Williamson documents, *Journal of the American Medical Association* **274**:219–24

Gordon, R., Hastings, G., McDermott, L., and Siquier, P. (2007). The critical role of social marketing. In Saren M (ed.) *Critical marketing: defining the field.* pp.159–77. London: Elsevier.

Grant, I., Hassan, L., Hastings, G., MacKintosh, A. M., and Eadie, D. (2007). The influence of branding on adolescent smoking behaviour: exploring the mediating role of image and attitudes. *International Journal of Nonprofit and Voluntary Sector Marketing.* Published online, early view: 11 September 2007.

Grocer, The (2001). 70cl for WKD Original Vodka Blue. *The Grocer* September 8: 72.

Grocer, The (2004). WKD shot in store. *The Grocer* **227**(7656):68.

Grube, J. W. and Wallack, L. (1994). Television beer advertising and drinking knowledge, beliefs, and intentions among schoolchildren. *American Journal of Public Health* **84**:254–9.

Hafez, N. and Ling, P. M. (2005). How Philip Morris built Marlboro into a global brand for young adults: implications for international tobacco control. *Tobacco Control* **14**:262–71.

Hastings, G. and MacFadyen, L. M. (2000). 'A day in the life of an advertising man: review of internal documents from the UK tobacco industry's principle advertising agencies', *British Medical Journal* **321**:366–71.

Hastings, G. and Saren, M. (2003). The critical contribution of social marketing: theory and application. *Marketing Theory* **3**:305–22.

Hastings, G., Anderson, S., Cooke, E., and Gordon, R. (2005). Alcohol marketing and young people's drinking: A review of the research. *Journal of Public Health Policy* **26**:296–311.

Kluger, R. (1996). *Ashes to ashes: America's hundred year cigarette war, the public health, and the unabashed triumph of Philip Morris.* New York: Alfred A. Knopf.

Lee, B. and Tremblay, V. J. (1992). Advertising and the US market demand for beer. *Applied Economics* **24**:69–76.

Lieber, L. (1996). *Commercial and character slogan recall by children aged 9 to 11 years: Budweiser Frogs versus Bugs Bunny.* Berkeley, CA: Center on Alcohol Advertising.

Lovato, C., Linn, G., Stead, L. F., and Best, A. (2003). Impact of tobacco advertising and promotion on increasing adolescent smoking behaviours. Cochrane Database of Systematic Reviews **4**:CD003439.

MacFadyen, L., Hastings, G. B., and MacKintosh, A. M. (2001). Cross sectional study of young people's awareness of and involvement with tobacco marketing. *British Medical Journal* **322**:513–17.

McDermott, L. and Angus, K. (2003). Preliminary analysis of food industry advertising documents. Memorandum to the House of Commons Health Select Committee, November. Available at: http://www.publications.parliament.uk/pa/cm200304/cmselect/cmhealth/23/23we62.htm (accessed 5 May 2008).

Maher, A., Wilson, N., Signal, L., and Thomson, G. (2006). Patterns of sports sponsorship by gambling, alcohol and food companies: an internet survey. *BMC Public Health* **6**:95.

Murphy, J. (ed.) (1987). *Branding: a key marketing tool.* New York: McGraw-Hill.

Pollay R. W. (2000). Targeting youth and concerned smokers: evidence from Canadian tobacco industry documents *Tobacco Control* **9**:136–47.

Prime Minister's Strategy Unit (2004). *Alcohol harm reduction strategy for England.* London: Stationery Office.

Silverman, D. (ed.) (1995). *Interpreting qualitative data.* London: Sage.

Smee, C., Economics and Operational Research Division, Department of Health (UK) (1992). *Effect of tobacco advertising on tobacco sponsorship: a discussion document reviewing the evidence.* London: Department of Health.

Snyder, L. B., Milici, F. F., Slater, M., Sun, H., and Strizhakova, Y. (2006). Effects of alcohol advertising exposure on drinking among youth, *Archives of Pediatrics and Adolescent Medicine* **160**:18–24.

Stacy, A. W., Zogg, J. B., Unger, J. B., and Dent, C. W. (2004). Exposure to televised alcohol ads and subsequent adolescent alcohol use. *American Journal of Health Behaviour* **28**:498–509.

The Leading Edge Consultancy (1997). *American Blends NPD Qualitative Debrief Presentation. Prepared for Gallaher Limited.* Submission to the House of Commons Health Committee. Available at http://www.tobaccopapers.com/PDFs/0400-0499/0479.pdf (accessed 5 May 2008).

World Health Organization (WHO) (2003). *Draft WHO framework convention on tobacco control,* *A/FCTC/INB6/5.* Geneva: WHO.

Part II

Public health branding case studies

5

Help: A European public health brand in the making?

Gerard Hastings, Jo Freeman, Renata Spackova, and Pierre Siquier

Summary

- *Help* is the first attempt to build a pan-European public health brand.
- Its progress is analysed in terms of three key branding constructs: recognition, promise and delivery.
- A mixture of qualitative and quantitative research suggests that it is making progress in all three areas.
- *Help* suggests that international public health brands can be successfully built and deployed.
- However, it also suggests that building these brands presents unique challenges. In particular, it is difficult to pull together like-minded but nonetheless independent government and non-governmental tobacco control stakeholders behind a cohesive brand strategy; a corporation, such as Philip Morris or BAT, with its more hierarchical and clearly defined structures does not face these problems.

Introduction

Smoking has a devastating effect on the health of the people of Europe. A survey by the International Union Against Cancer in 2000 showed that it kills over 655 000 Europeans every year, around 290 000 of whom die in middle age. One out of four deaths caused by cancer is directly attributable to smoking.

However there is also reason for optimism: Europe is gradually turning away from tobacco. According to findings from the recent 2007 EU Eurobarometer – the six-monthly public opinion survey conducted by the European Commission across all EU member states – smoking prevalence across the EU has decreased from 33 to 27 per cent between 2002 and 2007. These figures hide major disparities between countries: Sweden has fewer than 20 per cent smokers (though it also has a significant proportion of oral snuff users), and Slovenia has 23 per cent; at the other extreme are countries such as Greece (42 per cent) and Latvia, Hungary and Bulgaria (36 per cent each), while as many as 15 countries still have prevalence rates of over 30 per cent. Nonetheless the over-all trends are positive.

One way of encouraging these positive trends is through mass media campaigns. Six major reviews have looked at their effectiveness in recent years and concluded consistently – if sometimes cautiously – that they can both encourage quitting and prevent smoking onset (see Box 5.1). Thus, a recent systematic review by Jepson *et al.* (Jepson *et al.* 2006) for the UK National Institute for Clinical Excellence (NICE) suggests that they can be effective in encouraging cessation, and that new media such as mobile communications and the internet show particular potential. On the preventive side, Sowden and Arblaster (1998), Farrelly *et al.* (2003), Richardson *et al.* (2007) (another NICE review), Friend and Levy (2002) and the NHS Centre for Reviews and Dissemination (1999) have all concluded that media campaigns have a positive role to play.

However, success does seem to be dependent on *how* the media are used. Focusing on prevention in isolation can have mixed results (Friend and Levy 2002). It can backfire by suggesting the double standard that smoking is acceptable for adults but not children,

Box 5.1 Review evidence on media-based anti-smoking campaigns

There is evidence that mass media campaigns can prevent the uptake of smoking and also influence knowledge, attitudes and intentions of children and young people. (Richardson *et al.* 2007: 4)

Well-funded and implemented mass-media campaigns targeted at the general popu-lation and implemented at the state level, in conjunction with a comprehensive tobacco control program, are associated with reduced smoking rates. Youth-oriented interventions have shown more mixed results, particularly smaller, community-level media programs, but indicate strong potential. (Friend and Levy 2002: 95)

There is some evidence that the mass media can be effective in preventing the uptake of smoking in young people, but overall the evidence is not strong. (Sowden and Arblaster 1998: 1)

The success of the national truth campaign, Florida campaign before complementary programmes, and the impact of an antidrug media campaign in Kentucky suggest that an aggressive, targeted, and/or well funded media campaign alone may be suffi-cient to affect youth smoking. (Farrelly *et al.* 2003: 45)

When considered together, there is a high degree of consistency in findings, which provide good support for the notion that anti-smoking advertising can influence youth smoking. (Wakefield *et al.* 2003: 242)

Overall, there appears to be evidence that mass media interventions can have a posi-tive effect on quit rates. However the size of effect is difficult to determine given the lack of a control group in many of the studies. (Jepson *et al.* 2006: 5)

turning tobacco into a 'forbidden fruit'. In a similar vein, the best campaigns are based on formative research with the target audience (Sowden and Arblaster 1998). Jepson *et al.*'s NICE review (Jepson *et al.* 2006) suggests that successful efforts should use a mix of media. More broadly, it is increasingly apparent that effective campaigns need to link in with other intervention activities, most notably policy change (Friend and Levy 2002; Richardson *et al.* 2007). Hence recent moves to make public places smoke-free in Ireland and Scotland were accompanied by explanatory media efforts (Harrison and Hurst 2005). Finally, all but one of the reviews agree that media campaigns need to be well resourced and sustained to succeed.

It is this last point that takes us into the area of branding. As Evans and Hastings discuss in Chapter 1, brands are valuable to – and indeed have come to dominate – the commercial sector because they provide a company (or its offerings) with a presence and an identity. From this base, it is not just possible to generate ad hoc transactions with customers, but to build sustained relationships with them. The result is loyalty from the customer and longevity for the marketer. However, such benefits depend on a sustained presence in the market place.

Some of the most successful commercial branders have been the tobacco companies. Marlboro, Silk Cut and Benson & Hedges have flourished for decades, while Lucky Strike is a centenarian. The *Help* anti-smoking campaign set out to challenge this hegemony by building the first ever pan-European health brand.

The origins of *Help*

The *Help* campaign had its origins in an EC conference organized in Rome in November 2003. This brought together over 200 of the leading tobacco control professionals from across Europe to decide whether and how best to run an anti-smoking media campaign. The principal conclusions echo the evidence base summarized above, arguing that 'media campaigns' can 'play a key role to build knowledge, change attitudes and behaviour in support of a tobacco-free society' (Tobacco Youth Prevention and Communication Conference, 2003), and that future campaigns should follow the precepts laid down in Box 5.2.

As a result of this, the European Commission issued a call for tenders in 2004 for a multimedia campaign that met these criteria, and 'would contribute to changing the social norm from smoking to non-smoking in the European Union' (Tobacco Youth Prevention and Communication Conference, 2003). More specifically it should address the three key issues of tobacco control:

◆ prevention: targeting mainly 15–24 year-olds;
◆ cessation: targeting 25 and 35 year-olds;
◆ passive smoking: targeting the whole population.

This campaign was to be run in the then 25 European member states (this increased to 27 with the accession of Bulgaria and Romania in January 2007). It would be an important plank of the Commission's tobacco control strategy for the foreseeable future, with initial

---

Box 5.2 The Rome Precepts

Future EU anti-smoking mass media campaigns should:

1. Form part of a comprehensive tobacco control strategy

2. Address the whole tobacco control agenda, not just prevention

3. Be subject to careful pretesting and evaluation

4. Link in with national-level activity

5. Involve a partnership of all the stakeholders with an interest in European tobacco control – except the tobacco industry

6. Use a mix of traditional and new media

7. Be sustained

The overall aim of the campaign should be to:
'contribute to change the social norm from smoking to nonsmoking in the European Union'.
ASPECT Consortium (2004)

---

funding of €72 million. This made it the biggest ever European anti-smoking campaign – although when the budget was split between member states and over the four years of the initial funding period it was lightweight by commercial standards. Prior to the introduction of a tobacco ad ban, for example, it is estimated that the tobacco industry spent some €140 million annually on advertising in the UK alone (ASH 2006).

The *Help* campaign

The winning bid for the tender emphasized the opportunity not just for a standard health communication campaign, but the development of a pan-European public health brand to symbolize and encourage Europe's journey away from tobacco. To do this, as is noted many times elsewhere in this book, the brand would need to build a public profile, make a meaningful and attractive offer to potential customers and then provide satisfaction: the branding adage *recognition*, *promise*, *delivery* would apply as much to tobacco control as it does to tobacco promotion.

Recognition

This is a function of awareness and appreciation; the cognitive and the connative. In advertising terms this puts the emphasis on the creative approach and the media strategy.

Following the Rome conclusions, the creative approach set out to avoid preaching and patronizing. The aim was to try and engage with the audience as equals; to present scenarios, but allow them to draw their own conclusions; to get them onside in a collective rejection of tobacco. It would also need to appeal to smokers and nonsmokers alike.

The concept of 'Help – tobacco, you're not alone' emerged from this brief. This was intended to work at two levels: first, it could encourage the individual and collective efforts of citizens, offering both information and positive support (e.g. cessation guidance); second, it could complement activities at a national and regional level providing a link to anti-smoking organizations and services.

This would be presented through a series of executions designed to highlight the fact that smoking encourages us to engage in bizarre behaviour. The designers opted to illustrate this by creating a ridiculous parallel world where cigarettes were replaced by leeks (later changed to paper whistles). The absurdity was intended to encourage both smokers and nonsmokers to rethink their behaviour and to raise three parallel questions: Why would I want to start smoking? Why do I continue to smoke? and Why do I put up with other people's smoke?

Extensive pretesting was undertaken involving a total of 38 focus groups across 20 countries (Figure 5.1 presents the sample breakdown).

This revealed both strengths and weaknesses. On the plus side, the word *Help* was well understood by speakers of all languages. The concept of support and encouragement that it implied was also liked. The absurd scenarios successfully did the job of getting across the strangeness of smoking behaviours.

On the other hand, the 'tobacco, you're not alone' tagline did not work; the focus group participants could not see the logical link with the ads, and this lack of understanding made people uncomfortable with the line, sometimes triggering rejection. The tagline was therefore change to read 'for a life without tobacco', which was better liked and understood. The association between the words 'life' and 'without tobacco' was felt to be appropriate and realistic, and it focused on achievable solutions. The result was a personally relevant message. The message was developed into a brand logo (see Figure 5.2) that could be easily understood, and adapted well to all media and communication channels.

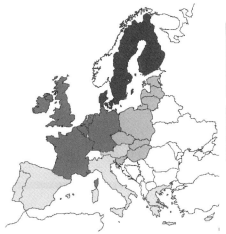

South			East		
Cyprus	2		Hungary	3	
Spain	3		Lithuania	2	
Greece	2		Poland	2	
Italy	3		Slovakia	2	
Portugal	3		Czech Rep	3	
Total	**13**		**Total**	**12**	

North			West		
Denmark	1		Germany	3	
Finland	1		Austria	1	
Sweden	1		Belgium	1	
Total	**3**		France	2	
			Ireland	1	
			Netherlands	1	
			UK	1	
			Total	**10**	

Total focus groups   38

Fig. 5.1 Groups per region.

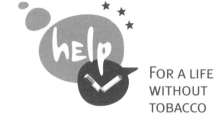

Fig. 5.2 The *Help* logo.
Reproduced with permission
from Ligaris.

FOR A LIFE
WITHOUT
TOBACCO

The pre-testing also revealed marked cultural differences about tobacco. Specifically, the north of Europe had (and still has) much more negative attitudes towards tobacco than the south and east. The Nordic countries felt that in the initial versions of the films there were too many smokers who showed too little regard for their fellow citizens; this meant that the depictions lacked credibility. The storyboards were modified to take these comments into account. However, this cultural divergence continues to be a challenge; tackling an issue like passive smoking is difficult when parts of Europe have complete bans on smoking in public places, where as others barely even acknowledge the problem.

This links into a perennial branding and advertising issue in business: to internationalize or to stay local. There are pros and cons either way, but in the case of *Help*, thinking was influenced by competitive analysis (see Chapter 4) which showed that tobacco companies have been very successful in building not just European, but global brands.

The media strategy for *Help* was designed to be both far-reaching and engaging. The reach would be provided by television – still the dominant advertising medium in Europe, especially for *Help*'s target group, even though its power has reduced in recent years (ANA/Forrester 2006, cited in *Marketing Today* 2007). For example, the latest phase of advertising in January and February 2007 reached 73 per cent of 15–34-year-olds across Europe and gave them an average 6.5 'opportunities to see'. Overall, the campaign has reached all 27 member states on 96 national channels. Over 46,700 television ads have been broadcast since 2005. Television also made it possible to run the same set of commercials in all 27 countries. At the same time, the use of the national television and sensitive translation added a local touch to this heavy media impact.

The engagement was sought through a combination of public relations and new media activity. The former was driven by a series of events across the EU designed to highlight key aspects of the campaign such as its launch, the harmful effects of smoking through carbon monoxide testing and link-ups with other agencies such as the European Youth Forum (see below).

Turning to new media, 16–24 year olds Europeans now spend, on average, 14.7 hours a week on the internet (Carat Global Management/Isobar data 2007). This makes it an important communication channel, which not only enhances the power of conventional channels like television, but also facilitates the development of more customized and even interactive content. This has encouraged the commercial sector to include new media in their media planning.

The *Help* campaign followed suit, using new media in two main ways. First, it uses its own website (www.help-eu.com), which has been developed and enhanced during the three years of the campaign, starting with simple facts and figures about tobacco control in each country and moving towards a complete range of guidance on how to quit smoking, avoid taking it up in the first place and address passive smoking.

Second, it has used a viral marketing campaign called www.nicomarket.com which uses the ruse of a phoney online shop selling bogus tobacco-based products, such as face cream and room fresheners, which highlight the social drawbacks of smoking.

Both the website and the viral campaign have been promoted by a combination of banner advertising on key target group websites such as MSN and Yahoo, and posting onto other key sites with youth content such as such as Meetic and TillLate, and placing the viral campaign videos on DailyMotion and MTV websites, triggering further dissemination.

Promise

The core of the *Help* promise is that it will not judge or patronise; it treats its audience as equals. This was a challenge for the *Help* creative concept, which had to portray smoking rather than smokers as bizarre, as demeaning smokers themselves could clearly backfire. It also meant that the campaign developers had to rescind some of the control of the campaign to the target group, as there had to be some element of joint ownership. Traditional media like television make this quite difficult; they typically comprise prefabricated messages devised by the sender – the audience's contribution is largely restricted to rejection or acceptance.

However, public events are much more interactive and flexible. Meanings can be negotiated and agreed.

New media take this flexibility onto a much larger scale. In particular, viral campaigns actually depend on the audience transmitting the message themselves. As a result they have to be both engaging and enjoyable. They also give the audience a lot of power; people can say whatever they like in their accompanying blogs. This is a bit nerve-wracking for public health, which is traditionally an expert-driven discipline.

The second element of the *Help* promise is that it offers help and support. This has to be genuinely useful and really available. This takes us on to the third element of branding: delivery.

Delivery

Having promised meaningful help, the campaign had to provide it. It could do this directly through its media efforts, and indirectly through partnership.

Taking the direct level first, at its simplest this means that the media activity has to attract attention, meet with approval and actually get people to reconsider the role of smoking in their lives. More fundamentally, it means offering genuinely useful help. The website has to be accessed and the guidance needs to be used and appreciated. In the case of *Help*, the website included an e-mail cessation coaching service. Perhaps equally challenging, the target has to get involved in owning and honing the brand; the viral campaign must spread while retaining its integrity.

Thus, as with all good social marketing, the ultimate test of *Help*'s success is behaviour change.

At an indirect level, delivery is all about partnership at both a national and regional level. The campaign had to link up with the many government and non-governmental organization (NGO) stakeholders involved in European tobacco control. Finally, in terms of delivery, recalling the need for media campaigns to link in with other tobacco control activity to maximize effectiveness, *Help* sought to advance policy change, especially in the area of smoke-free public places.

Judging delivery – and the success of the *Help* brand – requires formal evaluation.

Did it work?

Judging the success of any brand is difficult; and it is particularly so for a health brand where sales and shareholder value do not provide a ready calibration of progress. In the case of *Help*, following on from the discussion of delivery, four indicators will be examined:

- consumer awareness and appreciation;
- behaviour change (did people do anything as a result of *Help*?);
- partnership and stakeholder marketing;
- policy change.

Consumer awareness and appreciation

An annual evaluation survey for the television campaign was set up by the independent survey institute Ipsos to measure the effectiveness of the television campaign. Some 25 000 telephone interviews were conducted in 25 EU member states in each year through a representative sample of the national population aged 15 and over. These results were weighted for each country, based on their sociodemographic data. Overall European results were weighted through the demographic weight of each country, and then compared with previous waves.

This provides a useful overview of progress over a three-year period (see Figure 5.3). It suggests that the campaign has succeeded in creating a reasonably high profile. According to the third post-test, conducted in March 2007, 172 million Europeans (and 60 per cent of those under 25) said they had seen the campaign.

Table 5.1 Understanding and liking of campaign.

	Percentage of respondents answering 'yes'[*]	
	Young people (n = 3624)	Total (n = 24 161)
Generally speaking did you like this campaign?	83	77
Would you say the campaign:		
delivers a worthwhile message?	91	86
is an incentive to look for information?	74	68
is easy to understand?	91	86

*Includes respondents who answered 'yes, quite a lot' and 'yes, a little'

Table 5.2 Appreciation of *Help* campaign's message.

	Percentage of respondents who agree with statement*	
	Young people (*n* = 3624)	Total (*n* = 24 161)
To what extent do you agree that the advertisements are trying to convey the message:		
it is ridiculous to smoke to be like others?	85	82
there is help available to stop smoking?	81	77
you should not start smoking?	87	84
smoking harms the health of others around you?	86	84

*Includes 'agree somewhat' and 'strongly agree'

The campaign was also both understood and well liked (see Tables 5.1 and 5.2) *Help*, then, does seem to have succeeded in the first stage of developing a brand: Europeans know, understand and appreciate the campaign.

Behaviour change

Help did not aim to produce a mass exodus from smoking; this would have been unrealistic. However it does seem to have encouraged some more minor behavioural shifts:

- ◆ *Accessing and using the website.* Unlike conventional media, websites require deliberate efforts on the part of the user. Visits to the site can be measured and distinctions drawn between new and repeat visitors. It is also possible to assess the duration of these visits, giving some indication of degree of engagement. Between its launch in 2005 and mid-2007, just over 4 million people visited the site at least once, and on

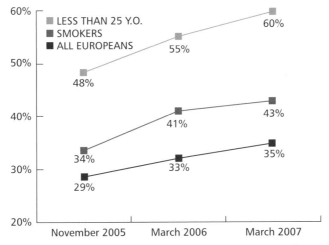

Fig. 5.3 Awareness of the *Help* television ads. Reproduced with permission from Ligaris. Source: IPSOS post-test results.

average they stayed on the site for 8–10 minutes. Furthermore, the traffic to the website correlates with the media campaign (see Figure 5.4)

◆ *The viral campaign.* As mentioned above, this is dependent for its success not just on people logging on to the site, but for them to be sufficiently engaged and intrigued by the material they find there to pass it on to their peers. Viral campaigns have demonstrated considerable success in recent years; for example, a message spread by Hotmail reached 11 million users in just 18 months (Kelly 2000) and Paypal succeeded in gaining over 3 million users in its first nine months through a viral campaign (De Bruyn and Lilien 2003). Early indications for the *Help* viral campaign are encouraging – of the 263 000 visitors in the first five weeks of the campaign, 15 per cent passed it on – a figure that compares favourably with commercial campaign results.

◆ *Cessation coaching.* Signing up to and using the e-mail cessation coaching service is perhaps the most complex behaviour change attempted by the *Help* campaign. To date, 91 000 smokers have signed up, a figure that is currently growing at 11 000 per week.

Partnership and stakeholder marketing

Three steps were taken to try and ensure involvement of the campaign among key stakeholders. First, because a number of countries were already running mass media campaigns on all three *Help* topics (prevention, cessation and passive smoking) it was crucial for the campaign to be complementary rather than competitive. Regular information was therefore exchanged with the health ministries of all European member states.

In addition, particular efforts were made to cooperate closely with all national and local NGOs and associations involved in the European network for tobacco control and smoking prevention. An advisory board was established with representatives from the key networks including the International Network of Women Against Tobacco (INWAT), the European Network for Smoking Prevention (ENSP), the European Network on Young People and Tobacco (ENYPAT), the European Heart Network (EHN), the European Network of Quitlines (ENQ), European Cancer Leagues (ECL) and the World Health Organization (WHO). The job of this board is to work closely with the Commission in order to elaborate the strategic content of the campaign, ensure message consistency with tobacco control themes and also to provide guidance on the communication plan.

Thirdly, a specific action plan was developed in conjunction with the ENSP, Europe's largest anti-smoking network, representing no fewer than 650 organizations, and the ENQ. Both organizations help with national and local implementation. In addition, *Help* provides grant support for national projects that would be linked to the *Help* campaign – a sort of franchise operation. To date, 16 national projects have been set up with the ENSP partners (see Table 5.3).

Beyond the tobacco control community, the *Help* campaign has also linked up with an industry partner in the form of MTV Europe, who funded the production of an additional television ad with a dedicated microsite. This was called 'Smoking, where do you stand?' and targeted young people, encouraging them to reflect on their tobacco behav-

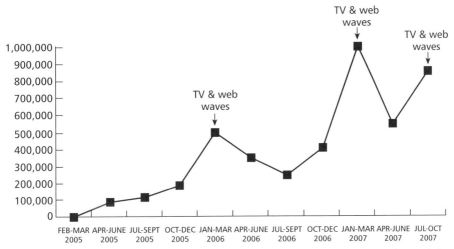

Fig. 5.4 Website visits correlate with waves of television advertising. Reproduced with permission from Ligaris.

iour via an interactive questionnaire on the website. The MTV 40-second TV spot was broadcast over 110 times during regular programmes. The online campaign delivered over 2 million impressions and generated a very positive average click-through rate (CTR) of 0.38 per cent, which is over three times the industry average. The UK was particularly successful with an impressive CTR of 1.90 per cent.

More direct efforts were made to link up with young people through a key youth association: the European Youth Forum. This is an umbrella organization that gathers together 94 international non-governmental youth organizations and national youth councils. In 2006, *Help* worked with them in the production of a European youth manifesto on tobacco. As with the viral campaign, much control of this was devolved to the young people themselves, who held a complex series of meetings in 25 member states (Bulgaria and Rumania were still to join the EU). Again there is danger in letting go like this; the resulting policy document could have been extremely problematic. In the event, however, the result was a radical agenda that called for both plain packaging and a complete ban on smoking in all public places. This ambitious manifesto has now been formally adopted by the European Commission.

Policy change

The smoke-free agenda addressed by the youth manifesto was picked up by the main *Help* advertising, with the most recent flight of ads focusing on this issue. The tagline for the last ad, for instance, emphasized the fact that in Europe, 19 000 *nonsmokers* die from tobacco-related diseases every year. This was seen by around 30 per cent of Europeans and over three-quarters (78 per cent) of them liked it. Importantly, this success was geographically patterned. In the north and west, where smoke-free is already a prominent issue and in some instances complete bans have been implemented, *Help* is

Table 5.3 National projects set up with partners from the European Network for Smoking Prevention.

Country	Project
Austria	Promotion of smoke-free schools and universities
Belgium	Belgium *Help* actions for smoking prevention
Czech Republic	Raising awareness on availability of treatment of tobacco dependence
Denmark	*Help* smoking cessation events on training schemes for teenagers
Estonia	Estonian *Help* actions for smoking prevention
France	Harmful effects of waterpipe smoking; smoke-free parties
Germany	Smoke-free working place
Hungary	Strengthening the local impact of the international *Help* campaign
Ireland	Smoking prevention and cessation in universities and colleges
Italy	Italian *Help* actions for smoking prevention
Portugal	*Help* campaign
Slovakia	*Help* campaign
Slovenia	02 belongs to you
Spain	Self-help computer program for smoking cessation in youth
Sweden	Reducing the use of oral smokeless tobacco in Sweden
UK	*Help* campaign

a more muted presence; but in the south and east – where it is typically the only voice raising this issue – the *Help* ad is both more prominent and appreciated.

Challenges

Help also provides some interesting lessons on the difficulties of international branding for public health. The European tobacco control community is a complex organism. It comprises a raft of government and NGO stakeholders who have in common an abiding desire to fight the harm being done by smoking, but also have many differences. At a country level, the variations in tobacco control culture across the EU are daunting – as noted in the introduction.

The NGO sector has similar variations. Some organizations see tobacco use in all its forms as the problem – smoking, oral tobacco and nicotine addiction need to be fought with equal dedication. For others the emphasis is on smoking, with the consumption of oral tobacco being seen as much less of a problem – indeed some feel its cleaner Swedish form may present a public health opportunity for harm reduction. Others again see the possibility of working with the more enlightened tobacco companies (e.g. Swedish Match) to produce a new generation of safer tobacco products and nicotine delivery devices.

These internal variations and complexities make the tobacco control movement quite unlike a corporation, which has a clear hierarchical structure, well-defined operating procedures and a shared vision. They also present particular challenges for brand development

Table 5.4 Raising the issue of smoke-free.

Region (*n* = 24 161)	Awareness (%)	Appreciation (%)
North	22	77
West	27	75
South	30	80
East	37	83

and management: decisions are debated and questioned, and alternative approaches are championed. The *Help* campaign has had to cope with robust debate throughout. The creative approach of ridiculing smoking, the hazards of working with youth organizations outside tobacco control and, most recently, the nicomarket viral campaign, have all been energetically criticized.

The last provides an interesting illustration of the challenges such debates present. On the one hand, some sections of tobacco control were anxious because they felt the viral campaign focused too much attention on nicotine rather than smoke, with the accompanying concern that it might put people off pharmaceutical cessation products such as nicotine replacement therapy (NRT) patches and gum. And the critics did not pull their punches: the initial e-mail launching the attack talked of 'tobacco control' being 'its own worst enemy' and the campaign being 'astonishingly counter productive' (B. Youdan, personal communication). Strong words indeed for someone writing purely on the basis of opinion, without any supporting evidence. Furthermore, there are equally strong opinions in the other direction: that we have a moral and pedagogical obligation to warn young people about nicotine – addiction to which is arguably driving the whole tobacco pandemic. Such debate presents obvious advantages: new ideas are often valuable and different points of view can add strength. On the other hand, it may also undermine the putative brand and create a culture where change is more likely – thereby threatening the longevity and steady progress that is so crucial to relationship and brand building.

In the event, the dispute was resolved in the best traditions of both public health and marketing: through research. A survey was conducted with 1000 young people (500 smokers and 500 nonsmokers), half of whom logged on to the site prior to interview (the test group) and half of whom had never done so (the control group). This showed that both groups were equally likely to agree that 'it is the nicotine in cigarettes that causes the harm' (63% vs. 62% respectively); that 'nicotine replacement products make it easier to give up smoking' (60% vs. 62% respectively); and (among smokers) 'If I wanted to give up smoking, I'd try nicotine replacement products' (63% vs. 62% respectively).

Working within a European political context can also present challenges. Many agendas have to be satisfied and unpredictable problems can arise just because of the complexities of the European Commission, an organization that incorporates 27 countries and deals with many other priorities not just beyond tobacco control, but beyond public health. The funding source for *Help* illustrates the sort of paradox that can result. The European Commission, through its Common Agricultural Policy, has for many years subsidized tobacco farmers; after many protests from public health and tobacco control, this funding is now due to cease, but in the meantime a very small percentage of it is allocated to anti-tobacco education – and thence to fund *Help*.

Thus *Help* has had to tread a precarious path between pharma and farming and faces an end to its principal source of funding. Meanwhile Philip Morris and its Marlboro brand have entered their sixth decade.

Conclusion: a brand is born

Help represents an ambitious attempt to build a public health brand across Europe that can begin to compete with the tobacco brands that wreak such harm. Brands are ultimately about generating recognition, making valued promises and, above all, delivering on these promises. This chapter has shown that *Help* has had successes at all three levels.

For public health, however, the key question is whether such brands can deliver behaviour change. The answer seems to be a cautious 'yes'. *Help* has not resulted in mass reductions in smoking prevalence, but it has got people to do some positive things about their health. Some 4.2 million Europeans have visited an anti-tobacco website – traffic driven by the television advertising; 15 per cent of those visiting the viral site have gone to the trouble of passing it on to their peers, and after just three months, some 91 000 smokers have signed up for e-mail coaching to help them quit. In this way it has edged towards its aim of denormalizing smoking.

The challenges of international branding have also become apparent, however. In particular, public health lacks the structures, coherence and funding streams that deliver the potential for great longevity to the private sector. Nonetheless, *Help* has succeeded in developing a putative brand and established itself as platform for future public health activity. Perhaps more importantly, it has shown that, notwithstanding the challenges, public health can seriously engage with branding at an international level; at long last the Marlboro Man has a bit of competition.

References

Action on Smoking and Health (ASH) (2006). Factsheet No. 16: The economics of tobacco. Available at: http://www.oldash.org.uk/html/factsheets/html/fact16.html (accessed 20 November 2007).

ASPECT Consortium (2004). *Tobacco or health in the European Union past, present and future.* Luxembourg: Office for Official Publications of the European Communities.

Carat Global Management/Isobar data. (2007). European Interactive Advertising Agency. Mediascope Europe Study Pan-European Results. Conducted by SPA, Synovate.

De Bruyn, A. and Lilien, G. L. (2003). Harnessing the power of viral marketing: A multi-stage model of word of mouth through electronic referrals. Working paper. Department of Business Administration, Pennsylvania State University. Available at: http://www.arnaud.debruyn.info/research/papers/viralmarketing.pdf (accessed 20 November 2007).

European Commission (2003). Tobacco Youth Prevention and Communication Conference. Rome 13–15 November, 2003. Availabe at: http://europa.eu.int/comm/dgs/health_consumer/index_en.htm. (accessed 5 May 2008).

Farrelly, M. C., Niederdeppe, J. and Yarsevich, J. (2003). Youth tobacco prevention mass media campaigns: past, present and future directions. *Tobacco Control* **12**:i35

Friend, K. and Levy, D. (2002). Reductions in smoking prevalence and cigarette consumption associated with mass-media campaigns. *Health Education Research Theory and Practice* **17**:85–98

Harrison, R. and Hurst, J. (2005). The unwelcome guest: how Scotland invited the tobacco industry to smoke outside. Available at: http://repositories.cdlib.org/tc/reports/Scotland2005 (accessed 20 November 2007).

Jepson, R., Harris, F., Rowa-Dewar, N., MacGillivray S. Hastings G. Kearney N *et al.* (2006). *A review of the effectiveness of Mass Media Interventions which both Encourage Quit Attempts and Reinforce Current and Recent Attempts to Quit Smoking.* London: NICE. Available at: www.nice.org.uk/ncemedia/pdf/SmokingCessationmassMediafullreview.pdf (accessed 4 December 2007).

Kelly, E. (2000). This is one virus you want to spread. *Fortune Magazine*, (online) 27 November (accessed 16 Dec 2007).

Marketing Today (2007). Beyond the 30 second spot: marketers adding alternatives to television advertising. Available at: http://www.marketingtoday.com/research/0306/tv_advertising_less_effective.htm (accessed 5 December 2007).

NHS Centre for Reviews and Dissemination (1999). *Preventing the uptake of smoking in young people. York: Centre for Reviews and Dissemination (CRD). Effective Health Care 5* (p 1–12). Available at: http://www.york.ac.uk/inst/crd/ehc55.pdf (accesed 2 Dec 2007).

Richardson, L., Allen, P., McCullough, L., Bauld, L., Assanand, S., Greaves, L., *et al.* (2007). *NICE RAPID REVIEW Interventions to Prevent the Uptake of Smoking in Children and Young People Full Report. 22 November* (accessed 8 December 2007). British Columbia Centre of Excellence for Women's Health. London: NICE. Available at: http://www.nice.org.uk/nicemedia/pdf/PreventingSmokingChildrenEvidence%20ReviewFullReport.pdf.

Sowden, A. J. and Arblaster, L. (1998). Mass media interventions for preventing smoking in young people. *Cochrane Database of Systematic Reviews* **4**: CD001006.

6

Branding play for children: *VERB*™ *It's what you do*

Marian Huhman, Simani M. Price, and Lance D. Potter

Summary

- The *VERB* campaign used a branding strategy closely modeled after the methods used to brand commercial products in the private sector.
- The *VERB* brand was the organizing element for the campaign's marketing approach and advertising platforms to reach its target audience of tweens.
- A continuous tracking survey monitored the *VERB* brand's performance, giving feedback about the reach, appeal and relevance of the brand and the television commercials.
- Requests to use the *VERB* brand for different behaviors and in different settings were examples of opportunities that were considered; some were implemented, with lessons learned for other public health campaigns.

Products are created in the factory. Brands are created in the mind.

(Walter Landor, founder Landor Associates)

In recent decades, public health has turned to the world of commercial marketing to find fresh ways to communicate health messages to large numbers of youths and adults. This has led to the emergence of social marketing and the development of communication campaigns that have adopted private sector methods such as using paid media to convey health-promoting messages to public health consumers (Evans *et al.* 2002; Smith *et al.* 2006). Social and commercial marketers put the consumer's needs and values at the center of their persuasive endeavor (Grier and Bryant 2005). Around those needs and values, they build a marketing mix – advertising strategies, distribution channels, segmentation to subgroups, balance of promotions, and advertising – to build a relationship with the consumer. The organizing element of the marketing mix in the commercial world, and increasingly in public health, is a brand.

A brand is a set of enduring and distinctive characteristics that are associated with the brand in the mind of the consumer (Aaker 1996). Although a logo may be a point of entry for a brand, the brand is much more than a logo, a trademark or a slogan. A brand transcends the material aspects of an emblem or graphic to convey an array of complex meanings as diverse as high quality, relaxed lifestyle, low fat, trustworthy or cute. Building on the notion of marketing as being about partnering with the consumer (Fournier 1995), marketers also refer to the brand as a relationship, with promises, ideas and expectations between the consumer and the company, product, idea or service (McDivitt 2003; Wheeler 2003).

The Centers for Disease Control and Prevention (CDC) turned to commercial marketing to design and implement *VERB. It's what you do*, a communication campaign based on social marketing principles to promote the benefits of daily physical activity to children aged 9–13 years (tweens) (Wong *et al.* 2004). In the authorizing legislation for *VERB*, US Congress specified that the same communication methods employed by the best kids' marketers should be used to communicate messages to help children develop healthy lifestyles. CDC chose to focus the campaign on physical activity because of the substantial evidence regarding the physical and psychological benefits to children of being physically active (CDC 1996; Williams *et al.* 2002; Strong *et al.* 2005) and because of concern for the growing appeal to children of screen-dominated sedentary pursuits (Roberts *et al.* 2005).

The creative teams hired to design the campaign advised unequivocally that the campaign messages and advertising should be built around a brand. The plan that they produced followed the same roadmap used for brands such as McDonald's, Verizon and Nickelodeon, and included extensive qualitative work with tweens to inform the development of the brand, the testing of all advertisements and promotions, the continuous gauging of the brand's performance, and refreshing the brand in response to feedback (Asbury *et al.*, in press). A brand manager with extensive experience with youth brands in the private sector was on the CDC team and directed the creative development.

Throughout the campaign, all aspects of the advertising and promotional materials, the products for schools, communities and the internet, were affixed with the *VERB* logo. The brand emerged from the combination of the *VERB* logo and the images, colors, text, and emotions that the advertising was eliciting. The advertising was essential to build understanding about what the brand meant, but eventually the brand took on the intended meanings of a bundle of benefits of being physically active – doing something that was fun, cool, and an opportunity to be with friends.

This chapter reports on *VERB* as a branded campaign. It summarizes the development of the *VERB* brand, detailing how the brand's distinctiveness and relevance were maintained, and how the brand was kept fresh. The methods to assess the brand's performance are shown and the results are reported. The brand concept occupies such a huge part of marketing that numerous tag words have sprung up to differentiate the multiple aspects of brands. Identity, equity, assets, brand extensions and co-branding are a few examples of tag terms from the commercial marketing world that are now appearing in the public health literature and will be discussed here in relation to *VERB*. We also discuss a challenge faced by *VERB* and one that will be an emerging issue for public health brands: helping public health practitioners in local communities use, but not dilute, brand assets that were being maintained by commercial marketers at the national level.

Story of the *VERB* brand

Branding is about making an emotional connection. People fall in love with brands – they trust them, develop strong loyalties, buy them, and believe in their superiority. The brand is shorthand. It stands for something and demonstrates it.

Wheeler (2003: 2)

Analyzing the competition

An early step in brand development is a careful analysis of rival forces. For a commercial product, obvious competitors would be similar products with well-recognized brands. Less obvious rivals could be new entrants into the marketplace, low-priced alternatives or online competitors looking to enlarge distribution. For a health behavior, the competition includes the behavior the target audience prefers to do or has become habituated to, and includes, in some cases, organizations that may be positioned in opposition to the desired behavior (Kotler *et al.* 2002). *VERB* wanted tweens to substitute active play for some of the behaviors they were doing in their discretionary time, including hanging out with friends, playing video and computer games, and watching television. A competitive analysis must drill down to discover the benefits a person gains from the rival behavior. In particular, what needs are being met by the rival behavior? The new brand has to signify meeting those needs. Meeting those needs and promising even greater benefits than the competing behavior is the emotional connection that is sought by the new brand.

Besides studying the competition for tweens' time and attention, the brand development phase included the study of other children's brands to examine the way that their meanings were communicated through visual and design elements. Organizations and companies that targeted youth were potential competitors, but were also potential partners because their brands were valued by the tween audience. Although *VERB* planners were well aware of the irony of building relationships with media icons such as Nickelodeon, Disney and AOL, it was felt that associating *VERB* with brands, magazines and television shows that were already well known and liked by tweens could boost *VERB*'s value to tweens.

From competitive analysis to the *VERB* brand

Extensive qualitative study with tweens on how they were spending their discretionary time and the benefits they were garnering from those pursuits revealed that their choices in sedentary activities were conferring benefits of familiarity, comfort, and, because they were good at them, increased self-esteem. Tweens reported that they had dreams and fantasies – from the everyday to the adventurous – and they believed they were possible. Many of them played out those dreams in the virtual world of video and computer games and television. Most tweens were not opposed to being physically active; indeed, many aspired to be more active, but were not confident in their athletic abilities and feared negative judgments by their peers. Both involved and uninvolved youth were attracted to notions of self-discovery and all wanted to feel good about themselves. The tweens revealed that having active peers increased their interest in physical activity, that competitive games could be fun but also scary, and that costs, time and family responsibilities, such as caring for younger siblings, were barriers (CDC 2000).

From the competitive analysis, positive emotions surrounding discovering something fun and active you are good at and can dream about merged into 'Freeing kids to turn dreams into action' as the brand's overall vision. The creative designers expanded this vision to build the brand identity – the values and uniqueness – that they wanted for *VERB*. Brand identity is a key concept in brand management (Wheeler 2003). The brand is an intangible in the minds of the consumer; the brand identity is the visual and verbal expression of the brand. Typical questions that marketers use to guide them as they develop the brand's identity (Kepferer 2004) include the following:

◆ What makes it different?

◆ What need is the brand fulfilling?

◆ What are the enduring characteristics of the brand?

◆ What are its values?

◆ What are the signs that make the brand recognizable?

What made the brand different from other brands was that it was not connected to a product and that the brand used a word that was familiar to tweens from schoolwork, but gave it a new meaning and association as a commercial on television that showed kids playing actively. The brand sought to fulfill children's needs to discover things they could be good at that are valued by their friends, to have fun with their friends, and to have choices about trying new activities. The enduring characteristic, or the tone that would characterize every *VERB*-affiliated advertisement or item, was a supportive rather than an oppositional (don't do) message. Such an approach has been used in some other public health branded campaigns (Farrelly *et al*. 2002a; Worden and Slater 2004). *VERB*'s designers wanted *VERB*'s promise to 'be there for you 24/7' and to be in all the places that tweens could encounter it – watching television, in magazines, at the mall, on the internet, in schools, at sporting events, and at community recreational centers, festivals and cultural events. Another consistent message was that active play can be done anytime and anywhere.

The core values of the *VERB* brand were fairness, empowerment, a level playing field, to be nonjudgmental, and to fuse all ages, sexes and cultures. These values were kept front and center to the creative team as they developed the visual, auditory and tactile elements of hundreds of materials throughout the five years of the campaign. To increase the visual impact and to make it easily recognizable, the *VERB* logo (Fig. 6.1) was created in all capital letters, giving the word prominence and differentiating it from the grammatical word, verb. Each letter is outlined in varying shades of blue so that the logo letters seem to vibrate, enhancing the conveyance of motion and action.

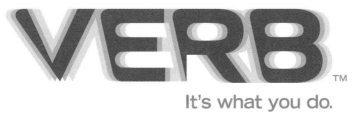

Fig. 6.1 *VERB* logo. Reproduced with permission from the Center for Disease Control and Prevention.

Marketers connect a tagline to a logo as a short phrase that captures the brand essence, personality and positioning (Wheeler 2003). Taglines carry different types of messages. *VERB*'s tagline 'It's what you do' is a blend of an imperative message (e.g. Nike: Just do it) and a descriptive message (e.g. Allstate: You're in good hands) and sprang from the *VERB*'s empowerment value to convey to tweens the freedom to choose their own way to be physically active.

Merging the desired brand identity to the *VERB* concept and logo was an iterative process in which various concepts, logos and sample ads were tested with children to determine their preferences. The brand positioning for *VERB* – the angle that would be developed to grab tweens' attention and get them to purchase the product of physical activity – also emerged from this process. Marketers refer to positioning as the way to break into the market and to generate market share (Kepferer 1997). Generating market share in this case meant getting tweens to add physical activity to their crowded schedules. One way to do this was for tweens to perceive *VERB* as their own brand, not connected to the adult world. Another way was to position active play as the easy, appealing choice for the tween (McKinnon 2007). The ads were designed to minimize the perceived barriers to physical activity and to motivate tweens to seek active play opportunities. Third, *VERB* aspired to become a lifestyle brand for tweens. For a tween to see himself/herself as a '*VERB* kid' would increase the likelihood that he or she would integrate physical activity into their lives, thus trumping other more sedentary pursuits.

Launching the brand

The *VERB* campaign was launched in June 2002; establishing the *VERB* brand was the campaign designers' first objective. The goal was to achieve 50 per cent awareness of the brand among tweens by the end of the first year. Breaking through the continuous bombardment of advertising with a new brand that will be noticed and understood by the audience is difficult and expensive. The cost of launching a new branded product is estimated to be $100 million or more (Aaker and Keller 1990; Kotler and Keller 2005). The first-year budget for *VERB* was $125 million, most of which went toward the creative development of the brand, the production of the advertising, and the purchasing of media. Due to government funding cycles, time was short. Contractors were hired, the brand was conceived and developed, the initial ads were produced (with animated characters because there was not time to produce ads with live actors), and the media were purchased, all in eight months, a process that typically requires three years.

To attract tweens' attention to the new brand, the creative team designed the brand launch as a 'teaser campaign', with ads that were fast-paced, visually riveting, and a little obscure about what the ad was really about (Fig. 6.2). The brand launch featured television spots with animated boys and girls being physically active and enveloped in verbs. For example, a girl was shown diving into a swimming pool full of water swirling with action words and emerging from the pool covered with verbs. The voiceover was inviting and inclusive: 'This summer, everywhere you go, everywhere you look, there are verbs out there, waiting for you to get into … *VERB*. It's what you do'.

Following the six months of the teaser campaign, new ads were shown that bridged the brand launch with the full roll-out of the campaign. Using the same animated characters from the brand launch, the characters morphed into real children who were 'finding their *VERB*'. *VERB*s were highlighted, such as 'bounce' or 'race'. 'Spin' showed skaters, dancers and a celebrity snowboarder doing spin moves on her snowboard.

Enriching the *VERB* brand

Marketers strive to increase the value of a brand because high value translates to greater power, usefulness and sales. A top brand such as Coca-Cola is estimated to have a value of $68 billion (*Business Week* 2004). A brand's value is often referred to as its assets or equity (Aaker 1991; Wheeler 2003). Brand equity is built through awareness, recognition and a loyal customer base. A quick route to building equity for a new brand is to link it or *co-brand* with a high-equity brand that is already popular and easily recognized by the target (Keller 2003). *VERB* co-branded with numerous media companies (e.g. Nickelodeon, the Cartoon Network and *Sports Illustrated for Kids*) as part of the added value gained from the media that *VERB* purchased from them. The children who visited Nickelodeon's 'Let's Just Play' tour at parks and zoos in the summer of 2005 saw banners co-branded with *VERB* and Nickelodeon. Similarly, celebrities with high recognition and popularity, such as

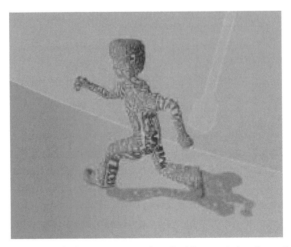

Fig. 6.2 Teaser ad: verb-covered character. Reproduced with permission from the Center for Disease Control and Prevention.

Tony Hawk, Donavan McNabb and Venus Williams, were featured in the *VERB* commercials and promotions as a way to spark interest in *VERB* and to enrich the *VERB* brand.

Relationship between the *VERB* brand and the advertising

Advertising is the vehicle of persuasion to drive the consumer to purchase the product, or here, to engage in physical activity. The ads illustrate and expand on the benefits that are promised by the brand, thus furthering the understanding of the brand. Advertising stimulates a person's cognitions (informational and awareness) and affect (emotional, likeability and attraction), which are then filtered through prior experiences with or memories of the product or brand (Vakratsas and Ambler 1999). How cognitions and affect about a product's advertising lead to trial behavior (buying the product or trying physical activity) and in what order is unclear (Vakratsas and Ambler 1999). The *VERB* designers believed that the sensory/affective dimension was particularly important for *VERB* because of the age of the target and the belief that children may follow more affective rather than analytic information processes (Zhang and Sood 2002).

The *VERB* designers believed that the ads were always brand building, but that the ads had to change to hold the tweens' interest. The *VERB* campaign's 4.5 years of advertising and promotional activities were divided into four phases. Each phase centered on an advertising theme, called a message platform. As shown in Table 6.1, all of the phases were under the vision of the *VERB* brand: 'Free kids to play out their dreams'. The message platform could be similar through some phases, as in *VERB* phases 2 and 3, but the advertising strategy changed. Phase 2 emphasized playing in the backyard while, in phase 3, the ads gave tweens ideas about making up their own games. Consistency between the advertising and the *VERB* brand was critical and was ensured by carefully considering that every ad, promotion, school kit and image that was part of any marketing activity was 'on brand'.

The *VERB* ads were shaped to affect the attitudes of different segments, such as the child with lower self-efficacy about physical activity; they could include a 'call to action',

Table 6.1 Overall strategy for reaching tweens with messages about physical activity: *VERB*, phases 1–4.

	Free kids to play out their dreams			
	Phase 1	**Phase 2**	**Phase 3**	**Phase 4**
Message platform	Put verbs into action as VERBs.	Infuse play with status of organized sports.	Infuse play with status of organized sports.	Ignite desire for physical activity.
Strategy	World of action words to discover and make yours.	Bring all that's good in organized sports to the backyard.	You don't have to be a pro to play.	Nothing replaces the rush and exhilaration of physical activity.
Main idea for the tween message	Find your VERB.	Everyday is game day: get out and go play.	Kids make up their own rules.	I can't NOT play.

such as directing the tween to visit the *VERB* website. Promotions, such as the *VERB* Activity Zone booth at cultural festivals, were opportunities to experience the brand (Heitzler *et al.*, 2008). *VERB*-branded items that were given away at events (e.g. wristbands, hacky sacks and Frisbees) were called 'brand in the hand'. Thus, the brand was reassuring in its constancy, while the advertising was kept fresh through new ads and promotions. The ads set out to grab the target audience's attention by being distinctive, novel, but still relevant and appealing.

Disseminating the *VERB* message

The *VERB* advertising and promotions reached tweens in their homes, in school and in their communities. The primary vehicle was paid advertising in the general market and in ethnic media channels. The *VERB* commercials aired on television and on radio channels that were popular with children, such as the Cartoon Network, Nickelodeon, The WB, Disney (including Radio Disney), Telemundo, and Black Entertainment Television (BET). The national television media market averaged 107 gross rating points (a measure of reach and frequency of advertising) per week over the life of the campaign. Print advertising was placed in dozens of youth publications, such as *Sports Illustrated for Kids*, *Teen People*, and *ELLEgirl*. A website, VERBnow, was created where children could get ideas about active games, watch tutorials from sports celebrities, and record their physical activity to become eligible to win prizes for being active.

VERB reached children in schools through advertising shown on Channel One in thousands of middle school classrooms and through classroom-based activity kits that included instructions, posters, rewards and activity incentives such as pedometers. During each semester beginning in the second phase of advertising, 1500 schools across the USA participated in the school promotions. In addition, book covers, day planners and customized lesson plans that incorporated physical activities were sent to schools across the country.

VERB reached children in their communities by sending activity-promoting kits similar to those used by schools to recreational centers, camps and daycare centers. Community-based events (e.g. cultural festivals, powwows and fairs) and guerrilla marketing (e.g. using college-aged young adults to engage tweens in being physically active at events and tween hangouts) spread the awareness of *VERB* and directly communicated the message that physical activity was fun, cool, and a way to play with friends.

The marketing activities were implemented at a fairly consistent level over the 4.5 years of the campaign. By this we mean that television commercials were always airing, except for several weeks during November and December when marketers typically do not try to compete with holiday-related products. School promotions occurred throughout the school year and were specifically designed to be short-term (e.g. one month) so that the *VERB*-branded poster that anchored the activity did not become part of the classroom wallpaper, thus jeopardizing the cool factor of the brand. When the children were out for the summer, community promotions and helping tweens find local places to play were weighted more heavily. Marketing activities also had to be responsive to changes in tween media use. For example, 'Cell phone 8372' was the organizing concept for the summer of 2005 and featured commercials about a cell phone that magically becomes active and leads its owner to the park to play. The numbers 8372 spell *VERB* on a phone keypad and the call to action in the ads was for tweens to go to the 8372 website to find places in their community to be active and to sign up to receive text messages prompting them to be active.

Decisions about the timing and the placement of advertising were driven by a desire to use resources wisely and were strategic for nurturing the brand and disseminating the *VERB*'s core message to get active. For example, by the third phase of the campaign, children's awareness of the brand (75 per cent awareness) was so strong and so consistent that the marketers directed a higher level of resources to the experiential marketing elements, such as mobile tours (*VERB* vans going to zoos, parks and sporting events to engage tweens in physical activity) and street teams, because they reasoned that the children needed support in experiencing being active and trying out activities, while still seeing the brand and messages through broadcast advertising, albeit at a lower intensity than at the beginning of the campaign.

Developing and using tracking data to inform the brand and advertising strategy

Strategic decision making required the campaign planners to keep a finger on the tween pulse, not only to keep up with the rapid changes in media and marketing to the children but to know intimately what tweens thought of the *VERB* brand and its advertising. Classic questions asked by brand managers include: does the audience have knowledge of the brand; do they comprehend the meaning of the brand and message; do the brand and the commercials using the brand have appeal for the audience; and do our commercials stand out so that they will be noticed (Aaker 1996; Evans *et al.* 2005; Value based management.net 2007). To answer these questions, *VERB* employed a classic brand management tool: a tracking survey. Tracking surveys are developed specifically for a company or a campaign to monitor the awareness and the reactions to the brand and product by continuously assessing knowledge and attitudes toward the brand and the advertising (Keller and Sood 1995). Wear in (i.e. acceptance and likeability of new ads) and wear out (i.e. the audience is tired of the ads) of the ads are also monitored.

The *VERB* Continuous Tracking Survey

The campaign planners developed the *VERB* Continuous Tracking Survey (VCTS) to monitor the performance of the *VERB* brand and advertising. The VCTS was a national cross-sectional telephone survey conducted over the five years of the campaign to help the advertising agencies manage the brand and give interim assessments of the campaign in support of the national outcome evaluation (Potter *et al.*, 2008). The VCTS collected data from 300 children nationally on a monthly basis from October 2002 through August 2004. Because the monthly assessments showed so much consistency in the performance of the brand, the VCTS switched to quarterly data collection from

November 2004 until the last administration in September 2006. Thirty-one rounds of data were collected over the course of the campaign, resulting in a total sample size of 9200 tweens.

Brand awareness

The VCTS tracked the awareness of *VERB*, the source of the awareness (television, radio and internet), message comprehension, and the appeal of the brand and television commercials (CDC 2007). The awareness of *VERB* was assessed by asking, 'Have you seen, heard, or read any messages or advertising about kids getting active?' Those who reported the *VERB* messages without further prompting were categorized as having 'unaided awareness' of the campaign. All of the other children were asked, 'Have you seen, heard, or read any messages or advertising about *VERB*?' The children who answered in the affirmative were categorized as having 'aided awareness' of *VERB*. Unaided and aided awareness were combined to create a total awareness measure. Understanding of the brand and messages was assessed by the open-ended question, 'What is *VERB* all about?' and 'What ideas did *VERB* give you?'

For each quarter of the campaign, the 31 waves of tracking data were aggregated for analysis to show the awareness of *VERB* and how tweens rated the brand and commercials. Figure 6.3 shows that 60 per cent of tweens reported awareness of *VERB* six months after the start of the campaign, the point that we started the tracking survey;

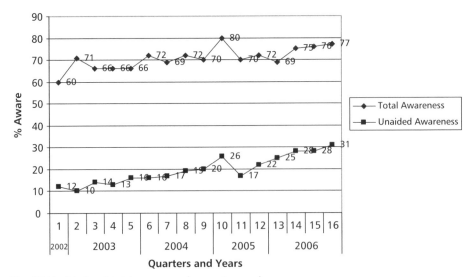

Fig. 6.3 Unaided and total awareness by quarters and years.
Awareness of *VERB* was assessed by asking, 'Have you seen, heard, or read any messages or advertising about kids getting active?' Those who reported *VERB* messages without further prompting were categorized as having 'unaided awareness' of the campaign. All of the other children were asked, 'Have you seen, heard, or read any messages or advertising about *VERB*?' The children who answered in the affirmative were categorized as having 'aided awareness' of *VERB*. Unaided and aided awareness were combined to create a total awareness measure.

this increased to 77 per cent awareness by the last quarter of the campaign. Unaided awareness or spontaneous recall of *VERB* by a tween when asked if they had seen any advertising or commercials about getting active is a more robust indicator of resonance among the target audience. Unaided awareness increased steadily throughout the campaign to the end when almost one of three tweens spontaneously named *VERB* when asked to recall any advertising about getting kids active.

In addition, 90 per cent of the tweens who were aware of *VERB* either aided or unaided were able to describe correctly a key message of the campaign, such as being about all kinds of sports, playing actively, or learning new outside games.

Brand awareness is one important dimension that brand managers need in order to assess market penetration. More nuanced and multidimensional assessments are obtained through questions regarding tweens' disposition to the brand itself and their reactions to the television commercials, the primary channel for *VERB* advertising. The tweens were asked to rate nine statements about the brand using a five-point Likert-type scale, where 1 = really disagree and 5 = really agree. For their reactions to the television commercials, the tweens rated their agreement on statements about recently viewed *VERB* commercials using a dichotomous scale (yes or no).

Figure 6.4 shows the mean values of the items for each quarter. Examples of brand dimensions and the items to tap those dimensions included (1) appeal of the brand (e.g. is cool, is fun), (2) relevance for them (e.g. is saying something important to me; gives me ideas about different activities; is for all kinds of kids), and (3) bridge to action (*VERB* makes me want to get more active). The tweens rated *VERB* very positively on these items, with averages above 4 on the five-point scale across all quarters.

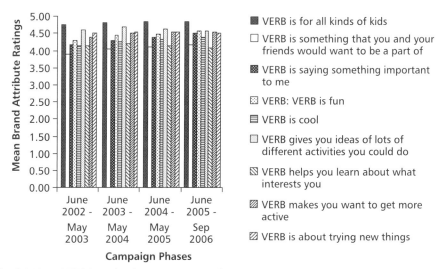

Fig. 6.4 Mean *VERB* brand ratings across campaign years.
Respondents rated the brand attributes using a five-point Likert-type scale, where 1 = really disagree and 5 = really agree.

The purpose of the VCTS was not only to assess *VERB*'s resonance with the target audience overall but to uncover the differences among the subgroups that could inform the needs for market segmentation. For example, the tracking data showed that brand appeal was very strong among all children. However, it was slightly, but significantly, lower among the older children (aged 12–13 years old) than the younger children (aged 9–10 years old); it was also lower among boys than among girls. Qualitative work with the boys showed that they liked the skill-building and competitive elements of physical activity; thus, advertising to boys was developed to emphasize these elements. Skill-building tutorials for tennis, soccer and football were developed for the *VERB* website featuring sports celebrities. To better reach the older boys, more advertising was purchased in magazines that targeted the older tween boys, such as *Game Pro* and *Boys Life*.

The VCTS was also used to inform needs for segmentation to tweens of different races and ethnicities. During the first year of the campaign, the VCTS indicated that the *VERB* brand awareness was higher among Caucasians (67 per cent) versus African-Americans (55 per cent) or Hispanics (58 per cent). Despite the lower awareness rates, the minority tween audiences found the brand appealing in the first year. During the first year, among the tweens who were aware of *VERB*, the brand was rated slightly higher overall by African-American ($M = 4.5$ 0.58) and Hispanic ($M = 4.5$ 0.62) tweens versus Caucasian tweens ($M = 4.3$ 0.68; $p < 0.05$). Of interest, there was no difference in the percentage agreement with the *VERB* brand attribute statement 'VERB is for all kinds of kids' by race or ethnicity (percentage 'really agree' ranged from 82 to 86 per cent) during the first year, suggesting that the brand was perceived as being multiethnic, as designed by campaign planners. These findings and focus groups with children of different ethnicities confirmed that the brand and advertising were relevant to them but were reaching fewer minority tweens compared with white tweens. To amend this disparity, more media were purchased in the outlets that reached these groups, such as BET and Telemundo. By the fourth year of the campaign, there were no differences in the overall appeal of the *VERB* brand by race or ethnicity.

VERB advertising

The primary vehicle for communicating about *VERB* to the target audience was commercials on cable television. Questions on the VCTS assessed the dimensions of the commercials that were similar to the dimensions of the brand itself, such as likeability (e.g. is cool; is exciting) and differentiation (e.g. is really different from other commercials out there). The VCTS data indicated that tweens' agreement with positive statements regarding the most recently seen *VERB* commercial was high from the beginning of the campaign and increased as the campaign progressed (Figure 6.5). The percentage of tweens who responded yes to the statement about the most recently seen *VERB* commercial, 'The commercial is exciting', increased from 65 per cent during the first year to 74 per cent by the fourth year of the campaign ($p < 0.05$). The item, 'Is the kind of ad you might talk to your friends about', is notable because, unlike the other items, it probes for the likelihood that the tween would take action about the commercial, if only to talk about it with a friend. While the levels of agreement on this item were lower than on

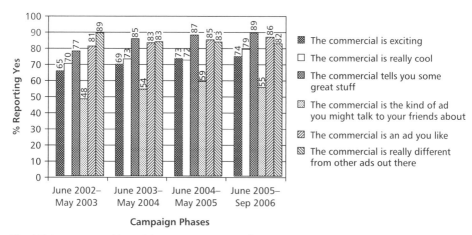

Fig. 6.5 Agreement with positive statements regarding most recently seen *VERB* ads by campaign phases.

Respondents rated their agreement regarding positive statements on recently viewed *VERB* commercials using a dichotomous scale (yes or no).

other items, we viewed the percentages of the tweens (more than half for phases 2-4) as a very positive sign that the ads might generate 'buzz' or a word-of-mouth spread of the *VERB* message – a highly desirable consequence of effective marketing (Thomas 2004).

Leveraging the *VERB* brand

The continuous tracking data informed strategic decisions and gave feedback that the brand was appealing to tweens and that the messages were resonating with them. Furthermore, the annual outcome evaluations were showing that tweens' attitudes and behaviors were changing as a result of the campaign (Huhman *et al.* 2005). This evidence of success prompted questions about leveraging the *VERB* brand for other purposes, including a brand extension. Companies can develop a brand extension when they use a successful brand name to launch a new product or product category (Kotler and Armstrong 2006). Examples are the expansion of the Liz Claiborne brand from clothing to bedding and fragrances and Apple's expansion from computers to handheld music devices and the iPhone.

The benefits of borrowing assets of a known popular brand to launch a new product and thus leapfrog ahead in the marketplace have made brand extensions for child and adult products a hot topic in marketing (Zhang and Sood 2002; Kepferer 2004). They can also carry risks. Product development can spread resources too thinly, and dilution of the parent brand or confusion about the brand identity can tarnish the parent brand. For example, an extension of *VERB* could have been to promote healthy eating – something we were, in fact, approached about. We declined this move for several reasons. Brand extensions should be attempted when the source or parent brand has well-established assets and sufficient resources exist to build a new product line (Aaker 1996; Kepferer 2004). The *VERB* brand was relatively young and sustained funding was uncertain. The brand identity has to transfer to the new product. Apple's brand identity is for electronics that are sleek, sophisticated and user-friendly; this represents a brand asset that can transfer to multiple electronic devices. *VERB*'s identity as active play being fun, cool and a social opportunity does not transfer to eating. Compared with physical activity, eating behavior has a hugely different set of motivators, barriers, values and competing behaviors; it was thus judged to be too different to place under the *VERB* brand.

Another opportunity to leverage the *VERB* brand came through requests by communities to use the *VERB* brand and advertising to build awareness and participation for their local programs, events and activities. These opportunities presented challenges that illustrated the differences between the commercial world culture and public health. On one hand, we knew the importance of fiercely protecting the brand's assets (cool, fun and social) but, on the other hand, we knew that the communities could leverage the cachet of the *VERB* brand to promote local activities. Long-term sustainability of the *VERB* effort depended on communities mobilizing resources for physical activity. However, the wrong associations (exercise) or distributions (an adult-oriented event) could confuse tweens and dilute the brand assets. Community-level partners also brought expectations of shared decision making that sometimes contrasted with the brand managers' need to carefully choreograph the presentation of *VERB*.

VERB faced these challenges carefully and achieved some remarkable successes. Brand guidelines were developed that mandated how and where the *VERB* logo could be used and what kinds of activities or events were appropriate; *VERB*-approved materials were provided. The *VERB* team members worked with the communities to ensure that maintaining the cool factor was in the forefront of their decisions. In particular, the *VERB* Summer Scorecard (VSS) was a community-based activity that evolved into an annual local promotional event for tweens (Farrelly *et al.* 2002b; Bretthauer-Mueller *et al.*, 2008). In their initial years, the VSS communities were carefully blending the essence of the *VERB* brand into their activity. In at least three of the communities, the VSS became a kind of brand extension with its own credibility and awareness level and appears to have become a sustainable offshoot of *VERB*.

Conclusion

The *VERB* campaign branded active play as an appealing and easy pursuit for every child and as a lifestyle choice that all children aged 9–13 years could aspire to adopt. The *VERB* designers applied the branding tactics that marketers use for youth-directed brands in the commercial world to a behavior that is important for the health of America's children. Methods to build brand equity, maintain the brand identity, and measure the brand's performance were applied in a fashion that was typical of the marketing industry and worked well for *VERB*.

We believe the branding was an enormously important building block to the rest of the campaign activities and a cornerstone of the campaign's success. The brand was an anchor to the message publicizing the benefits of physical activity and was a shortcut to reaching ubiquity with the message. We offer the tracking data shown here as evidence that the brand's assets (e.g. appeal, relevance and coolness) gained strength early and remained robust throughout the campaign phases. The levels of awareness of *VERB* were similar to the awareness levels found for the *truth*® brand (Farrelly *et al.* 2002b) and the anti-drug brand (Harmatz 2004).

The campaign used the awareness and favorable attitudes about the brand as a springboard to getting tweens active in campaign-sponsored events, promotions, school activities, websites and engagement of communities. Outcome evaluations have shown favorable results in a number of areas, including tweens' beliefs about the benefits of physical activity and their engagement in physical activity during their free time (Huhman *et al.* 2007).

Another advantage of a branding strategy that we realized with *VERB* is that the brand functions as an organizing concept, helping the team bring order to decision making (e.g. is the idea on brand?), to categorize relationships (e.g. brand partners), and to simplify communications to the stakeholders. Once the brand was established, using the term 'VERB' was a vehicle for precision (the CDC's social marketing of physical activity to tweens) and conciseness (promoting the fun, cool and sociability of physical activity) that transcended the health message itself.

National public health campaigns wishing to develop a brand among a population of Americans, in this case, children aged 9–13 years, can learn from the experiences of *VERB* we have described here. Capturing children's attention and imagination with a branded health message is possible, but it requires investments of creative personnel, time and financial resources. Investment is especially critical up front to bring the brand to the marketplace in a way that will truly compete with other sophisticated, professionally produced, and well-financed commercial products. *VERB* benefited greatly from the expertise of private sector marketers hired to develop and maintain the brand, to create the brand-associated activities and materials, and to negotiate the media contracts to deliver the branded messages.

Children are savvy consumers; a successful brand needs to be relevant and appealing to them, to be distinctive, and to communicate that it fulfills a need for them. We also discovered ways to maximize the brand's potential by bringing it to the unique setting of a community where local citizens could mobilize to create the options and opportunities for children to be active. These community efforts to leverage the *VERB* brand demonstrated that the best of the world of commercial marketing can be combined with the core mission of public health to advance efforts to produce a nation of physically active children.

Disclaimer

The findings and conclusions in this paper are those of the authors and do not necessarily represent the views of the Centers for Disease Control and Prevention.

References

Aaker, D. A. (1991). *Managing brand equity: capitalizing on the value of a brand name*. New York: Free Press.

Aaker, D. (1996). *Building strong brands*. New York: Free Press.

Aaker, D. A. and Keller, K. L. (1990). Consumer evaluations of brand extensions. *Journal of Marketing* **54**:27–41.

Asbury, L.D., Wong, F.L., and Price, S.M., Nolin, M.J. (2008). The VERB™ campaign: applying a branding strategy in public health. *American Journal of Preventive Medicine*. **34**(65):S175–S182.

Bretthauer-Mueller, R., Berkowitz, J. M., Thomas, M., McCarthy, S., Green, L. A., Melancon H., *et al.* (2008). Catalyzing community action within a national media campaign: *VERB*(tm) community and national partnerships. *American Journal of Preventive Medicine*. **34**(65):S204–S215.

Business Week. (2004). The world's most valuable brands. *Business Week*, 2 August, 64–71.

Centers for Disease Control and Prevention (1996). Surgeon General's report on physical activity and health. *Journal of the American Medical Association* **276**:522.

Centers for Disease Control and Prevention (2000). Aeffect. Life's first great crossroad. Available at: http://www.cdc.gov/youthcampaign/research/PDF/4 4 02-LifesFirstCrossroadsRes.pdf (accessed 24 August 2007).

Centers for Disease Control and Prevention (2002). Formative Research Reports. Executive summaries for brand development. Available at: http://www.cdc.gov/YouthCampaign/research/resource (accessed 30 July 2007).

Centers for Disease Control and Prevention (2007). Continuous Tracking Survey. Available at: http://www.cdc.gov/youthcampaign/research/PDF/ContinuousTrackingSurvey.pdf (accessed 30 July, 2007).

Courtney, A. H. (2004). Using community-based prevention marketing to promote physical activity among tweens. *Social Marketing Quarterly* **10**:58–61.

Evans, W. D., Wasserman, J., Bertolotti, E., and Martino, S. C. (2002). Branding behavior: the strategy behind the *truth* campaign. *Social Marketing Quarterly* **7**:17–29.

Evans, W. D., Price, S., and Blahut, S. (2005). Evaluating the truth brand. *Journal of Health Communication* **10**:181–92.

Farrelly, M. C., Healton, C. G., Davis, K. C., Messeri, P., Hersey, J. C., and Haviland, M. L. (2002a). Getting to the truth: evaluating national tobacco countermarketing campaigns. *American Journal of Public Health* **92**:901–7.

Farrelly, M. C., Davis, K. C., Yarsevich, J. M., Havilad, M. L., Hersey, J. C., Girlando, M. E., *et al.* (2002b). *Getting to the truth: assessing youths' reaction to the truth and 'Think. Don't Smoke' tobacco countermarketing campaigns.* Legacy First Look Report 9. Washington, DC: American Legacy Foundation.

Fournier, S. 1995. *A consumer-brand relationship perspective on brand equity*. Report No.: 95–111. Cambridge, MA: Marketing Science Institute.

Grier, S. and Bryant, C. A. (2005). Social marketing in public health. *Annual Review of Public Health* **26**:319–39.

Harmatz, V. (2004). The importance of branding in the national youth anti-drug media campaign. *Social Marketing Quarterly* **10**:59–61.

Heitzler, C.D., Asbury, L.D., and Kusner, S. (2008). Bringing 'play' to life: experiential marketing in the *VERB*™ campaign. *American Journal of Preventive Medicine*. **34**(65):S188–S193.

Huhman, M., Potter, L. D., Wong, F. L., Banspach, S. W., Duke, J. C., and Heitzler, C. D. (2005). Effects of a mass media campaign to increase physical activity among children: year-1 results of the *VERB*™ campaign 2002–2004. *Pediatrics* **116**:e277–e284.

Huhman, M., Potter, L. D., Duke, J. C., Judkins, D. R., Heitzler, C. D., and Wong, F. L. (2007). Evaluation of a national physical activity intervention for children: *VERB* campaign 2002–2004. *American Journal of Preventive Medicine* **32**:38–43.

Keller, K. L. (2003). Brand synthesis: The multidimensionality of brand knowledge. *Journal of Consumer Research* **29**:595–600.

Keller, K. L and Sood, S. (1995). *Developing a brand equity measurement system: current practices and recommended approaches*. Report No. 95. Cambridge, MA: Marketing Science Institute.

Kepferer, J. N. (1997). *Strategic brand management: creating and sustaining brand equity long term.* London: Kogan Page.

Kepferer, J. N. (2004). *The new strategic brand management: Creating and sustaining brand equity long term.* London: Kogan Page.

Kotler, P. and Armstrong, G. (2006). *Principles of Marketing* (11th edn). Upper Saddle River, NJ: Pearson Prentice Hall.

Kotler, P. and Keller, K. L. (2005). *Marketing Management* (12th edn).

Kotler, P., Roberto, N., and Lee, N. (2002). *Social marketing: Improving the quality of life* (2nd edn). Thousand Oaks, CA: Sage.

McDivitt, J. (2003). Is there a role for branding in social marketing? *Social Marketing Quarterly* 9:11–7.

McKinnon, R. (2007). Lessons from *VERB*: A case for branding in nutrition education. *Journal of Nutrition Education and Behavior* 39(Suppl. 2):S53–S54.

Potter, L. D., Judkins, D.R., Piesse, P., Nolin, M.J., and Huhman, M. (2008). Methodology of the outcome evaluation of the *VERB*™ campaign. *American Journal of Preventive Medicine.* 34(65):S224–S234.

Roberts, D. F. and Foer, U.G., Rideout, V. (2005). *Generation M: Media in the lives of 8 to 18 year-olds.* Menlo Park, CA: Kaiser Family Foundation.

Smith, B. J., Bauman, A. E., Chen, T., Loveday, S., Costello, M., Mackie, B., *et al.* (2006). Hepatitis C in Australia: impact of a mass media campaign. *American Journal of Preventive Medicine* 31:492–8.

Strong, W. B., Malina, R. M., Blimkie, C. J., Daniels, S. R., Dishman, R. K., Gutin, B., *et al.* (2005). Evidence based physical activity for school-age youth. *Journal of Pediatrics* 146:732–7.

Thomas, G. M. (2004). Building the buzz in the hive mind. *Journal of Consumer Behavior* 4:64–72.

Vakratsas, D. and Ambler, T. (1999). How advertising works: What do we really know? *Journal of Marketing* 63:26–44.

Value based management.net. (2007). Brand Asset Valuator. Available at: http://www.valuebasedmanagement.net/methods_brand_asset_valuator.html (accessed on 16 July, 2007).

Wheeler, A. (2003). *Designing brand identity: a complete guide to creating, building, and maintaining strong brands.* Hoboken, NJ: John Wiley.

Williams, C. L., Hayman, L. L., Daniels, S. R., Robinson, T.N., Steinberger, J., Paridon, S., *et al.* (2002). Cardiovascular health in childhood: a statement for health professionals from the Committee on Atherosclerosis, Hypertension, and Obesity in the Young (AHOY) of the Council on Cardiovascular Disease in the Young. American Heart Association. *Circulation* 106:143–60.

Wong, F., Huhman, M., Heitzler, C., Asbury, L., Bretthauer-Mueller, R., McCarthy, S., *et al.* (2004). *VERB* – a social marketing campaign to increase physical activity among youth. *Preventing Chronic Disease* 1(3).

Worden, J. K. and Slater, M. D. (2004). Theory and practice in the national youth anti-drug media campaign. *Social Marketing Quarterly* 10:13–27.

Zhang, S. and, Sood, S. (2002). 'Deep' and 'surface' cues: Brand extension evaluations by children and adults. *Journal of Consumer Research* 29:129–41.

7

Case studies of youth tobacco prevention campaigns from the USA
Truth and half-truths

Matthew C. Farrelly and Kevin C. Davis

Summary

- For decades, cigarette companies have successfully harnessed the power of branding to transform a simple product into a powerful tool that projects a complex set of images and personality traits to its user.
- Beginning with California's large-scale anti-smoking campaign in 1990 – the first in 20 years – tobacco control efforts began to counter and deconstruct cigarette brand imagery.
- In 1998, the Florida *truth* campaign extended earlier efforts by California and Massachusetts to counter tobacco brands by developing a tobacco control brand aimed at youth and intended to take market share away from cigarette brands.
- The Florida and national *truth* campaign (launched in 2000) developed counter brands that served as an outlet for teen expression and rebellion with messages that countered tobacco brands and challenged manipulative tobacco company marketing.
- Evidence shows that tobacco countermarketing campaigns are effective in reducing youth and adult smoking. In addition, an emerging literature suggests that the brand equity of youth tobacco counter brands adds value to the campaigns.
- However, branding in tobacco countermarketing campaigns remains uncommon.

Introduction

Efforts to reduce tobacco use worldwide have gained significant momentum in the past two decades. Although the US Surgeon General Report on smoking in 1964 concluded that smoking caused lung cancer, it was not until the early 1990s that the US government began to provide meaningful funding to states to implement programs to reduce tobacco use. It was not until the late 1990s that substantial funds were available to combat tobacco use as a result of settlements with the tobacco industry. Florida, Minnesota, Mississippi and Texas negotiated separate multi-billion dollar settlements with the tobacco industry, while in November 1998, the remaining 46 states collectively negotiated the Master Settlement Agreement (MSA) for $206 billion dollars to be paid over 25 years. Although there was no firm commitment in these settlements to dedicate funds to tobacco control efforts, many states did use these funds to mount large, comprehensive tobacco control programs, including large anti-smoking campaigns. The MSA also restricted tobacco companies from advertising on outdoor billboards and efforts to market tobacco to youth.

On the worldwide stage, the idea for an international framework convention on tobacco control was conceived in the mid-1990s and was later adopted in 2003 by the World Health Assembly. Some of the major elements of this convention include increasing the price of tobacco products, prohibiting sales to minors, passing laws that prohibit smoking in public places to reduce exposure to secondhand smoke, banning all tobacco advertising, and engaging in public education.

In this chapter we review the history of US anti-smoking campaigns, including the emergence of counterindustry campaigns that preceded branded tobacco countermarketing campaigns. We then describe recent countermarketing campaigns, their use of branding, their effectiveness, and the contributions of branding. As part of this discussion, we will also describe and review the evidence for industry-sponsored youth 'prevention' campaigns. We conclude with a summary of the evidence and implications for the future. Before we discuss anti-smoking campaigns, we describe how Philip Morris developed the Marlboro brand to illustrate the techniques of branding and the images that later countermarketing campaigns attacked. Philip Morris developed the Marlboro brand to build a relationship with smokers, to add value to a product that inherently has little value, and to implicitly counter emerging government warnings about the health effects of smoking.

For nearly all American adults as well as millions of others worldwide, the Marlboro Man conjures up the masculine image of a rugged cowboy, riding a horse in the western USA. The advertisements said little and relied on images of real cowboys at work in wide open country to evoke freedom and simplicity at a time when society was becoming increasingly complex. In fact, their simple slogan, 'Come to where the flavor is … Come to Marlboro Country' was so successful, it survives to this day (Kluger 1997). The imagery of the campaign beckoned '… Americans to an earlier, simpler, morally unambiguous time, to the frontier irretrievably lost to the encroachment of thronged modernity' (Kluger 1997: 296). Indeed, the Marlboro brand is one example of how tobacco companies harnessed the power branding to sell a product. After all, cigarettes are little more than a commodity and yet, many smokers are very loyal to their brands because of the image their brand communicates to others.

The image of the cowboy may have been the nearly perfect foil against the mounting evidence of the dangers of smoking. In the 1950s, epidemiologists conducted the first large-scale case-control and prospective studies examining the link between smoking and lung cancer. These studies demonstrated that smoking caused cancer and became the central studies in the first US Surgeon General Report on smoking in 1964. This report was a major milestone in government efforts to highlight the dangers of smoking and discourage smoking. The report concluded that:

> [the] risk of developing lung cancer increases with duration of smoking and the number of cigarettes smoked per day, and is diminished by discontinuing smoking. In comparison with non-smokers, average male smokers of cigarettes have approximately a 9- to 10-fold risk of developing lung cancer and heavy smokers at least a 20-fold risk.
>
> (US Public Health Service 1964)

In 1965, the Federal Cigarette Labeling Act was passed, requiring labels on cigarette packs that stated 'Caution: Cigarette Smoking May Be Hazardous to Your Health' (e.g. see CDC 2007).

Although cigarette sales decreased following the 1964 Surgeon General Report, Marlboro fared better than its competitors and steadily gained market share in the decades to come (Kluger 1997). In 1967, the Federal Communications Commission ruled that the Fairness Doctrine, which required broadcasters allow for contrasting viewpoints on controversial issues, called for a balance between cigarette and anti-smoking advertisements on television and radio. As a result, the first national anti-smoking campaign in the USA ensued in July 1967 and continued until 31 December 1970, when cigarette television advertisements were banned by Congress (Farrelly *et al.* 2003). Because there were no longer cigarette advertisements on television, the anti-smoking commercials also went off the air. The last Marlboro commercial aired right before midnight before the deadline and Philip Morris' advertising director Jack Landry 'watched four of his beloved cowboys gallop off into the sunset for the last time, and wept' (Kluger 1997: 335). However, Marlboro billboard advertisements continued until 24 April 1999, when they were banned by the MSA, along with all other outdoor cigarette advertisements. Marlboro continued print ads until 2006 when Philip Morris' voluntarily ceased print advertising (Johnson 2007); a final ad showed a cowboy riding a horse into the sunset.

Although government-sponsored anti-smoking efforts in the USA began with this first Surgeon General Report and the Fairness Doctrine period of anti-smoking advertisements, it would take over 25 years before anti-smoking efforts began to try to knock the Marlboro Man off his horse with campaigns that directly challenged tobacco industry images and marketing. Throughout the years, anti-smoking campaigns have used a variety of approaches, including more recent campaigns that directly counter the tobacco industry and others that brand their campaigns. Systematic reviews of the evidence show that anti-smoking campaigns are effective in reducing youth smoking and promoting cessation (Siegel 1998; Hopkins *et al.* 2001; Farrelly *et al.* 2003, forthcoming; Wakefield *et al.* 2003). What is not clear is whether or not developing branded anti-smoking campaigns makes a contribution above and beyond the content of the campaign.

A brief history of anti-smoking campaigns and the development of countermarketing campaigns

Anti-smoking campaigns in the USA have evolved over time, beginning with messages in the late 1960s that highlighted the health effects of smoking, but made little mention of the cigarette makers that aggressively promoted their products. This was a sensible start as very few Americans recognized the long-term health consequences of smoking. In the 1980s and early 1990s, campaigns began to counter the images of smoking and cigarette advertising by attempting to recast the social imagery of smoking, painting it as a nasty habit. Then, in the mid to late 1990s, campaigns began to challenge the tobacco industry more aggressively with the help of previously secret industry documents, pointing out their deceptive marketing and their efforts to conceal the truth about the health consequences of smoking. Then, nearly 30 years after tobacco companies used branding to position their product, countermarketing campaigns began to add branding techniques to their arsenal.

The first anti-smoking advertisements in the USA began during the Fairness Doctrine, were valued at $75 million of free air time, and featured messages that focused on the long-term health consequences of smoking. The advertising effort, spearheaded by the American Cancer Society, included advertisements with statements such as 'Have you ever wondered what happens when you smoke a cigarette? [pause] We have ... American Cancer Society' (Kluger 1997: 111). These advertisements have been credited for reducing per capita cigarette consumption (Warner 1977, 1979; Schneider *et al.* 1981) and youth smoking (Lewit *et al.* 1981). From 1970 to 2000, there were no large-scale national anti-smoking campaigns on television (Siegel 1998).

During the interim, states began to mount their own campaigns. These began in Minnesota from 1986 to 1991, followed by campaigns in California (1990), Massachusetts (1994), Arizona (1996), Oregon (1997) and Florida (1998). Following successful lawsuits against major tobacco companies in Florida, Minnesota, Mississippi and Texas, further campaigns followed the landmark MSA in November 1998.

As anti-smoking campaigns became more numerous, the message strategies have become more varied. Campaigns aimed at preventing youth from smoking stressed short-term consequences of smoking such as bad breath, stained teeth, wrinkles, shortness of breath, and inability to perform well in sports (Farrelly *et al.* 2003). The Arizona youth smoking prevention campaign was tagged 'Tobacco, the tumor-causing, teeth staining, smelly, puking habit', while Texas' pilot campaign that began in 2000 was tagged 'Tobacco is Foul'. Other campaigns aimed at youth have focused on social norms and have attempted to correct youth's misperceptions that smoking is common (Farrelly *et al.* 2003).

In April 1990, California took a bold new approach to anti-smoking campaigns, attacking the tobacco industry head on and drawing attention to its manipulative marketing. The campaign's opening salvo stated in a full-page print ad, 'This is going to be a media campaign about a media campaign – as much about hype as hygiene. It's going to talk about a shared community opportunity and a shared community menace' (Balbach and Glantz 1998: 398). The campaign's first television commercial, 'Industry Spokesman', portrayed tobacco industry executives joking about recruiting new smokers (Balbach and Glantz 1998). This campaign defined the struggle as a head-to-head battle for market share and they aimed at countering tobacco industry influences by deglamorizing tobacco, deconstructing cigarette brands, and revealing the industry's deceptive

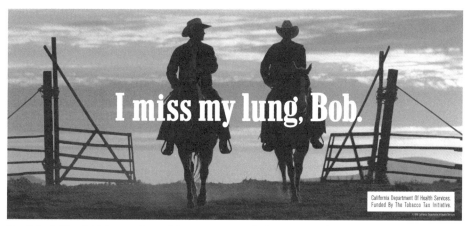

Fig. 7.1 California Tobacco Control Program counterindustry campaign 'I miss my lung, Bob' billboard advertisement. Reproduced with permission from the California Department of Public Health.

marketing tactics. California's counterindustry advertisements included direct attacks on the imagery of the Marlboro Man (Figs. 7.1 and 7.2). However, the California campaign struggled to maintain its initial strong edge due to political pressures (Balbach and Glantz 1998). In fact, Glantz (1997) presents data suggesting that the declines in cigarette sales that followed the onset of the campaign were slowed when the campaign was temporarily suspended and later when the counterindustry messages were weakened. Despite these challenges, a number of studies have documented the success of the California Tobacco Control Program and its media campaign (Hu *et al.* 1995; Pierce *et al.* 1998; DHHS 2000; Farrelly *et al.* 2003).

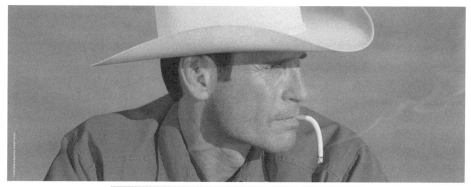

Fig. 7.2 California Tobacco Control Program counterindustry campaign 'smoking causes impotence' billboard advertisement. Reproduced with permission from the California Department of Public Health.

Although California was well into its counterindustry campaign by 1994, an event that year would have a profound effect on tobacco control and anti-smoking campaign strategies. In May of 1994, Professor Stan Glantz received a box of tobacco company internal documents that summarized the results of industry research and public relation strategies. These documents, sent with a return address of 'Mr. Butts' were also shared with members of the press (Glantz *et al.* 1996). In contrast to their public statements, these documents disclosed the tobacco companies' knowledge of the addictive and damaging nature of tobacco. Glantz quotes industry memos with statements such as, 'We are … in the business of selling nicotine, an addictive drug …' (Brown & Williamson 1963, in Glantz *et al.* 1996: 15), and 'In most cases, the smoker of a filter cigarette was getting as much or more nicotine and tar as he would have gotten from a regular cigarette' (Brown & Williamson 1976, in Glantz *et al.* 1996: 16).

Glantz *et al.* also report a Brown & Williamson advertisement for Vantage cigarettes printed in *Time* magazine. The advert, printed in 1977, implied that smoking low-tar cigarettes was less harmful for one's health: 'I hear the things being said against high-tar smoking as well as the next guy. And so I started looking. For a low-tar smoke that had honest-to-goodness taste' (Glantz *et al.* 1996: 16).

These and similar documents that later became available through lawsuits with major tobacco companies provided ample fodder for state and national campaigns that would increasingly focus on tobacco companies' manipulative marketing strategies and denials of the true health effects of tobacco.

Following California, Massachusetts was the second state to mount a large-scale tobacco control program with an aggressive mass media campaign. The Massachusetts campaign launched in October 1993 and initially focused on youth prevention messages that high-lighted the short-term health effects of smoking (e.g. wrinkles) and deglamorized tobacco use. The campaign then took a more aggressive approach by using personal testimonials to highlight the ravages of smoking and manipulative industry tactics. One series, all tagged 'The Truth', involved graphic, emotionally charged advertisements. In the first advertise-ment, images of Wayne MacLaren, the former Marlboro Man, are juxtaposed with images of him dying of lung cancer in a hospital room. The advertisement is narrated by MacLaren's brother, who describes how he used to love cigarette ads with a rugged, inde-pendent cowboy. He goes on to say that the industry used his brother in ads 'to create an image that smoking makes you independent. Don't believe it' (Earle 2000: 235).

Another set of Massachusetts ads chronicles the life of Pam Laffin who developed emphysema and had a lung removed at age 26 and died at 31, leaving behind two young girls. The advertisements show graphic images of her in a wheelchair, breathing through a respirator, her face bloated from the medicine she must take. Subsequent advertise-ments take the industry to task for advertising the good things it has done for the victims of abuse, while doing nothing to help 'the victims of tobacco' or the children of parents like Pam Laffin who died from tobacco-related diseases. Other advertisements feature celebrities with lung cancer, including a former radio personality who sings happy birth-day to the tobacco industry through an electronic voice box. Biener *et al.* (2000) found that the Massachusetts advertisements that elicited strong emotions (e.g. sadness and fear) were rated more effective than humorous or entertaining advertisements by smokers that quit, nonsmokers and smokers who planed to quit soon.

Arizona's anti-smoking campaign began in 1996 and focused on youth prevention. Rather than focus on the tobacco industry, this campaign deglamorized tobacco use, using messages with the tagline 'tobacco: a tumor-causing, teeth-staining, smelly, puking habit'. Oregon's public education campaign that began in 1997 highlighted the dangers of tobacco use and exposure to secondhand smoke, drawing on advertisements developed by other states (e.g. California and Massachusetts).

The next state to take on a counterindustry approach was Florida's well-known *truth* campaign that began in 1998 and was followed by the national *truth* campaign in 2000. The Florida campaign marked the beginning of branded anti-smoking campaigns, which we discuss below.

Branded tobacco countermarketing campaigns

Prior to the launch of Florida's *truth* campaign, anti-smoking messages aimed at youth focused on deglamorizing tobacco use and highlighting the health effects of tobacco. For example, Arizona's campaign focused on tobacco as a disgusting habit while that of Massachusetts highlighted short-term effects such as wrinkles, yellow teeth, bad breath, and poor performance in sports, along with graphic images of longer-term health effects. These approaches were attempting to recast the social image of smoking as unattractive, as positive social images of smoking increase the likelihood that people will experiment with smoking (Burton *et al.* 1989). The previous campaigns also confronted the tobacco industry, but stopped short of using a branded campaign as a tool to weave together these various efforts to deglamorize tobacco and confront the tobacco industry. Then came *truth* – the first branded countermarketing campaign. This campaign, which began in Florida, developed a logo that was on all of its advertisements. It was more than a tagline, it was a brand like other commercial brands and was intended to be the mechanism by which the campaign would develop an identity and develop a relationship with its target audience of teens.

As we noted when discussing Marlboro and the Marlboro Man, a brand and its associated images is a powerful tool to communicate one's identity to others quickly. A man who smokes Marlboro wants others to think that he too is rugged and independent and cannot be bothered by what the government has to say about the dangers of smoking. With decades of ubiquitous and powerful tobacco advertising and attractive portrayals of smoking in the movies, youth understand that the act of smoking sends a powerful message – a message of rebellion. Successful youth prevention requires campaign planners to grapple with these powerful social images and to harness teen rebellion against tobacco use and the tobacco industry. That was what the Florida *truth* campaign aimed to do.

The Florida *truth* campaign

Thanks to an $11.3 billion settlement between the State of Florida and major tobacco companies in 1997, the Florida Tobacco Pilot Program was established in 1997 with

$23.2 million to plan the program in the first fiscal year (1 July 1997 to 30 June 1998). It received $70 million in FY 1999, $39.1 million in FY 2000 and 2001, and $29.8 million in FY 2002. Although the average funding over this period was less than funding for the California and Massachusetts programs, the fact that all of the Florida funds were aimed at youth prevention meant that Florida would spend more money per youth than any other campaign, past or present. This unprecedented level of funding enabled Florida to mount a large-scale, professionally developed anti-smoking campaign targeted to youth aged 12–17 in the context of a comprehensive tobacco control program aimed at youth smoking prevention.

The campaign was developed by an agency that had never developed a social marketing campaign. According to the agency's president, their clients included 'a bicycle company, a basketball shoe company, and a fast-food restaurant, among others' (Hicks 2001). They modeled their approach after other successful youth brands such as Nintendo, Mountain Dew and Skechers. Their goal was to understand their target audience by getting into the heads of youth. Hicks (2001) describes how the agency's qualitative research indicated that youth disliked anti-tobacco efforts that passed judgment on smokers and did not want to be told what to do. From this research they came to a number of conclusions:

◆ youth had a complete understanding of the health effects of smoking;

◆ tobacco was a way for youth to signal that they were in control;

◆ tobacco was a tool of rebellion – precisely because it is deadly.

Their research also suggested that previous efforts with directive (possibly preachy) messages may have had the potential to backfire with some youth by making smoking an even more powerful tool for rebellion. The agency focused on this latter notion, aiming to create a brand that provided an alternative outlet for this rebellion. They wanted to show rebellious youth confronting the tobacco industry and exposing the industry's deceptive marketing practices and efforts to recruit youth to supply future generations of smokers. The agency accomplished this with ample funding, an understanding of their audience, and campaign messages that featured humor, rebellion, satire and stark facts about the death toll of tobacco. They sought to avoid messages that came across as preachy. Instead, they created an attractive brand that would draw youth in and deliver the facts about the industry and tobacco use, letting the youth make their own decisions about tobacco use.

In the first few years of the campaign, many of the advertisements involved questioning tobacco company statements. For example, the 'No More Addictive' series questioned tobacco company statements suggesting that cigarettes were no more addictive than carrots, gummy bears or television. In one ad from this series, a man is shown putting on what look like nicotine patches as he tries to resist the temptation to eat gummy bears. Another series called 'Awards' involved teens visiting tobacco companies to deliver awards such as the 'Fish Hook' for successfully luring kids to smoke and the 'Golden Sloth' award for taking 50 years to figure out that smoking causes lung cancer. The most aggressive advertisement, 'Demon Awards', shows a spoof award show where tobacco wins the 'Most Deaths in a Single Year' award for killing more people in a year than suicide, illicit drugs and murder combined. The 'Cinema' series produced what looked like movie trailers for action-packed films. One such trailer shows a suburban father who puts corporate profits above the health and safety of his family, his daughter and her friends. He sees his daughter's friends as a source for future smokers. He supports the tobacco industry's practice of targeting youth with marketing and advertising strategies.

One final commercial that illustrates the Florida *truth* campaign's humorous and irreverent side is a musical entitled 'Focus on the Positive'. It stars dancing and singing tobacco executives, and opens with teens questioning tobacco executives about tobacco products. The executives then burst into song, urging the teens to focus on the positive:

> So why destroy the research?
>
> You think that they're afraid?
>
> Naw, we're just getting ready for a tickertape parade!
>
> …
>
> Let's try to focus on the positive.
>
> Sure they may kill 4 million folks a year.
>
> But let's stay focused on the positive-
>
> There's plenty of us still here.
>
> So what if we remove a lung
>
> You shouldn't be depressed.
>
> It's really for the best.
>
> It's something off your chest.
>
> And yes we know that tobacco causes cancer of the bladder! It doesn't really matter – they make diapers for adults!

Overall, the campaign set out to position *truth* as an attractive brand that was humorous, rebellious, skeptical, and not preachy. By showing youth sticking it to the (tobacco executive) man, they were trying to paint tobacco-free youth as cool and confrontational.

The national *truth* campaign

Building on the Florida *truth* experience, the American Legacy Foundation developed the national *truth* campaign with several agencies, including the one that developed the Florida *truth* campaign. Like the Florida campaign, the national campaign began with a series of morbidly humorous advertisements entitled 'Kills 1/3' to draw attention to the fact that one-third of youth that try smoking eventually die of tobacco-related diseases. One of these, called 'Splode', shows three edgy-looking teens bungee jumping off a bridge and grabbing a can of soda when they reach the bottom of their jump. As the third teen bounces back up, the camera pans out to show a big explosion. The following statement then appears on the screen: 'Only one product kills one-third of the people who use it. Tobacco'. Possibly the most controversial series of *truth* ads, known as 'Body Bags', was released early in the first year of the campaign. The first in the series showed teens unloading 1200 body bags outside a major tobacco company in New York City. The teens use a bull horn to call out to tobacco company employees in the offices above, asking them if they know how many people die every day from tobacco-related diseases. The teens then leave the body bags on the sidewalk so they can see what 1200 people looks like. The commercial ends with a chilling aerial view of 1200 body bags. Other television advertisements continued this theme, such as the advertisement that shows teens building a memorial in Washington, DC with 1200 body bags. The campaign also used print advertisements such as the one in Fig. 7.3 that leaves readers with the question, 'What if cigarette ads told the truth?'

These advertisements represented an evolution of the campaign, combining stark facts about the death toll of tobacco, with confrontation of the industry and graphic images. These advertisements caught the ire of tobacco companies that claimed that the advertisements went too far and violated the terms of the MSA not to 'vilify' tobacco companies (NPR 2000).

Like the Florida *truth* campaign, the national *truth* campaign describes itself as 'an outlet [for teens] to express themselves; *truth*® provides an alternative … As a brand, *truth*® directly counters messages from the tobacco company brands …' (American Legacy Foundation 2007). The campaign aims to use 'challenging, thought-provoking ad contexts and images of teens in control, rebelling against [the tobacco industry]' (Evans *et al.* 2002: 19). In the over seven years that the campaign has been on the air,

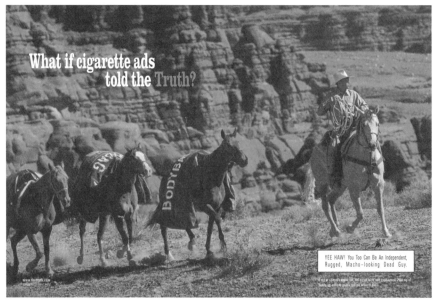

Fig. 7.3 American Legacy Foundation truth® campaign. Reproduced with permission from the American Legacy Foundation.

it has used a similar style and approach, while varying the specific messages. As the campaign has evolved, it has made frequent use of industry documents and memos to expose manipulative marketing practices and denials of the true health effects of tobacco. For example, in the 'Orange Curtain' series from 2002 and 2003, one advertisement featured a homeless man pulling back an orange curtain to show an industry memo describing project 'SCUM' or 'sub culture urban marketing', an effort to market cigarettes to street people and other 'subcultures'. Other campaigns such as 'Crazyworld' and 'Connect truth®' remarked that the tobacco industry plays by a different set of rules than other companies that recall products that are harmful. These advertisements also highlight the manipulation of tobacco products, such as the addition of ammonia to increase the delivery of nicotine in cigarettes. Throughout its history, the campaign worked to keep the information relevant and salient to youth audiences and to balance serious facts and information with an irreverent style that would connect to youth. This was also accomplished by placing the advertisements on popular teen television programs, websites and concert tours. The goal was to position the brand like other popular teen brands.

Summary of the potential benefits of branding for youth smoking prevention

Existing branded tobacco countermarketing campaigns share a number of common elements. First, by focusing on a brand rather than sponsors (e.g. government, foundation, adults), the campaigns avoid overtly representing authority figures. This also makes teen spokespeople more prominent and more credible. In essence, a brand begins as an empty vessel; it appears independent of its sponsors, and campaign planners can build it from the ground up. The brand can then attract teens and in the process, serve as an outlet for campaign messages without coming across as a 'preachy' authority figure. Goldman and Glantz succinctly summarize the benefits of the counterindustry approach that is integral to the *truth* campaigns:

> By making youth aware of the industry's calculated attempts to manipulate them, these advertisements tell young people that they are not acting independently. They also transform a low-interest topic, smoking, into an attention-getting, emotional issue, and reconfigure the parent–rebellious child dynamic by giving both youth and adults a common enemy – the tobacco industry.
>
> (Goldman and Glantz 1998: 774)

The branded campaigns above also made efforts to get to know their target audiences with qualitative research. This understanding enabled them to create campaigns that would address youth needs and aspirations for social acceptance, independence and rebellion. Below we present evidence on the effectiveness of these campaigns and the contribution, if any, from the brands.

Tobacco industry-sponsored 'prevention' campaigns

In 1999, Philip Morris launched its own campaign entitled 'Think. Don't Smoke'. In stark contrast to the risk-taking edgy-looking teens from the *truth* advertisements, the Philip Morris advertisements featured clean-cut teens. With titles such as 'Choice' and 'My Reasons', the Philip Morris advertisements are focused on messages highlighting personal choice. In 'Choice', an African-American teen on a bus is asked if he has ever tried cigarettes. He responds, 'Nope', providing the rationale that 'I don't know, I just never wanted to, you know what I mean'. The advertisements never discuss the deadly and addictive nature of tobacco, they are preachy, and they direct teens not to smoke with their 'Think. Don't Smoke' message. As Earle notes, this campaign is reminiscent of a scene in the book *Thank You for Smoking* where the creative director for the industry campaign says how he wants 'to speak to them with the voice of despised authority ... You know what I love about it? Its dullness ... kids are going to look at this and go "Puuke"' (Earle 2000: 215).

Not to be outdone by Philip Morris, the Lorilllard tobacco company created its own campaign entitled 'Tobacco is Whacko, if You're a Teen' (Fig. 7.4) – in other words, it is fine if you are an adult or want to act grown up. This campaign also uses a strategy that directly contradicts the strategy used by the Florida and national *truth* campaigns by sending directive 'don't smoke' messages to teens. However, in contrast to the 'Think. Don't Smoke' advertisements, the Lorillard advertisements featured risk-taking teens and stronger prevention messages. For example, in one advertisement a teen enters a dark tattoo and piercing parlor to get his tongue pierced. After a graphic shot of the procedure itself, the elderly, yellow-toothed piercer asks the teen if he wants to smoke a cigarette

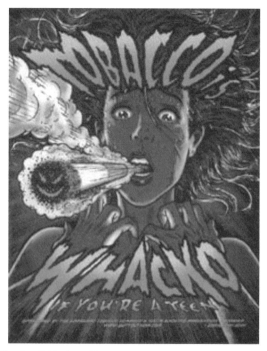

Fig. 7.4 Tobacco is Whacko, if You're a Teen.

with him. The teen responds, 'What do you think? I'm crazy?' In other words, he is crazy enough to suffer a tongue piercing but not to subject his body to smoking. Although this campaign was also silent on the role of tobacco in marketing tobacco, the content of the messages attempted to appeal to risk-taking teens. Compared with Philip Morris, Lorillard spent significantly less on their campaign and as a result, awareness of the campaign was quite low (Farrelly *et al.* 2002).

A number of studies have shown that the types of advertisements featured in Philip Morris' campaign do not resonate with teens and are associated with more favorable attitudes toward the industry and an increased likelihood of smoking in the future – possibly what the industry intended if the satirical *Thank You for Smoking* was a close approximation of reality. Although it is debatable whether or not Philip Morris deliberately created a bad campaign, the fact that the same company produces Marlboro, the most popular cigarette among teens and adults, suggests that they have the sophistication to create an effective youth prevention campaign.

In a study of the influence of the national *truth* campaign on beliefs and attitudes towards tobacco and the tobacco industry after the first ten months of the campaign, Farrelly *et al.* (2002) found that recall of the Philip Morris 'Think. Don't Smoke' (TDS) advertisements was associated with greater intentions to smoke and more favorable attitudes toward the tobacco industry. This study was later extended to include three years of data and found similar results (Farrelly *et al.*, forthcoming). The TDS campaign has also been found to be ineffective in changing youths' perceptions of smoking prevalence among their peers. A study by Davis *et al.* (2007) analyzed the relationship between confirmed recall of TDS and perceived smoking prevalence among youth and found no evidence of an association. A published report using similar data also found that youths who saw the TDS ads had significantly less favorable reactions to TDS compared with youths' reactions to the *truth* campaign (American Legacy Foundation 2002). This latter study is consistent with a qualitative study of various youth prevention messages that indicated that youth disliked the TDS advertisements (Goldman and Glantz 1998).

These findings are consistent with a recent controlled experiment showing that tobacco industry-sponsored anti-smoking ads provoked more favorable attitudes toward tobacco (Henriksen *et al.* 2006). In addition, a school-based study of US youth found that exposure to tobacco company youth smoking prevention advertising had no effect on youth smoking outcomes, whereas exposure to the Philip Morris 'Talk. They'll Listen' parent-focused youth smoking prevention campaign was associated with lower perceived harm of smoking, stronger approval of smoking, and stronger intentions to smoke (Wakefield *et al.* 2006).

Evaluating the effectiveness of tobacco countermarketing brands

The Taskforce on Community Preventive Services has concluded that a mass media campaign, combined with other interventions, is effective in preventing youth smoking initiation and promoting cessation (Hopkins *et al.* 2001). However, since the time of that review, a number of additional studies have found that tobacco countermarketing campaigns aimed at youth are effective. For example, a number of studies have shown that the Florida *truth* campaign was effective in changing youth's attitudes and in reducing youth smoking (Sly *et al.* 2001, 2002; Niederdeppe *et al.* 2004). Both Sly *et al.* (2001) and Niederdeppe *et al.* (2004) found that tobacco-related beliefs and attitudes and smoking behavior were significantly different in Florida versus the remaining USA after *truth* campaign. In addition, although the Florida Tobacco Control Program included components other than the media campaign, these activities did not begin until the second year of the campaign, after *truth* had shown an impact (Farrelly *et al.* 2003). Sly *et al.* (2002) examined the impact of *truth* on smoking initiation with two measures of initiation: (1) whether the youth smoked at all in the past 30 days at follow-up and (2) whether the youth was an 'established' smoker at follow-up, defined as smoking on six or more days in the past month and more than five cigarettes per day. They measured campaign exposure with a complex index that combined three different measures: (1) recall of up to two campaign advertisements, (2) cognitive reactions to these advertisements, and (3) agreement with a campaign-related belief – 'You feel tobacco companies are just trying to use you'. The index equaled 0 if the youth could not confirm awareness of any advertisements; it equaled 2 if the respondent confirmed awareness of two advertisements and said that both advertisements made them 'stop and think about whether or not they should smoke' and if they responded 'some' or 'a lot' in response to the belief described above; for all other respondents it equaled 1. These values were determined based on the follow-up survey measures. These analyses indicate that those who scored higher on the exposure index were less likely to become smokers and established smokers. These results are consistent with a longitudinal study of the earlier Massachusetts campaign that showed that exposure to that campaign was associated with decreased initiation (Siegel and Biener 2000).

Whether or not the *truth* brand itself contributed something above and beyond the messages themselves is difficult to conclude from the available evidence. Awareness of the brand logo was, however, quite high in the early years of the campaign. After a year of the campaign, two-thirds of youth could recognize the *truth* logo and nearly 90 per cent recalled at least one campaign advertisement (Sly *et al.* 2001).

There is also a growing evidence base that the national *truth* campaign is effective. Ten months after the campaign launched, approximately three-quarters of youth in the USA could recall at least one of the campaign's advertisements. In addition, recall of these advertisements was associated with changes in campaign-targeted beliefs and attitudes early in the campaign's history (Farrelly *et al.* 2002; Hersey *et al.* 2003; Evans *et al.* 2004; Thrasher *et al.* 2004). More recent studies have confirmed these results three years into the campaign (Farrelly *et al.*, forthcoming) and show that recall of *truth* is associated with lower perceptions of the prevalence of smoking among youth (Davis *et al.* 2007). Another study that used differences in market-level delivery of the national *truth* campaign found that two years into the campaign that *truth* was associated with lower smoking rates among youth (Farrelly *et al.* 2005). They found that the greater the number of advertisements that aired in a given market, the less likely youth were to smoke.

This analysis accounted for a number of demographic factors and state-level cigarette prices and funding for tobacco control programs.

Despite this considerable evidence base for tobacco countermarketing campaigns in general and the *truth* campaign specifically, there are very few studies that specifically examine the contributions of brands. Evans and colleagues proposed a series of constructs to capture the value or 'brand equity' of the national *truth* campaign (Evans *et al.* 2002). In the case of *truth*, higher brand equity would indicate a greater interest or likelihood of adopting a smoke-free lifestyle (Evans *et al.* 2002). What is unique in the case of a countermarketing campaign is that there is no product to evaluate, but rather the adoption of a set of beliefs, attitudes and behaviors. Evans *et al.* (2002) adapted Aaker's brand equity model to the *truth* campaign. The constructs include concepts such as brand awareness, loyalty, perceived quality, popularity and personality. These questions were asked of youth in a nationally representative survey of 12–17-year-olds in June of 2001, roughly a year and a half into the campaign. The authors found that more than three-quarters of youth agree (or strongly agreed) with each of the constructs with the exception of brand personality (68 per cent agreement). The highest agreement was for brand awareness at 90 per cent.

The measures were used to create a brand equity scale (Blahut *et al.* 2004), which was subsequently used in another study that tested whether or not brand equity mediated the relationship between *truth* campaign exposure and smoking behavior (Evans *et al.* 2005). In this latter study, the authors found that higher campaign exposure is associated with higher brand equity and that while simple exposure is associated with reduced smoking uptake, brand equity is associated with reductions in smoking uptake beyond campaign exposure alone (Evans *et al.* 2005). Although this analysis relies on cross-sectional data, it suggests that a brand can have a unique contribution. However, this latter finding would need to be confirmed in a longitudinal study that can better isolate the causal mechanisms.

To address this limitation, Evans *et al.* (2007) examined whether brand equity for Ohio's *Stand* campaign was associated with decreased smoking initiation in a prospective study of youth. A baseline telephone survey of 1657 11–17-year-olds was conducted in the summer of 2003. Longitudinal follow-up surveys of all of the baseline participants who agreed to be recontacted were conducted in the spring of 2004 and 2005. The analysis was restricted to youths who were nonsmokers at baseline, but were either open to smoking or had tried smoking in the past. To augment the sample, a random sample of youths who were closed to smoking at baseline was also included. The first follow-up survey sample size was 1010 youths; 673 completed the second follow-up survey. Of the initial eligible sample, 75 per cent participated in the first follow-up survey and 67 per cent participated in the second follow-up. Non-respondents were more likely than respondents to be white and older. The brand equity scale was constructed in a manner that was similar to the scale developed in Evans *et al.* (2002), with modifications to reflect the specifics of the *Stand* brand.

The results show that overall brand equity was associated with decreased smoking initiation. The authors also found that the brand equity subscales of brand loyalty, popularity and awareness were also all significant in both the first and second follow-up surveys. The brand personality was significant only in the first follow-up survey. Although it is possible that attrition influenced their results, these findings suggest that brand equity served as a protective factor against smoking. What was not clear in this study is the contribution of branding above simple awareness. However, the combined results of Evans *et al.* (2007) and Evans *et al.* (2005) suggest that branding may have contributed to decreased initiation above and beyond simple exposure.

Discussion and conclusion

During the 20th Century, tobacco companies have convinced millions of Americans to smoke a product that most at least intuitively knew would harm their health. By the 1950s, careful epidemiological studies clearly linked smoking to cancer. Later, the 1964 Surgeon General Report on smoking reinforced this message. Tobacco companies responded forcefully with clever advertising to address growing concerns among smokers. The Marlboro brand and the Marlboro Man is an example of how branding was success- fully used as a foil against the mounting evidence of the dangers of smoking. Marlboro used images of a rugged cowboy and wide open country to evoke freedom and simplicity. Although the Surgeon General Report and national anti-smoking advertisements from 1967 to 1970 did drive down smoking rates and sales, there were no large-scale anti- smoking campaigns until the 1990s to counter cigarette advertising.

Beginning with California's campaign in the 1990s, anti-smoking campaigns began to directly counter cigarette advertising and tobacco company marketing. California defined its campaign as a head-to-head battle for market share. Their advertising aimed to deglamorize tobacco, deconstruct cigarette brands and reveal the industry's deceptive marketing tactics. For example, California had billboards with cowboys suffering from tobacco-related diseases. In the mid-1990s, internal industry documents were found that contradicted public statements by tobacco companies denying the addictive nature of tobacco and health effects of smoking. These documents provided considerable fodder for counterindustry campaigns and ultimately led to the 1998 Master Settlement Agreement and other settlements in the late 1990s between states and major tobacco companies. State campaigns became increasingly aggressive with graphic images of the ravages of smoking, emotional testimonies from those suffering from tobacco-related diseases, and challenges to the tobacco industry.

Building on these initial campaigns, the State of Florida and the American Legacy Foundation developed tobacco countermarketing campaigns aimed at youth prevention, using branding as a central element. Rather than delivering directive, preachy messages about the health effects of tobacco, these campaigns featured empowered, edgy-looking teens confronting the tobacco industry. A goal of these campaigns was to develop brands that youth could relate to and that could be used to channel youths' desire to counter authority. These campaigns were in stark contrast with ineffective industry-sponsored youth prevention campaigns that ultimately failed and may have been counterproductive.

The available evidence shows that anti-smoking campaigns have been effective in reducing youth and adult smoking. Studies have also found that the Florida and national *truth* campaigns have been effective in changing beliefs and attitudes and reducing youth smoking. In addition, an emerging literature suggests that branding youth countermarketing campaigns has added value beyond simple campaign exposure.

Campaign planners developed these brands by using formative research to understand the target audience's relationship with tobacco and existing anti-smoking campaigns. This research pointed to criticisms and gaps in existing campaigns that could be addressed by developing a branded countermarketing campaign that would appeal to the target audience and serve as a vehicle through which the campaigns could project an identity. This identity was built in a number of ways – through advertisements on television shows and sponsorship of concerts and events that appealed to the target audience; through careful selection of credible-looking actors in advertisements; and through unpredictable and attractive advertisements. These efforts were intended to communicate to the target audience that the campaign understood them.

Although preliminary evidence suggests that branding has been successful, the use of branding has been limited to date. In fact, no campaign in the USA aimed at smoking cessation has used branding. Moving forward, anti-smoking campaigns should continue to explore the possible benefits of branding as a way to connect with their audience. For example, in an era when smokers are increasingly stigmatized and socially isolated, it may be all the more important to develop a branded campaign that can connect with smokers. Otherwise, it is possible that remaining smokers, numb to the barrage of health warnings, will tune out anti-smoking messages. While the evidence in tobacco control is limited for branding, its longtime and widespread use in cigarette advertising suggests that it has been a powerful tool for marketing tobacco.

References

American Legacy Foundation. (2002). Getting to the truth: Assessing youths' reactions to the truth and 'Think. Don't smoke' tobacco countermarketing campaigns. First look report. Washington, DC. Available at: http://www.americanlegacy.org/PDF/truth_Fact_Sheet.pdf (accessed 21 September 2007).

Balbach, E. D. and Glantz, S. A. (1998). Tobacco control advocates must demand high-quality media campaigns: the California experience. *Tobacco Control* **7**:397–408.

Biener, L., McCallum-Keeler, G., and Nyman, A. L. (2000). Adults' response to Massachusetts antitobacco television advertisements: impact of viewer and ad characteristics. *Tobacco Control* **9**:401–7.

Blahut, S., Evan, D., Price, S., and Ulasevich, A. (2004). A confirmatory test of a higher order factor structure: brand equity and the Truth campaign. *Social Marketing Quarterly* **10**:1–13.

Burton, D., Sussman, S., Hansen, W. B., Johnson, C. A., and Flay, B. R. (1989). 'Image attributions and smoking intentions among seventh grade students. *Child Development* **52**:1499–511.

Centers for Disease Control and Prevention. (2007). Federal policy and legislation. Available at: http://www.cdc.gov/tobacco/data_statistics/by_topic/policy/legislation.htm (accessed 2 March 2008).

Davis K.C., Nonnemaker, J.M., Farrelly M.C. (2007). Association between national smoking prevention campaigns and perceived smoking prevalence among youth in the United States. *Journal of Adolescent Health* **41**:430–436.

Department of Health and Human Services. (2000). *Reducing tobacco use: a report of the Surgeon General*. Atlanta, GA: US Department of Health and Human Services, Centers for Disease Control and Prevention, National Center for Chronic Disease Prevention and Health Promotion, Office on Smoking and Health.

Earle, R. (2000). *The Massachusetts Tobacco Control Program, the art of cause marketing*. NTC/contemporary publishing group. Chicago, IL.

Evans, W. D., Wasserman, J., Bertolotti, E., and Martino, S. (2002). Branding behavior: The strategy behind the truth[sm] campaign. *Social Marketing Quarterly* **8**:17–29.

Evans, W. D., Price, S., Blahut, S. (2004). Social imagery, tobacco dependence, and the *truth* campaign. *Journal of Health Communication* **9**:425–41.

Evans, W. D., Price, S., and Blahut, S. (2005). Evaluating the truth[®] brand. *Journal of Health Communication* **10**:181–92.

Evans, W. D, Renaud, J., Blitstein, J., Hersey, J., Ray, S., Schieber, B., and Willett, J. (2007). Prevention effects of an anti-tobacco brand on adolescent smoking initiation. *Social Marketing Quarterly* **13**:2–20.

Farrelly, M. C., Healton, C. H., Davis, K. C. (2002). Getting to the truth: evaluating national tobacco countermarketing campaigns. *American Journal of Public Health* **92**:901–7.

Farrelly, M. C., Niederdeppe, J., and Yarsevich, J. (2003). Youth tobacco prevention mass media campaigns: past, present, and future directions. *Tobacco Control* **12**:i35.

Farrelly, M. C., Davis, K. C., Haviland, M. L. (2005). Evidence of a dose-response relationship between 'truth' antismoking ads and youth smoking prevalence. *American Journal of Public Health* **95**:425–31.

Farrelly, M. C., Crankshaw, E., and Davis, K. C. (in press). 'Assessing the effectiveness of the mass media in discouraging smoking behavior. In *The role of media in promoting and discouraging tobacco use*. Bethesda, MD: National Cancer Institute.

Farrelly, M. C., Davis, K. C., Duke, J., Messeri, P. (in press). Sustaining 'truth': Changes in youth tobacco attitudes and smoking intentions after three years of a national antismoking campaign. *Health Education Research*.

Glantz, S. A. (1997). Glantz responds. *American Journal of Public Health* **87**:870–1.

Glantz, S. A., Slade, J., Bero, L. A., Hanauer, P., and Barnes, D. E. (eds.) (1996). *The cigarette papers*. Berkeley, CA: University of California Press.

Goldman, L. K. and Glantz, S. A. (1998). Evaluation of antismoking advertising campaigns. *Journal of the American Medical Association* **279**:772–7.

Hersey, J. C., Niederdeppe, J., Evans, W. D. (2003). The effects of state counterindustry media campaigns on beliefs, attitudes, and smoking status among teens and young adults. *Preventive Medicine* **37**:544–52.

Hicks, J. J. (2001). The strategy behind Florida's 'truth' campaign. *Tobacco Control* **10**:3–5.

Henriksen, L., Dauphinee, A. L., Wang, Y., *et al.* (2006). Industry sponsored anti-smoking ads and adolescent reactance: test of a boomerang effect. *Tobacco Control* **15**:13–18.

Hopkins, D. P., Briss, P. A., Ricard, C. J., Husten, C. G., Carande-Kulis, V. G., Fielding, J. E., *et al.* (2001). Reviews of evidence regarding interventions to reduce tobacco use and exposure to environmental tobacco smoke. *American Journal of Preventive Medicine* **20**(S2):16–66.

Hu, T. W., Sung, H. Y., and Keeler, T. E. (1995). Reducing cigarette consumption in California: tobacco taxes vs. an antismoking media campaign. *American Journal of Public Health* **85**:1218–22.

Johnson, B. (2007). Marlboro Man rides into the sunset. *Advertising Age*. **78**:1–50.

Kluger, R. (1997). *Ashes to ashes: America's hundred-year cigarette war, the public health, and the unabashed triumph of Philip Morris*. New York: Vintage Books.

Lewit, E. M., Coate, D., and Grossman, M. 1981. 'The effects of government regulation on teenage smoking. *Journal of Law and Economics* **24**:545–69.

Niederdeppe, J., Farrelly, M. C., and Haviland, M. L. (2004). Confirming 'truth': More evidence of a successful tobacco countermarketing campaign in Florida. *American Journal of Public Health* **94**:255–7.

NPR. (2000). Olympic anti-tobacco ads. Available at: http://www.npr.org/templates/story/story.php?storyId=1105913 (accessed 3 March 2008).

Pierce, J. P., Gilpin, E. A., Emery, S. L. (1998). Has the California tobacco control program reduced smoking?' *Journal of the American Medical Association* **280**:893–9.

Public Health Service, Office of the Surgeon General. (1964). *Smoking and health: Report of the Advisory Committee to the Surgeon General of the Public Health Service*. US Public Health Service: Washington, DC.

Schneider, L., Klein, B., and Murphy, K. M. (1981). Governmental regulation of cigarette health information. *Journal of Law and Economics* **24**:575–612.

Siegel, M. (1998). Mass media antismoking campaigns: a powerful tool for health promotion. *Annals of Internal Medicine* **129:128–32.**

Siegel, M. and Biener, L. (2000). The impact of antismoking media campaigns on progression to established smoking: results of a longitudinal youth study in Massachusetts. *American Journal of Public Health* **90**:380–86.

Sly, D. F., Hopkins, R. S., Trapido, E., *et al.* (2001). Influence of a counteradvertising media campaign on initiation of smoking: the Florida 'Truth' campaign. *American Journal of Public Health* **91**:233–8.

Sly, D. F., Trapido, E., and Ray, S. (2002). Evidence of the dose effects of an antitobacco counteradvertising campaign. *Preventive Medicine* **35**:511–18.

Thrasher, J. F., Niederdeppe, J., Farrelly, M. C. (2004). The impact of anti-tobacco industry prevention messages in tobacco producing regions: evidence from the US truth campaign. *Tobacco Control* **13**:283–8.

Wakefield, M., Flay, B. R., Nichter, M., and Giovino, G. (2003). Effects of anti-smoking advertising influence youth smoking? A review. *Journal of Health Communication* **8**:229–47.

Wakefield, M., Terry-McElrath, Y., Emery, S. (2006). Effect of televised, tobacco company-funded smoking prevention advertising on youth smoking-related beliefs, intentions, and behavior. *American Journal of Public Health* **96**:2154–60.

Warner, K. E. (1977). The effects of the antismoking campaign on cigarette consumption. *American Journal of Public Health* **67**:645–50.

Warner, K. E. (1979). Clearing the airwaves: the cigarette ad ban revisited. *Policy Analysis* **5**:435–50.

8

High brand recognition in the context of an unsuccessful communication campaign
The National Youth Anti-Drug Media Campaign

Lela Jacobsohn and Robert C. Hornik

Summary

- The brand name associated with the National Youth Anti-Drug Media Campaign was highly recognized, but this brand name awareness did not translate into the intended change in cognitive or behavioral marijuana use outcomes.

- There are several approaches to brand name recognition measurement, including the comparison of recognition rates of true and false brand phrases, and their association with ad exposure; here they provide parallel support to claims of substantial brand name learning. However, recognition measures comprise only one aspect of overall brand evaluation measures.

- Strong brand name recognition can link together the ads of a public health communication campaign; this connectedness, or aggregating, of the messages may lead to positive or negative consequences for the campaign.

Introduction

The National Youth Anti-Drug Media Campaign was launched by the US Office of National Drug Control Policy (ONDCP) in 1998. This campaign, currently ongoing as of June 2007, is driven by three main goals: to empower youth to reject illegal drugs, to prevent initiation of youth drug use, and to persuade occasional drug users to cease use. In the 1998 to 2004 period covered by this chapter, the campaign primarily intended to prevent drug use initiation among 9–18-year-olds and predominantly focused these efforts on prevention of marijuana use. US Congress dedicated nearly $1 billion toward the funding of this campaign. The initiative's centerpiece was a large-scale health communication campaign; it included paid media advertising and employed a multimedia approach with a heavy emphasis on television. Through these media, the campaign tried to reach both parents and youth, with separate components for each. Targeting these audiences included a substantial effort to associate a brand name with each component of the campaign.

The evaluation of the campaign concluded that it had had no positive impact on youth cognitions, intentions or behavior with respect to marijuana use. In other words, no consistent intended downstream effects were observed. Moreover, the results of the evaluation indicated the possibility of unintended boomerang effects on youth such that higher levels of exposure were associated with more pro-drug outcomes (Hornik *et al.* 2008).

Thus, the campaign represents a branded initiative that did not achieve the desired public health outcomes. Despite these results, the brand name achieved high levels of recognition, as this chapter will detail. The following section of the chapter will describe the campaign's branding effort, present the methods used for assessing it, and report those results. The chapter concludes with a discussion of why it might be that apparently positive outcomes in brand recognition were not associated with positive behavior change.

Branding in the campaign

The campaign's communication strategy included use of a brand to build a unifying identity for the campaign (National Youth Anti-Drug Media Campaign 2001). The over-riding goals of branding were to integrate diverse media messages using a shared campaign signature and to connect print, radio and television advertising, as well as non-advertising components of the campaign, via a brand name or signature that would take the place of the 'Office of National Drug Control Policy' as the predominant name on ads for both youth and parents. Moreover, given recognition of and positive associations with the brand, the familiarity with the brand name might generate an initial positive response to new campaign ads and strengthen the perception that each ad was part of a larger initiative which might desirably affect acceptance of the campaign's messages (Hornik *et al.* 2001).

Consequently, beginning in 2000, the advertising began to feature brand signatures as a way to connect the discrete ads to one another. The 'Anti-Drug' brand name was included on all campaign messages and customized for both parent ('Parents: The Anti-Drug') and youth ('_ _ _ _ _: My Anti-Drug') audiences.

This branding effort was first launched with the parent campaign. The brand was designed in response to research indicating that parents saw themselves as ineffective and inconsequential in their children's lives, but children saw them as the most critical influ-ence in their lives (National Youth Anti-Drug Media Campaign 2001). Accordingly, the brand tried to position parents as a powerful and effective force against drugs in their children's lives. While some ads used the basic phrase: 'Parents: The Anti-Drug', other ads paired the phrase with a specific value that best represented the theme and ideas conveyed in the ad to create the brand signature, such as 'Communication: The Anti-Drug' and 'Action: The Anti-Drug'.

The youth brand was introduced in a comparable manner in the fall of 2000. The branding research indicated that youth disliked messages that told them what to do and were looking for a brand and messages that gave them a sense of ownership and treated them respectfully as individuals (National Youth Anti-Drug Media Campaign 2001). The youth brand signature 'My Anti-Drug' was developed to address these needs. In the initial series of ads, youth were asked to name their own anti-drug, that is, what kept them away from drugs. In some of these ads, youth were asked 'What's Your Anti-Drug?', and in others, the brand phrase was comprised of a series of blanks preceding the brand, '_ _ _ _: My Anti-Drug', designed to allow for the youth audience's wide variety of interests and values. Youth were then encouraged to submit their own 'anti-drug' by mail or via the web, in an effort to promote involvement and ownership by the individual youth respondent. These responses were used in subsequent ads, where the blanks had possible or submitted responses filled in, such as 'Music: My Anti-Drug' or 'Soccer: My Anti-Drug' (Hornik *et al.* 2002a).

The goal of these initial groups of branded messages was to 'create and reinforce anti-drug norms by identifying positive alternatives in young people's own words' (Hornik *et al.* 2002b), other ads focused on other arguments, and the brand signature was customized accordingly. Indeed, during the campaign, different message themes were used for periods of time and then alternated, for example, positive alternatives, negative consequences and resistance skills. Different sub-brands were associated with such themes. Although the original brand signature fit easily with the important message theme that encouraged youth to focus on positive alternatives to drug use, it was adapted to other themes as the campaign changed focus. For example, 'Courage: The Anti-Drug' was linked to ads that discussed the individual's obligation to help friends who are using drugs.

Additional sub-brands were introduced with the onset of the Marijuana Initiative. (A shift in the campaign was initiated after a review of the campaign in spring 2002. Beginning in October 2002, the majority of ads focused on the negative consequences of using marijuana in order to portray marijuana use as a risky behavior. (National Youth Anti-Drug Media Campaign 2006)) Youth advertisements offered variations on the brand signature, which were focused on negative consequences of use, such as 'Harmless? Facts: The Anti-Drug' and 'Responsibility: The Anti-Drug'. These ads often depicted scenarios with implied marijuana use by multiple teens and showed immediate detrimental outcomes, such as harming an innocent child while driving and using marijuana. More recently, the campaign has shifted brands using the brand signature, 'Above the Influence' with the goal of portraying the difference between those who are using and not using, and the superior advantage of those who live above the influence of drugs. The analyses and discussion presented below cover the time period prior to the onset of the 'Above the Influence' portion of the campaign.

Methods used to establish brand name awareness

In the context of the multi-faceted measurement of brand equity laid out earlier in this volume by Evans, Blitstein, and Hersey in Chapter 3, the campaign evaluation's assessment of the brand focused on the aspect of brand name awareness. To evaluate the extent to which youth and parents were aware of the brand name, beginning in 2001, the evaluation instrument, the National Survey of Parents and Youth (NSPY) included questions focused on brand name recognition. In Chapter 3 of this volume, Evans, Blitstein, and Hersey, identify two types of brand exposure and recall measures – self-report and environmental – and also distinguish between recall and recognition measures. The campaign's brand awareness measures were based specifically on self-report recognition responses. The evaluation data revealed that self-report measures of campaign ad exposure matched with environmental indicators such as ad gross rating points (Southwell *et al.* 2002.)

Questions measured recognition of the brand signature used in particular ads. The youth questionnaire included the question, 'We want to ask you about some brief phrases that might or might not have appeared in the media around here, as part of ads against drug use. In recent months, have you seen or heard the following phrases?' followed by the showing of '_ _ _ _: My Anti-Drug' in addition to one of two slogans or phrases (chosen randomly) that were not the youth campaign brand signature but rather were made up; these were 'ringer' brand phrases. In 2001, parents were asked only about the actual brand signature: 'In recent months, have you seen or heard any ads containing phrases such as 'Communication: The Anti-Drug' or 'Parents: The Anti-Drug?' Starting in 2002, parents were also asked about their recall of one of two ringer slogans or phrases that were not the parent campaign brand signature.

Three main criteria were used to evaluate the branding efforts. First, it was important to establish increasing recognition of the brand signature over time. To do this, recognition rates between prior and subsequent waves were compared. This could establish that the continuing broadcast of the brand signature produced increasing recognition. However, given that the NSPY instrument began to include these questions only after the brand signature had been launched, no pre-branding estimate for recognition was available. It was possible then that reports of brand phrase recognition were exaggerated from the beginning. A portion of the youth and parent respondents could have provided the 'yes' answer – that they had seen or heard the brand phrase – in order to seem knowledgeable or 'in the know'. Alternatively, they might have mistakenly thought the phrase was one they had heard before. To deal with this, the evaluation employed two additional approaches.

The second criterion was to establish the relationship of brand phrase recognition with campaign ad recall. Accordingly, brand phrase recognition rates were compared across levels of the specific ad exposure measure. The NSPY measured specific exposure to campaign ads aired on television or radio. On laptop computers, respondents saw or heard ads playing in the previous two months and were asked whether and how often they had seen each ad (see Southwell *et al.* 2002 for evidence of the validity of this measure). If the advertising was producing brand recognition, there should have been a strong association between brand phrase recognition claims and specific campaign ad recall claims, given that the ads predominantly featured the brand. Certainly, those respondents with higher levels of exposure to anti-drug ads had many more opportunities to see or hear the brand signature than those less exposed. (The brand phrase recall questions were positioned in the NSPY instrument prior to questions regarding campaign ads recall as the replay of the ads could have revealed the brand signature.)

The third criterion was to compare recognition of true and false brand phrases, as referenced above. Was recognition less for slogans that sounded as if they could potentially have been a campaign brand phrase but in fact had not been used in the campaign's ads? The importance of comparing true and false phrase recognition rates is to establish that parents and youth are differentiating their respective campaign 'Anti-Drug' brand name from other anti-drug propaganda in the media environment, schools and community. This point builds on Evans, Blitstein, and Hersey's discussion of competing media messages (Chapter 5), in that social marketing messages directed toward the same behavioral goal may contribute complementarily (and thus not competitively) toward cognitive and behavior change, but may compete for recall, encoding and storage space and confound measurement of ad and brand exposure for a specific campaign. Therefore, when evaluating constructs related to a behavior that is commonly the target of public health or social marketing messages (e.g. drug use prevention or smoking cessation), demonstrating the audience's ability to distinguish the studied brand from other brands or unbranded ads that target the same behavior further builds the case for brand recognition and awareness. As mentioned above, this approach was used starting in 2001 with the youth questionnaire and in 2002 for the parent questionnaire.

The question wording for the parent questionnaire was then slightly revised with the addition of the ringer brand phrases: 'We want to ask you about some brief phrases that might or might not have appeared in the media around here, as part of ads against drug use. In recent months, have you seen or heard either of the following phrases?'

The false brand phrases that were included in the parent questionnaire were: 'If parents use, you lose' and 'Drugs? Not on my watch!' The two false brand phrases that were used in the youth version of the questionnaire in 2001 were 'I'm drug free and I'm doing just fine' and 'Drugs – I don't need them'. In the last half of 2002 a different ringer phrase was used for youth: 'Drugs: one word – dead'.

To complement the simple comparison of recognition rates for true and false phrases, we also looked at the association of true and false phrase recognition with campaign ad recall. It was expected that campaign ad recall would be associated with true but not false brand phrase recall.

Thus, several indicators of brand signature recognition are used in the campaign's evaluation of the brand. These measures of brand awareness focus on recognition of brand phrases, in contrast to the brand associations featured in the brand awareness subscale items described earlier in this volume (Evans, Blitstein, and Hersey 2008; Evans et al. 2007). The campaign evaluation's measures of branding are also narrower than the brand equity measures discussed in Chapters 1 and 3. For example, there were no questions in the NSPY asking how the audience perceived the personality of the brand or whether the brand was well liked by youth (popularity). These differences reflect the NSPY focus on evaluation of outcomes rather than on formative research.

Evidence for brand name awareness

Interestingly, the same evaluation that declared the campaign unsuccessful found that the brand signature was highly recognizable. The first marker was clearly met: recognition

Table 8.1 Percentage of youth and parent respondents reporting true brand phrase recognition over campaign waves 2001–2004.

Brand recognition	Jan–Jun 2001	Jul–Dec 2001	Jan–Jun 2002	Jul–Dec 2002	Jan–Jun 2003	Jul–Dec 2003	Jan–Jun 2004
Youth (%)	61	76	84	85	88	87	88
Parent (%)	46	63	62*	71	82	84	90

*In January to June 2002, parents responded to a newly worded question. Parent recognition of brand increased to 71 per cent in the following six-month period, from July to December 2002.

of youth and parent brand phrases was increasing as the campaign advanced (Hornik *et al.* 2003; Orwin *et al.* 2006). While recognition after rollout of the brand signature was relatively high even at the initial measurement (60 per cent and 46 per cent among youth and parents respectively), rates of recognition increased steadily and sizably, until only approximately 10 per cent of each sample was not reporting brand phrase recognition, as shown in Table 8.1.

This increasing pattern in brand phrase recognition reports is consistent with the campaign accumulating gross rating points for the brand and its diffusion into the population. The campaign and its associated brand were in the media environment for a longer period of time, and this likely resulted in a greater number of youth and parents who had seen or heard the brand signature, as intended. However, because there is no pre-launch estimate, these recognition data do not allow an absolute judgment of how high the recognition level was. Moreover, even absent exposure to the campaign's anti-drug messages, the brand phrases may have become more familiar to youth and parents with repeated completion of the questionnaire and thus driven affirmative answers to the brand phrase recognition questions (Hornik *et al.* 2003). Increasing recognition helps make the case, but it is open to challenge.

The second marker of recognition, the association between brand phrase recognition and specific ad exposure, was also well met: the greater the campaign exposure reported by respondents, the greater their likelihood of recognizing the brand phrase (Hornik *et al.* 2003; Orwin *et al.* 2006). Early in the branded campaign, the association between brand phrase recognition and cued recall of (exposure to) specific ads was quite strong. Between 2001 and the middle of 2003 among youth in the lowest exposure group, only 50 per cent reported recognizing the brand signature in contrast to 81 per cent of those youth respondents who had seen the campaign ads more than 12 times per month, the highest exposure group. The distinction was even greater among parents. In 2001, there was brand phrase recognition among only 34 per cent of the parents in the lowest exposure group, whereas 74 per cent of parents in the highest exposure group said that they had seen or heard the brand signature. In the first half of 2002, the wording was revised in the parent questionnaire, and similar differences were still evident: 40 per cent of the lowest exposure group in contrast to 71 per cent of the highest exposure group reported recognition of the brand signature. These differences for youth and for parents were substantial and statistically significant.

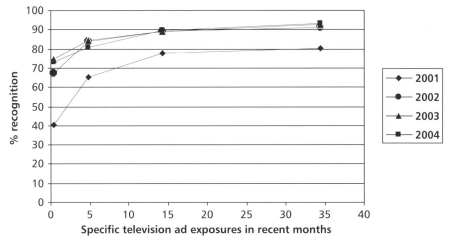

Fig. 8.1 Youth brand phrase recognition by exposure level and year.

Over time, into the years of 2003 and 2004, the relationship between ad exposure and brand phrase recognition grew to be less robust. It is likely that by the end of 2002, even those with little exposure to the campaign's messages had so many chances to become acquainted with the campaign brand signature that they were likely to be somewhat familiar with it. Therefore, the association became weaker, but this is mainly attributable to the growing likelihood that the low exposure group recognized the brand phrases. This relationship and the pattern over time for youth starting in 2001 are shown in Fig. 8.1.

Overall, there is strong support that the higher the respondent's exposure to the campaign, the more likely they were to recognize the brand signature, as expected. This result suggests that reports of brand phrase recognition reflected familiarity with the brand signature that was acquired through exposure to the campaign messages and thus was learned – rather than reflecting a tendency to try to appear knowledgeable or familiarity gained from repeated completion of the questionnaire, the concerns described above.

The third marker of recognition was to compare recognition rates of the real brand signature with rates of recognition of a false brand phrase, or ringer. These ringers, described earlier, were designed to sound as if they might have been used in the campaign's anti-drug messages, although they had not.

Initially, the youth recognition rates of true and false brand phrases were unpredictably similar, both at around 60 per cent, as shown in Table 8.2. Moreover, between the years of 2001 and 2004, the rate of recognition of the youth ringer brand phrases was surprisingly high. Approximately 58 per cent of youth reported recognizing one of the original false brand phrases, either 'I'm drug free and I'm doing just fine' or 'Drugs – I don't need them'. At first glance the high recognition of ringers and the similar recognition rates of true and false brand phrases seemed to suggest no brand phrase learning by youth. This conclusion was however inconsistent with the abovementioned evidence that true brand phrase recognition was significantly associated with ad recall and thus, brand signature learning was resulting from exposure to the ads.

Table 8.2 Percentage of youth respondents reporting brand phrase recognition over campaign waves 2001–2004.

Brand recognition	Jan–Jun 2001	Jul–Dec 2001	Jan–Jun 2002	Jul–Dec 2002	Jan–Jun 2003	Jul–Dec 2003	Jan–Jun 2004
True brand (%)	61	76	84	85	88	87	88
False: I'm drug free … (%)	59	53	56	59	59	60	61
False: Drugs – don't need them … (%)	60	53	N/A	N/A	N/A	N/A	N/A
False: One word – dead (%)	N/A	N/A	36	34	43	43	51

N/A: This brand phrase was not included in the NSPY questionnaire during this wave.

An alternative explanation was suggested: could it be that the ringer phrases for the youth were so conventional sounding that many thought they were legitimate, and decided mistakenly that they might have heard them? In contrast, the true phrase '_ _ _ _ _: My Anti-Drug' was entirely unconventional; if respondents did not actually recognize it, they were unlikely to mistakenly think they had. To address this possibility, a 'new' fictitious brand phrase was developed for youth which was purposefully designed to sound less standard. Youth respondents were asked about their recognition of this new ringer brand phrase starting in 2002, and the speculation about the false brands seemed to find support. Fifty-six per cent of the youth who were randomly asked about the original ringer brand phrase ('I'm drug free and I'm doing just fine') reported to have been seen or heard it; only 36 per cent of youth reported having seen or heard the new ringer brand phrase for youth, 'Drugs: one word – dead' (see Table 8.2). The new phrase had significantly lower recognition rates. In addition, both recognition rates were quite different from that of the true youth brand phrase in the same period of time (January to June 2002) which had climbed to 84 per cent. Discrepancy in youth recognition between true and false brand phrases increased over time from January 2001 through June 2002 and then remained relatively constant through June 2004. Thus, there is clear evidence from this analysis as well as the previous criteria that there was substantial learning of the true youth brand signature, and that the high level of recognition of the original ringer phrase was an artifact of the phrases chosen (and how easy it was to mistakenly 'recognize' the false phrase compared with the true phrase).

For parents, there was a somewhat more straightforward interpretation of true and false brand phrase recognition rates. At the initial measurement of false brand phrases, only 39 per cent of parents reported that they had seen or heard the false phrase, a substantially lower rate of mistaken recognition than the initial rates (60 per cent) for youth. Moreover, parents' recognition of the true brand phrase was approximately 25 per cent higher than that of the ringers; more than 60 per cent of parents stated that they had seen or heard the 'Parents: The Anti-Drug' signature. Although reported recognition of both true and false brand phrases increased over time from 2001 to 2004 by approximately 30 per cent, the rates of increase were similar. Thus, the sizable discrepancy between recognition of true and false phrases remained relatively constant, indicating the real brand signature learning from exposure to campaign ads.

However, one might question why recognition of false brand phrases increased over time at a similar rate to the real brand phrase, if true phrase recognition increases over time were due to brand signature learning. In the case of the parents, repeated exposure to brand phrases in the questionnaire and/or or parents' instinct to appear knowledge-able may have contributed to their reports of seeing or hearing the phrases and thus be responsible for the similar rates of increase in recognition over time of true and false brand phrases. The sizable absolute differences in their recognition rates however can be attributed to real exposure to the branded campaign messages, as can be the 90 per cent recognition rate, as of June 2004. These results are shown in Table 8.3.

There is a final piece of evidence that the true brand phrase was being learned from campaign exposure and that the false brand phrase recall was a reflection of other influences. As presented in Fig. 8.1, there was a substantial relationship between campaign ad recall and true brand phrase recall for youth. There is no evidence for the false brand phrase comparable to the strong association between true brand phrase recognition and ad exposure. The relationship between the measures of cued recall of specific ads and the recognition of false brand phrases is not significant for either youth or parents; the percentage of youth and parents reporting that they had seen or heard the ringer brand phrases does not vary with their level of reported exposure.

Given the high level of initial recognition of the true phrase along with the high levels of ringer recognition, it is not possible to know the absolute level of true phrase recognition. However, the growing recognition of the true brand phrase over time, sizable growing differences between false and true brand phrase recognition, and the association of ad exposure with recognition of only true but not false brand phrases together make a strong argument that considerable brand recognition occurred and was attributable to actual exposure to and learning of the brand signature.

Discussion

The methods used to establish brand awareness focused exclusively on recognition of the brand name. Multiple indicators were used to demonstrate that the campaign brand signature was being learned via exposure to the campaign messages. Indicators

Table 8.3 Percentage of parent respondents reporting brand phrase recognition over campaign waves 2001–2004.

Brand recognition	Jan–Jun 2001	Jul–Dec 2001	Jan–Jun 2002	Jul–Dec 2002	Jan–Jun 2003	Jul–Dec 2003	Jan–Jun 2004
True brand	46	63	62*	71	82	85	90
False – kids lose (%)	N/A	N/A	40	42	57	55	67
False – watch (%)	N/A	N/A	37	39	55	58	68

*In January to June 2002, parents responded to a newly worded question.

included growth in brand phrase recognition over time; that brand phrase recognition was significantly related to specific ad recall; and that in contrast false brand phrases did not increase in recognition over time and were not significantly related to specific ad recall. By many counts, the campaign clearly taught its brand signature, if recognition is the criterion for judging this.

Even with these strengths, there are limitations to how much this high brand recognition conveys about the success of overall brand. It may be that the youth and parent brand phrases were learned, but the impact of the brand signature on the campaign's target audiences may not have been as intended. The campaign had specified reasons for using the brand and the ideas for what it would represent. One reason was to shift the attention to the name of the Office of National Drug Control Policy to a brand name (National Youth Anti-Drug Media Campaign 2001). Was this aspect of the effort successful? Did people disassociate ads from the government organization and associate them simply with the brand? These questions are difficult to answer with the available data used for the evaluation of the campaign. They were not included as part of the branding evaluation. In addition, the campaign's communication strategy (National Youth Anti-Drug Media Campaign 2001) had made clear that the brand would try to position parents as an effective and critical force in their children's lives and would try to give youth a sense of respectfulness and individual ownership of the campaign's messages. However, accomplishment of these branding goals by the campaign was not measured. Indeed, we do not know how parents and youth interpreted their respective 'Anti-Drug' brands or how they liked them. Other chapters in this volume provide elaboration of these other perspectives on brand evaluation.

Instead, given the overall evaluation results of the campaign, we can speculate in the context of the campaign's lack of positive effects on cognitive and behavioral outcomes on the impact of the brand. More pointedly, we can consider why a highly recognized brand was not associated with a successful public health communication campaign.

One factor that may be critical in understanding the juxtaposition of these effects is that the actual brand in effect was not the same as the campaign-defined 'Anti-Drug' brand. That is, people may have absorbed a different common trait and point of view from the campaign ads they had seen or heard. It is possible that this actual brand and link across ads was not found in the brand signature, '_ _ _ _ _ _: (the/my) Anti-Drug'. Even more, it is possible that the brand signature was interpreted in an unintended manner. For example, the youth brand may have been translated to a need to have protection or a guard, *an anti-drug*, from the use of drugs, especially marijuana, thus underscoring that youth *do* use these drugs. In other words, the brand may have inadvertently communicated a message of normative use. Consider public health communication to youth about condom use analogously: you need to use a condom to protect yourself from HIV and other STDs. The evident message is that one needs a condom for protection when engaging in sexual intercourse; the protection is necessary when the behavior is going to take place and because the behavior is common and thus, assumed. Similarly, in this campaign, youth may have interpreted the brand to be suggesting that protection is necessary because the behavior will 'undoubtedly' take place as it is common, and even, assumed. Therefore, the brand associations may have been counter to the campaign's anti-drug message and thus, the high brand recognition could have been a contributing factor in the unintended effects. Again, without additional measures of brand perception and associations, this speculation can be neither validated nor eliminated. Moreover, this problematic interpretation may not be due to the language of the campaign brand signature at all. Rather, this perception of youth drug use as normative may be caused by the sheer presence of the anti-drug messages in the media environment, potentially amplified by the connective link of a brand signature. This is discussed below.

This argument is consistent with one possible explanation for the campaign's effects – a meta-message explanation. It is possible that higher levels of exposure to campaign messages may have boosted the visibility and attention given to youth drug use and inadvertently led to the development and intensification of the belief that marijuana use is widespread and thus prevalent among the respondents' peers due to the large-scale nature of the campaign. In other words, the total, or aggregate, effect of the campaign ads may have been to develop a belief in peer marijuana use prevalence and that 'everyone is doing it'. Such descriptive normative beliefs in turn may have led to more pro-drug outcomes of norms, intentions and initiation, as indicated in social norms theory (Perkins and Berkowitz 1986). Past research has established evidence that supports the notion of a meta-message of the campaign in accounting for its unintended effects (Hornik *et al.* 2003; Jacobsohn 2007). Youth who saw many messages (despite their anti-drug content) were more likely to believe that their peers were using marijuana; the belief that peers were using marijuana in turn predicted subsequent use of marijuana. In trying to understand how this meta-message effect occurred, the role of branding is worth some discussion.

It is possible that the branding may have served to connect the diverse ads to one another, creating a more aggregated campaign (indeed, this was one of the campaign's goals of using a branded approach). The aggregate effect of the campaign's anti-drug ads was to create a meta-message or normative implications resulting in increased perceptions of the prevalence of peer marijuana use. In other words, it is possible that, even with the high levels of exposure, the meta-message effect would not have occurred had the campaign ads not been linked together by the brand but rather been seen as discrete ads. Thus, the brand may have accomplished one of the strategic communication goals – to bring together the discrete ads – but this 'success' may have translated into undesirable overall effects of campaign exposure.

Another possible explanation for why high brand recognition was not associated with a successful campaign in terms of positive cognitive and behavioral outcomes may be driven by psychological reactance to a government authority. Brands help consumers connect products and their marketing to company names such as Nike and the Coca-Cola Company. Given this framework, it may have been that repeated exposure to the ads created not only a familiarity with the 'Anti-Drug' brand signature but also an association of the brand with the 'Sponsored by the Office of National Drug Control Policy' label on each ad. Therefore, as brand phrase recognition increased, so too may have awareness of the government sponsor. The high rates of brand recognition may have been tied to youth reactions to a government authority directing them what to do and what not to do. If these reactions were negative, due to what may have seemed to youth like authoritarian directions, youth may have rejected the anti-drug message by adopting more pro-drug beliefs, intentions, and even initiation of behavior. Indeed, psychological reactance theory (Brehm 1966, 1972; Brehm and Brehm 1981) predicts boomerang effects when youth resent being told what to do and perceive a threat to their freedom to engage in behaviors of their own choosing. Indeed, the campaign's formative branding research, described above, had already established that youth had reported that they were tired of being told what to do and wanted individual respect. Thus, the reactance explanation seems a viable way to connect the highly recognized brand signature with unintended campaign effects.

However, this explanation is less likely given the lack of compelling evidence that psychological reactance phenomena account for the campaign effects. Past research has tested this proposition and been unable to find convincing evidence with the available data that reactance, approximated by measurement of the audience evaluation of the ads, was responsible for the campaign's effects (Jacobsohn 2004, 2002). The effect of exposure on drug-related outcomes has not been shown to be contingent upon high or low reactance to the ads over time.

While only one of these explanations has empirical support, discussion of both brings attention to the fundamental point that the high brand name awareness and learning evident in the campaign, measured by brand phrase recognition, may have both positive and negative effects. It is also clear that the measurement of brand response was likely to have been insufficiently comprehensive to capture the overall impact of the brand. We have offered possible reasons for this juxtaposition of a highly recognizable brand in the context of an unsuccessful campaign. Moreover, the outcomes here suggest the need to employ additional measures of the brand, conventionally used in commercial marketing and referenced throughout this text, including brand attributes and attitude toward the brand.

Conclusions

Brand recognition may not always convert to campaign success. This disconnect may be because (1) other significant factors need to be taken into account, (2) messages are unpersuasive regardless of how well recognized the brand name may be, or (3) the brand name, alone or in conjunction with the ads, creates an unintended message which operates against the campaign goals. Concerning this last factor, branding can effectively serve to connect discrete ads together, resulting in a more aggregated campaign; however, the aggregate ad exposure effect may be consistent with or counter to the goals of a given campaign. The lessons from the branding experience with the National Youth Anti-Drug Media Campaign may encourage the inclusion of a baseline measurement of pre-launch brand recognition in addition to a broader range of measures to evaluate the branded aspects of campaigns. These lessons also suggest the need to pre-test and evaluate campaigns for their aggregate messages and consider the operation of the brand in its aggregate or cumulative effects.

Acknowledgement

The evaluation of the campaign was overseen by the National Institute on Drug Abuse (NIDA), and was contracted to and conducted by Westat and the Annenberg School for Communication at the University of Pennsylvania. The research and writing associated with this chapter is also supported by NIDA Grant #1-R03-DA-020893-01.

References

Brehm, J. W. (1966). *A theory of psychological reactance.* New York: Academic Press.

Brehm, J. W. (1972). *Responses to loss of freedom: a theory of psychological reactance.* Morristown, NJ: General Learning Press.

Brehm, S. S. and Brehm, J. W. (1981). *Psychological reactance.* New York: Wiley.

Evans, W. D., Renaud, J., Blitstein, J., Hersey, J., Ray, S., Schieber, B., and Willett, J. (2007). Prevention effects of an anti-tobacco brand on adolescent smoking initiation. *Social Marketing Quarterly* **13**:2–20.

Evans, W.D., Blistein, J., and Hersey, J. (2008). Evaluation of public health brands: design, measurement, and analysis. In: Evans, W.D. and Hastings, G., eds. *Public Health Branding: applying marketing for social change.* Oxford University Press, 43–72.

Hornik, R., Maklan, D., Orwin, R., Cadell, D., Judkins, D., Barmada, C., *et al.* (2001). *Evaluation of the National Youth Anti-Drug Media Campaign: third semi-annual report of findings.* Report prepared for the National Institute on Drug Abuse (Contract No. N01DA-8–5063), Washington DC: Westat.

Hornik, R., Maklan, D., Cadell, D., Barmada, C., Jacobsohn, L., Prado, A., *et al.* (2002a). *Evaluation of the National Youth Anti-Drug Media Campaign: fifth semi-annual report of findings.* Report prepared for the National Institute on Drug Abuse (Contract No. N01DA-8–5063).

Hornik, R., Maklan, D., Cadell, D., Prado, A., Barmada, C., Jacobsohn, L., *et al.* (2002b). *Evaluation of the National Youth Anti-Drug Media Campaign: Fourth semi-annual report of findings.* Report prepared for the National Institute on Drug Abuse (Contract No. N01DA-8–5063), Washington DC: Westat.

Hornik, R., Jacobsohn, L., Orwin, R., Piesse, A., and Kalton, G. (2008). Effects of the National Youth Anti-Drug Media Campaign on youth. *American Journal of Public Health.* Forthcoming.

Hornik, R., Maklan, D., Cadell, D., Barmada, C., Jacobsohn, L., Henderson, V., *et al.* (2003). *Evaluation of the National Youth Anti-Drug Media Campaign: 2003 report of findings.* Report prepared for the National Institute on Drug Abuse (Contract No. N01DA-8–5063), Washington DC: Westat.

Jacobsohn, L. (2002). Audience evaluation of anti-drug advertisements and its relationship to advertising effectiveness. Unpublished Masters thesis, University of Pennsylvania.

Jacobsohn, L. S. (2004). Psychological reactance and audience evaluation of anti-drug advertisements: explaining unanticipated communication effects. Paper presented at the Annual Conference of the National Communication Association, November 12, 2004, Chicago, IL.

Jacobsohn, L. S. (2007) Explaining the boomerang effects of the National Youth Anti-Drug Media Campaign [PhD Dissertation]. Philadelphia, PA: University of Pennsylvania.

National Youth Anti-Drug Media Campaign (2001). *Communication strategy statement supplement.* Washington, DC: Office of National Drug Control Policy.

National Youth Anti-Drug Media Campaign (2006). *Marijuana initiative fact sheet*. Washington, DC: Office of National Drug Control Policy.

Orwin, R., Cadell, D., Chu, A., Kalton, G., Maklan, D., Morin, C., *et al.* (2006). *Evaluation of the National Youth Anti-Drug Media Campaign: 2004 report of findings*. Report prepared for the National Institute on Drug Abuse (Contract No. N01DA-8-5063) Washington DC: Westat.

Perkins, H. W. and Berkowitz, A. D. (1986). Perceiving the community norms of alcohol use among students: Some research implications for campus alcohol education programming. *International Journal of the Addictions* **21**:961–76.

Southwell, B., Barmada, C., Hornik, R., and Maklan, D. (2002). Can we measure encoded exposure? Validation evidence from a national campaign. *Journal of Health Communication* **7**:445–53.

9

Branding through cultural grounding
The *keepin' it REAL* curriculum

Michael L. Hecht and Jeong Kyu Lee

Summary

- Culture plays an important role in commercial as well as public health branding.
- A cultural grounding approach to branding appeals to the cultural/social elements of the target population and nurtures a relationship with audiences by calling up their own meanings, messages and identities.
- A cultural grounding approach was used to develop the *keepin' it REAL* curriculum, an efficacious, multicultural, substance abuse prevention program for middle schools.
- The *keepin' it REAL* curriculum culturally grounded its branded health promotion messages through narratives and community-based participatory research.
- Cultural grounding can be used to develop a culturally grounded health brand and provides useful insights for health message design centered on social and cultural forces.

Introduction

Health message design theory has long recognized the role of culture and the social marketing approach of branding seems particularly attuned to this viewpoint. This approach recognizes the need to build strong brands in the globalized market. However, brands are not easily transportable across cultures. For example, China's new open-door policy has created an attractive new market for western companies. Yet, many western organizations rushed into China without considering cultural differences between the Chinese and domestic markets. As a result, many failed to build successful brands in the emerging Chinese market because they adopted marketing strategies that had proven successful in the western market and applied them to the Chinese market. Many companies now realize these approaches were problematic and are blending their brands with regional and cultural concerns (Melewar *et al.* 2004; Keller 2007).

This leads to the question, 'What is culture?' Although no single definition of culture is universally accepted in social science, there is generally agreement that culture is learned, shared and transmitted from one generation to the next, and it can be seen in a group's values, norms, practices, systems of meaning, ways of life, other social regularities and so on (Kreuter *et al.* 2003; Baldwin *et al.* 2006). Some specific examples illustrate how global brands have successfully capitalized on cultural elements in foreign markets. Coca-Cola adapted one of its brand names, 'Diet Coke' to 'Coke Light' or 'Coca-Cola Light' when it found that the word *diet* connoted the need for weight-reduction rather than minimizing weight gain in some countries (Dana and Oldfield 1999). In Indonesia, home to the world's largest Muslim population, KFC used Ramadan-themed outdoor advertising to encourage consumers to come to the restaurants during that holiday season (Keegan and Green 2005). Lastly, McDonald's advertising has been successful in Japan during the past several years. Their advertising has mainly focused on various aspects of fatherhood and relationship with family members. By doing so, McDonald's has encouraged Japanese consumers to associate the restaurant with family members interacting in various situations (Ono 1997).

Elaborating on this basis premise, we define culture as *code* (a system of meanings or rules), *conversation* (a way of interacting) and *community* (a sense of membership) (Philipsen 1992). These dimensions provide the basis for developing tailored and targeted health promotion messages because they help us to describe the cultural experiences and voices of group members as well as identify cultural similarities and differences across groups. Based on this definition, designers of health messages need to consider how members of a group will interpret a message (code), the best medium or form for conveying the message (conversation) to them, and the most salient identities of the target audience (community). In this chapter we explicate these ideas, describing a cultural approach to branding that we call *cultural grounding* (Hecht and Krieger 2006).

Culturally grounded branding is an audience-driven approach to understanding the 'culture' of groups as a starting point for health message design rather than adding culture to messages. The culturally grounded approach is predicated on the essential role of codes, conversations and communities in health message processing. Instead of universal messages focusing on dominant cultural values or even the modification of universal messages to 'other' cultures, an approach we call cultural sensitivity, a culturally grounded intervention creates a brand that involves cultural/social elements of branding because it utilizes the symbolic representations, norms and values of each identity group and communicates in a form and style that reflects those found within the culture. Cultural grounding attempts to make these branding elements into a network of associations (Mooij 1998) through multi-delivery strategies such as videos, billboards, product ancillaries, etc. In turn, it creates positive imagery associated with a brand and builds up strong relations with audiences. These networks emerge from the cultural code and are transmitted through social interaction among members of a community. As a result, brands can be developed *from* the codes, conversations and communities in order to make them more accessible to the target audience and promote identification and loyalty. Cultural grounding nurtures a relationship with the audience by calling upon their own meanings, messages and identities.

This chapter introduces the *keepin' it REAL* curriculum as an example of a culturally grounded approach to branding health promotion messages. At the heart of this process is the community-based participatory formative research used to derive the brand from the culture. Thus, the chapter describes the principle of cultural grounding as a method for developing a health brand and the ways that the curriculum was developed and implemented for multicultural, school-based substance use prevention.

The role of culture in branding

Grounding means starting with the basic elements of culture articulated in our definition. Various cultural groups differ in their systems of meanings (codes), ways of interacting (conversation), and sense of memberships/identity (community). In public health branding, culture plays an important role in branding because it provides a framework for targeting or tailoring messages for identity groups and their members as well as identifying the means of communicating messages that will appeal to local meanings and values. Thus the chapter discusses branding through the lens of code, conversation and community.

Code

Effective brands have significance that goes beyond their physical properties, utilitarian character and commercial value (Aaker *et al.* 2001) that largely rests upon their symbolic representations and expressions of cultural meanings and values (Richins 1994; Aaker *et al.* 2001). Shavitt has asserted that culture-specific meaning typically resides in the abstract qualities of the brand that provide primarily symbolic or value-expressive functions to the consumers (Shavitt 1990), what is commonly known as 'brand image'.

For instance, the National Pork Board launched the '*El cerdo es bueno* (Pork is Good)' campaign for the Hispanic market. Due to the experiences brought from their home countries, where pork-related illnesses are pervasive, many Hispanics, particularly among those who are immigrants or first-generation Americans, have health-related concerns regarding pork. The campaign was effective because it addressed key barriers to pork consumption based on their cultural experiences with a simple and straightforward message – 'Pork is Good' – conveying the meaning that US pork is safe, delicious and healthy (Korzenny and Korzenny 2005).

The *truth* campaign is another example of how effective branding utilizes cultural codes and images. The campaign builds a positive and anti-smoke identity through hard-hitting advertisements that feature teens confronting the tobacco industry (Farrelly *et al.* 2002). A well-known *truth* advertisement, called 'Body Bag', features teens piling body bags in front of a tobacco company's headquarters and, broadcasting loudly through a megaphone, explaining that these represent the 1200 people who die daily from smoking. This example demonstrates that the series of ads, including 'Body Bag', tells how risky smoking is using images such as the piling of body bags.

Conversation

Effective branding also must consider the messages and the channels through which they are presented. Brands tell stories or narratives that must resonate with cultural identities through culturally appropriate media. Cultures differ in their style of communicating (Hecht *et al.* 2003a) and this necessitates different branding messages. For example, Kishii (1988) identified several message characteristics that differ between Japanese and American culture. According to his findings, indirect rather than direct forms of expression are preferred in Japanese messages. This roundabout way of expression is pervasive in all kinds of communication in Japanese culture. Usually only brief dialogue or narration is used in television commercials in Japan; this is because in Japanese culture, the more a person talks, the less they are perceived as trustworthy (Keegan and Green 2005).

Cultural differences also exist in media use among cultural groups. The use of billboards is extremely effective in reaching African-American consumers in central cities. Large billboards deliver specific messages to an entire neighborhood, playing off the sense of community that is a high priority among African-Americans (Campanelli 1991). A recent innovation in outdoor advertising has been increasing the use of smaller posters in African-American urban communities. Compared with the large highway billboards, the main advantage of the small posters is that they can be placed low and close to the street, thus facilitating greater accessibility to passersby of all age groups (Williams and Tharp 2001).

Another example is the radio soap opera, termed *telenovela*, which was a culturally appropriate way to broadcast AIDS prevention messages to the intended audience in Tanzania. In 1993, over half of Tanzanian households owned a radio and about 60 per cent of them regularly listened to radio when the campaign was launched. The radio telenovela was an especially effective way to reach truck drivers who were most at risk of AIDS infection because it was the primary communication source for the drivers on the road. With the culturally preferred medium, the entertainment-education radio soap opera was a successful AIDS prevention strategy in Tanzania (Vaughan and Rogers 2000).

Community

Successful brands also create a sense of membership or loyalty that builds on identities in the community (Keller 2007). In the commercial domain, brand communities are organized and facilitated based on a structured set of relationships among admirers of a brand (Algesheimer *et al.* 2005). The *truth* campaign provides an excellent example of a health campaign that built a brand community. The campaign created a sense of membership in a rebellious youth culture around the code or image of 'truth'. It branded nonsmoking adolescents with the appealing label of 'truth teens', establishing an idealized social image to which youth could then aspire (Evans *et al.* 2005). As youth were exposed to the truth messages, they were expected to have a sense of membership as 'truth teens' combined with positive social imagery of not smoking. This membership led community members to resist adult influence and decrease the progression to established smoking.

Another example is the Philip Morris 'anti-smoking prevention' campaign. This campaign created an image of the nonsmoker that at-risk kids would not want to hang out with so that the 'models' being presented in the campaign were negative examples (see Chapter 7 in this book). This message almost invites a boomerang effect by creating a community of nonsmokers that many adolescents would not want to join. This is a kind of challenge to branding approaches, which build alternative identity for intervention. We will discuss this issue later.

Cultural grounding is a method for developing brands

Culture and the culturally sensitive approach

Culture is important for health-promotion interventions because the norms, attitudes and behavioral repertoires that adolescents use to make and enact decisions about risky behaviors are derived, at least in part, from their cultural backgrounds and identities. Effective health messages, like all communication, require adaptation to the intended audiences. It has long been recognized among communication scholars that the adaptation must reflect the situation, topic, context and other communicators (Street and Giles 1982). Despite this, many prevention messages are not suited to the groups for which they are intended. For example, a major criticism of the US 'Just Say No' campaign that began in the 1980s is that it promotes a singular resistance strategy at odds with the language practices of mainstream US youth culture (Hecht and Krieger 2006).

Cultural sensitivity is essential to the efficacy of interventions because it targets their cultural characteristics and broader sociocultural values of the intended target group (Kreuter *et al.* 2003). According to Resnicow *et al.* (1999), cultural sensitivity consists of two primary dimensions: surface structure and deep structure. Surface structure may include using certain colors, images, fonts or pictures of the group members (Kreuter *et al.* 2003). Resnicow *et al.* (1999) label these elements as 'superficial' characteristics of a proposed population and suggest that by matching materials to the superficial characteristics of the target group, the group's receptivity and acceptance of messages can be enhanced. Deep structure of cultural sensitivity reflects the broader sociocultural aspects and it conveys salience to a priority group. Using this approach, the target group's cultural values, beliefs and behaviors are recognized, reinforced and built upon to provide context and meaning to messages about a health problem or health behavior.

Castro and colleagues have suggested a three-part method for classifying accommodation strategies to achieve cultural sensitivity. The first is cognitive information processing characteristics, such as language and age or developmental level. The second is affective-motivational characteristics, such as gender, ethnic background and socioeconomic status. Finally, environmental characteristics should be considered, such as the ecological aspects of local community (Castro *et al.* 2004).

Kreuter *et al.* (2003) have proposed a more specific classification of the ways that prevention messages can be made culturally sensitive. First, peripheral strategies refer to 'packaging' the program to reflect the intended cultural group through the use of appropriate colors, images, fonts and pictures. Second, evidential strategies enhance the perceived relevance of a health issue for a group by presenting evidence about how it affects the group. Third, linguistic strategies make programs more accessible by providing them in the dominant or native tongue of the intended audience. Fourth, constituent-involving strategies draw on experiences of the group, such as involving lay community members in planning and decision making for the program. Fifth, sociocultural strategies are similar to Resnicow *et al.*'s (1999) concept of deep structure, and refer to strategies that discuss health issues in broader context of social and cultural values and characteristics of the intended audience (Hecht and Krieger 2006).

Defining cultural grounded approach

Typically, cultural sensitivity is concerned with how to transport an existing prevention program to a new culture through the introduction of superficial characteristics of the target group. Other times it involves infusing culture into a predetermined, transcultural health message. Cultural grounding incorporates the processes discussed in the cultural sensitivity approaches but it diverts philosophically through the assumption that prevention interventions are developed from within the culture, with cultural group members as active participants in message design and production.

This theoretical move is a 'difference of kind' or degree because those adopting the related sensitivity and adaptation approaches also enlist cultural members and incorporate their insights (Hecht and Krieger 2006). The principle of cultural grounding goes beyond modifying existing messages to a culture by assuming that the code, conversation and communities of the culture are the starting points for message design rather than an *a priori* often mainstream US or western message (Hecht and Krieger 2006). From this perspective, prevention interventions invoke symbolic representations and preferred communication modes across and within the variability in identities inherent within each culture by building on their narratives, cultural values and norms.

Cultural grounding as a method for developing a brand

In the traditional marketing perspective, brand is defined as the association of favorable imagery created by messages. A brand image is created that reflects what people think, feel and visualize when they see the brand's symbol or name. Effective brands evoke richer, stronger and more consistent favorable meanings and associations (Batra *et al.* 1996). In this chapter, we suggest that in order to develop strong brand, brand images must be interpretable within the symbolic system of the culture, communicated in a form that is consistent with cultural practices, and invoked within the nexus of identities that characterize group memberships. The cultural grounding approach develops brands that are grounded in the salient identities by reflecting the symbolic representations, norms and values of each identity group and communicating in a form and style that reflect those found within the culture.

Narratives

Narratives are an essential part of the grounding process. Narrative theory conceptualizes human thoughts and behaviors based upon narratives or stories. Narrative is both a way of coding or storing information (Howard 1991) as well as a method for expressing or communicating a meaning (Hecht and Miller-Day, in press). Narratives serve as the primary means for making sense of experiences and provide models for adolescent behavior (Bandura 1986). Several studies indicate that people see narrative messages as more realistic than statistical evidence (Greene and Brinn 2003) and that messages that combine narrative and statistical evidence are more persuasive than those presenting either type of evidence alone (Allen *et al.* 2000). They have proven effective in health promotion (Green 2006).

The cultural grounding approach utilizes the narratives/stories of the group members as reflections of the values, beliefs and implicit assumptions of their culture (Gosin *et al.* 2003). These narratives provide good reasons, which justify actions based upon the dominant stories within the group (Fisher 1987). Effective narratives have fidelity, or 'ring true' to cultural group members, and are coherent, or hold together as a narrative or story (Fisher 1987; Hecht and Miller-Day, in press). Different cultures are characterized by different narratives, both as a way of thinking as well as a style of expression. For example, Native American narrative is typically organized nonlinearly, like the spokes of a wheel, reflecting a central organizing element (the hub) and various storylines (the spokes) rather than a chronological progression (Lake 1997). In contrast to western linearity expressed in deductive or inductive organization, this nonlinear narrative starts with a basic premise and then can go off in multiple directions, all held together by their common premise. Branded messages targeting this culture should reflect this narrative style.

The Joe Camel campaign provides an excellent example of narrativity. Joe is not just a 'cool-looking' hippodrome who smokes, but a story about what it means to be a cool guy – hanging out in bars, with lots of girlfriends, dressing stylishly and so forth. Cultural grounding allows a brand to draw upon culturally shared symbol systems that express membership while making stories meaningful to the intended audience.

Identity

Identity is a second aspect of grounding. Identity reflects a sense of membership in a group, be it national, religious, ethnic or other basis in origin. For example, racial/ethnic identity includes several elements such as ethnic pride, affinity for in-group culture (e.g. food, media and language), involvement with in-group and out-group members and so on (Resnicow *et al.* 1999). These identities provide a powerful basis for communication. Recent theorizing argues that messages and relationships, themselves, are often manifestations of identity (Hecht 1993; Hecht *et al.* 2004).

Culturally grounded branding emphasizes group membership in a number of different ways. Brands can call upon existing identities, linking to those ways of being to establish a positive image or bond people to the message or product by developing new identities that connect people together around produce usage. In the first approach, the images and narratives created by culturally grounded approach are derived from within the community, enhancing community involvement and engagement (Algesheimer *et al.* 2005). If cultural group members recognize their identities and accept their association with the product or idea, a strong brand loyalty toward their community will be created. For example, Hallmark Cards launched its Afrocentric brand, Mahogany, to meet the needs of African-American ethnic consumers. In 1987, Mahogany started with only 16 cards but it offers about 1000 cards by 2002 (Kotler 2002).

On the other hand, brands also can create an identity group. This is very similar to brand community, which shares common values, norms and rituals among the brand community members. Brand community leads to greater community engagement and brand loyalty (Algesheimer *et al.* 2005). Harley-Davison's Harley Owners Group is a prototypical example of a brand community. As previously discussed, the *truth* campaign established an ideal social imagery to which teens aspire, leading them to membership of the 'truth teens', an identity group that resists the social influence of smoking (Evans *et al.* 2005).

Developing effective brands through the active participation of group members

We also argue that cultural grounding requires the active participation of the group members in health message design and production. Active participation increases the chances that culturally grounded brands will be consistent with the values and norms of the culture and reflect their members' cultural identities, meanings and values. These voices can be incorporated in many ways. Many use a 'community-based participatory approach' (Gosin *et al.* 2003) to gain the perspective of group members during formative research. In cultural grounding, the messages themselves emerge from this process with group members participating fully in message production so that accommodation of the prevention message occurs through the process of message development (Hecht and Krieger 2006).

Our approach utilizes community-based participatory research (Hecht and Miller-Day 2007). We believe that the fidelity and coherence of the narratives are enhanced when group members participate in designing and producing the materials and messages themselves. To us this means engaging the community as partners in the process, not just 'informants' or message evaluators. Partnership involves active participation in message creation, a process that often starts with narrative interviews to capture the stories of the target group members. Other methods include descriptions of existing narratives in the oral, written and mediated traditions of the group.

Evidence for a cultural grounding approach to branding

In some senses, cultural grounding parallels cultural sensitivity in that it is essential to general communication effectiveness (Hammer 1989) as well as interventions (Koss and Vargas 1992). Communication which adjusts to and accommodates culture is more effective (Hecht *et al.* 1993). Effective messages must be based on the underlying world views that develop through enculturation, and this is particularly true of interventions that seek to promote change (Koss and Vargas 1992). Schinke and his associates have argued that interventions targeting minority youth should emphasize ethnic pride and cultural identity (Schinke *et al.* 1990).

Some researchers assert that the targeted media are most effective when the symbols, characters and values depicted in the media are drawn from the intended audience's cultural background (McGuire 1984; Appiah 2001). Culturally-specific ads allow the audience to better identify with the message and the source of the message (Appiah 2001).

Furthermore, people who are more likely to identify with media characters and perceive themselves to be similar to media characters, are more influenced by media content in which those characters are portrayed (Huesman *et al*. 1983). For example, black viewers are more likely to identify with, and evaluate more favorably, ads depicting black characters than ads featuring white characters (Whittler 1991). This tendency is also observed in other ethnic groups such as Hispanics who seek out representations of their own culture (Stevenson and McIntyre 1995).

In recent years, new technology has enhanced the efficacy of culturally matched messages. Appiah investigated the effect of culturally targeted messages on the internet. The results showed that black audiences with strong ethnic identities respond more favorably to black-targeted online media and less favorably to white-targeted media, whereas black audiences with weak identities responded no differently to the online media based on the ethnic target of the internet site (Appiah 2004). Prior empirical studies have demonstrated that cultural grounding often produces better outcomes than mismatched or half-matched culturally grounded programs because people are more likely to accept targeted messages reflecting their cultural narratives, values and norms (Hecht *et al*. 1993; Hecht *et al*. 2003).

The Drug Resistance Strategies Project: a case study in the culturally grounded branding approach

The Drug Resistance Strategies (DRS) Project is the name of a venture that involved research into the social properties of adolescent substance use and the development of a school-based substance use curriculum. The DRS project was among the first to systematically investigate the social processes involved in drug use among adolescents. The project created a culturally grounded prevention program from this research using a participatory action approach to message design (Gosin *et al*. 2003; Hecht and Miller-Day, in press). The curriculum was built around understanding the narratives reflecting youth, gender and ethnic/racial identities in the urban middle schools of Phoenix, Arizona, an area that was used to develop a branded, school-based substance use prevention curriculum. These narratives provided access to their shared experiences, knowledge and values. The voices of target group members are essential to design a culturally grounded intervention that incorporates traditional ethnic values and practices that promote protection against drug use.

Strong brands include various elements, such as brand name, logo, slogan, attributes, images, user identity and so on. Branding strategies make associations between and among these elements that are consistent with consumers' values, norms or identity, thereby building strong relationships with consumers. To create culturally targeted branded prevention curricula, the DRS team considered not only symbolic representations of culture, such as visual image and language reflecting that of the participants, but also the variability inherent within a specific cultural group.

Finally, to ensure that the brand emerged from the culture rather than having culture added to it, community-based participatory research was used to develop the curriculum.

Teams of students, teachers and community members developed the lessons with us in an iterative process. We believe that fidelity and coherence are enhanced when group members participate in designing and producing the materials and messages themselves (Fisher 1987). We now describe these processes in more detail.

The role of narratives and identity in *keepin' it REAL*

The *keepin' it REAL* curriculum is a culturally grounded approach utilizing branding concepts and techniques to infuse cultural elements into the curriculum. First, the curriculum was developed based on cultural narratives. Narratives or stories were collected from adolescents in each ethnic group through narrative interviews (Hecht and Miller-Day, in press) and used to create the performance-based elements of the curriculum. As mentioned above, brand is not just image, but also stories or narratives associated with products/services. Narrative interviews are designed to elicit stories through questions that are not easily answerable in yes or no or didactic responses. For example, asking about what goes on in someone's neighborhood is more likely to elicit a narrative response than asking if people know each other in their neighborhood. Other techniques (e.g. 'tell me a story about …', 'recall a time when …') also are used.

Since the mid-1980s the DRS project has conducted extensive research using a variety of techniques to identify drug resistance narratives in order to design, implement, and evaluate a substance abuse prevention program, *keepin' it REAL* (*kiR*). This research identified the ways that offers were made (i.e. who, how and where) as well as how they were resisted and why. While the unique focus of this research was on describing the set of strategies adolescents use to refuse drug offers, it also helped us understanding their decision-making process. The narratives collected in this process not only provided the content of the prevention messages (i.e. examples of how to assess risks, make decisions and refuse drug offers) but they determined what the curriculum was about. In the process of this research, the lead author's brother, Albie Hecht, who had vast experience branding while president of television and film for Nickelodeon (e.g. SpongeBob SquarePants) and creator of Spike TV (the first network for men), suggested that the refusal strategies needed to reflect a brand. Examining our preliminary descriptions, he suggested 'REAL' as an acronym to brand the refusal strategies in a term in common parlance in youth culture ('get real', 'be real'). REAL summarizes four strategies we found used among youth from elementary through college ages: *refuse* (simple no), *explain* (no with an explanation), *avoid* (avoid the situation or offer), and *leave* (remove yourself from the situation).

REAL became the central brand image of the curriculum and was used to teach strategies for resisting drug offers and other skills. The narratives formed the basis of an award-winning series of five videotapes and public service announcements created by students at South Mountain High School in Phoenix, Arizona, teaching the resistance skills that form the core of the curriculum. The students developed scripts from proto-typical narratives for each resistance strategy and produced videos that provided an overview of the program and taught each resistance skill through enactments or models

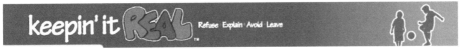

Fig. 9.1 *keepin' it REAL* logo. Reproduced with permissin from *keepin'it REAL*.

of successful drug resistance in recognizable locales, by youth similar to the students in age and ethnicity. Classroom-based materials and activities (e.g. role-plays created from the narratives) provide practices for assessing risk, making decisions and using the strategies (Gosin *et al.* 2003). Branding continued with focus groups of teachers and students. These groups suggested content and form for the lesson and led to the adoption of the phrase, 'keepin' it REAL' as our curriculum name and logo (Fig. 9.1). Focus groups also were used to pilot test the lessons.

The result was three versions of the curriculum that ethnically matched each of the main ethnic groups in the school population (i.e. Mexican-American and white/black versions) and a multicultural version that cut across these groups. As a result, *kiR* consists of three parallel versions of a ten-session classroom curriculum: a Mexican-American centered version targeting the largest ethnic group in the schools; a non-Mexican-American centered version that targeted the second and third largest ethnic groups in the schools (black/white); and a multicultural version that incorporated five lessons each from the first two versions and appealed to all three of the primary ethnic groups. The emphasis on Mexican-American youth culture responds to the needs of an under-researched community and at the same time provides a useful example of a specific culturally grounded program.

The *keepin' it REAL* curriculum: multi-delivery strategies

One of the aims of branding is to build relationships between consumers and products by reflecting consumer voices and adding meanings and values to their objects. The *kiR* curriculum used multi-delivery strategies and tactics to reach the target audience effectively so that they could interpret cultural elements in light of their motivations and aspirations.

Brand name or logo is an important branding element because it captures the central theme of the curriculum and effectively connects it to the target audience. Seventh-grade students in Phoenix, Arizona participated in creating the name, logo and slogan of the curriculum. The students determined that the best name for the curriculum was *keepin' it REAL* because 'it sounded like something we would say' and recommended the use of 'bubble letter' artwork and skits because the graffiti style of writing related to their urban environment (Gosin *et al.* 2003). The curriculum used incentives with program name and logo such as pens, baseball caps etc. to reward involvement and reinforce the brand image.

The *kiR* curriculum was implemented with multiple delivery methods such as videos, role-plays, billboards, boosters and so forth based on the belief that effective communication tools that are consistent over different media and over time should be developed for building and maintaining a strong brand (Aaker 1996). Similar information was included in each communication tool to offer consistency and facilitate building a strong and favorable brand (Keller 1998). The strategies were taught through the videos and class discussions. Other examples and exercises such as role-playing using culturally appropriate techniques and scenarios provided practice in using the strategies (Gosin *et al.* 2003). Billboards, radio and television public service announcements were created from the in-class videos to reinforce the program's content (Hecht and Krieger 2006). Research suggests, however, that it is primarily the classroom videos that account for the success of the intervention (Warren *et al.* 2006)

Evaluations of *keepin' it REAL*

A randomized trial was conducted among 35 middle schools (6035 students) that were randomly assigned to one of four conditions: Mexican-American curriculum, white/black curriculum, multicultural curriculum or control. A pretest was administered prior to the intervention and three posttests administered during an 18-month follow-up to examine the efficacy of the cultural grounding approach by examining its effects on substance use and comparing the effects of cultural matching (Mexican-Americans in the Mexican-American oriented program; African-Americans and European-Americans in the black/white program), inclusion or partial matching (all three groups in the multicultural program), and mismatches (Mexican-Americans in the black/white program; European-Americans and African-Americans in the Mexican-American program). Results supported the overall efficacy of the intervention but provided little substantial support of the cultural matching hypothesis (Hecht *et al.* 2003, 2006). The tests demonstrated that the Mexican-American and multicultural versions both produced significant effects relative to the control group (standard/existing intervention), indicating that it is not necessary to ethnically segregate students into narrowly matched programs. Instead, the process of incorporating a representative level of relevant cultural elements into the prevention message appeared critical (Hecht *et al.* 2003, 2006). In addition, the intervention proved effective even for those who had initiated use prior to the pretest (Kulis *et al.* 2007a) and was equally effective for males and females (Kulis *et al.* 2007b). Based on these findings, *kiR* was selected as a model program by the US Substance Abuse and Mental Health Services Administration's National Registry of Effective Prevention Programs.

Comparing cultural grounding and branding

There are several ways in which branding and cultural grounding diverge. First, branding is typically developed by marketing and advertising practitioners while the cultural grounding approach is more interactive and participatory (e.g. community-based participatory research). In the marketing domain, marketers recognize the important role of culture and they attempt to develop culturally specific programs, a practice commonly known as *diversity marketing*. The diversity marketing program has grown out of careful marketing research to identify different ethnic needs (Kotler 2002).

However, many culturally tailored marketing approaches seem to be superficial because they appear to be simple modifications of messages developed for a dominant culture (e.g. in the USA, European-American culture). For example, many African-American targeted programs have simply employed the images of black superstars such as Michael Jordan, Shaquille O'Neal, Halle Berry and so on (Kotler 2002).

The culturally grounded approach typically employs community-based participatory research or a comparable method. With the findings of the research, it moves beyond the superficial dimensions of culture (changing the ethnicity or appearance of role models) to the fundamental aspects of culture such as cultural narratives, values, beliefs and norms (Resnicow *et al.* 1999; Kreuter *et al.* 2003; Castro *et al.* 2004; Hecht and Krieger, 2006). The culturally grounded approach requires health message designers to engage cultural group members and work with them to develop culturally targeted messages reflecting the deep structure of each culture (Gosin *et al.* 2003; Hecht *et al.* 2006). As Kreuter and his colleagues have argued, socioculturally-based programs and materials should understand culturally normative practices and beliefs – the inner workings of culture rather than just outward appearances (Kreuter *et al.* 2003).

Another difference is that branding often creates something new or unique to differentiate the brand from other competitors, whereas cultural grounding tries to have the brand emerge from the culture. Marketers attempt to associate brands with favorable images and build unique identities to differentiate their brands from other competitors (Kotler 2002: 326). They can differentiate their brand images using symbols, colors, slogans and special attributes. For instance, the image of Apple Computers was built around its unique symbol, the apple. Some companies employ color identifiers such as blue (IBM) or yellow (Kodak), or a specific piece of sound or music. In contrast, the cultural grounding approach to branding tries to identify values, norms and identities embedded in the culture and derive the brand from those cultural elements. Cultural grounding does not necessarily create something new; instead, it tries to understand the existing thoughts and ideas embedded in each culture to derive the brand from them. For example, the phrase 'keepin' it REAL', was developed by students to explain or brand the *REAL* program. The phrase, itself, was in common use within the culture and has (fortunately) remained in use.

Finally, branding often is associated with favorable images (how a person should be) while cultural grounding is more than just images. In the commercial sector, branded messages create the associations with the brand. Brand image encompasses all the associations that a consumer holds for the brand. These include colors, sounds, smells, thoughts, feelings and imagery (Batra *et al.* 1996: 321). For instance, McDonald's advertising connects to an image of a 'typical user' with the character, Ronald McDonald, and a feeling of having fun with the symbol, golden arches (Kotler 2002).

Cultural grounding involves telling a story that reflects cultural elements based upon formative research with group members. As mentioned above, the *kiR* drug prevention curriculum is culturally grounded and derived from narrative theory and research. The program drew upon the stories that are salient to adolescents through the active participation of high school and middle school students (Hecht and Miller-Day, in press). Formative research was conducted to explicate adolescents' experience of drug use and drug offers (Hecht and Krieger 2006). The findings of this research led to the development of the *kiR* curriculum with students, teachers and community members utilizing narratives in which peer models of adolescents refuse drug offers to redefine the story of drug use norms and risk, as well as to develop communication competence and life skills (Hecht and Miller-Day, in press).

Challenges to cultural grounding to branding

Branding in the public health arena is inherently different from that in commercial marketing arena. Commercial branding typically suggests a benefit or an incentive, building the brand by presenting positive images of the product. However, while some health messages encourage the adoption of health behaviors, many stress avoidance of unhealthy behaviors. Members of the culture may not recognize the health brand as an incentive. Many health campaigns fail because what the campaigns ask the target audience to do is in opposition to their own self-interest or benefit and does not provide an explicit payback to compensate for what should not be done (e.g. quitting smoking) (Rothschild and Andreasen 1998). Health messages are challenged to show people being healthy as something to which people aspire. HIV/AIDS testing in Africa is the case for that issue. HIV/AIDS prevention campaigns are using advertising and mass media to emphasize the benefits of HIV testing such as a user-friendly, high-technical service, and support for those infected, yet people may refuse HIV testing, sometimes as a result of the threatened stigma, abandonment, violence or murder. The potential for negative consequences hinders them from obtaining the desirable treatments needed to combat the disease (Cock *et al.* 2002).

This raises the question of 'how health branding messages can deliver a promise or incentive (e.g. quitting smoking makes you healthier) that encourages healthy behaviors and/or discourages unhealthy ones. The cultural grounding approach suggests calling upon cultural identities and narratives that represent desirable health practices. For instance, peer pressure (e.g. norms) plays an important role in drug use among adolescents. The most common narrative among them presents drug users as mature and glamorous – cool guys in peer groups. This is reinforced in much of the media (DiFranza *et al.* 1992). Branding approaches are challenged by this narrative. However, peer influence may also be involved in drug abstinence (Robin and Johnson 1996; Elek *et al.* 2006). Kids who see their friends using drugs are more likely to follow whereas kids who believe their friends are anti-drug are more likely to abstain (Strasburger 2000). Narratives in which teens do not misuse substances and still have fun can be powerful means to shaping behavior. Here is the possibility that alternative identities and narratives may change normative behavior (e.g. drug use), if health messages are grounded in group members' experiences.

To overcome the challenges to culturally grounded branding, we propose the following solutions for health implementers. First, they have to consider people's perceptions of the identities and meanings in health messages. There has been a lack of understanding in cultural meanings and the preferred mode of communication at the level of message design.

Health message designers can use various methods (e.g. community-based participatory research) to understand how members of a group identify with health messages. Particularly, message designers need to focus on developing benefit-based messages so that their intended audiences are more prone to change than resistant to change. For instance, the *Small Step* campaign conducted qualitative research to identify barriers to healthy habits (US DHHS and The Advertising Council 2004). Based on the findings, the campaign encouraged adoption of healthy lifestyles to prevent obesity and consequent health risks. The campaign emphasized that a 'small step' in everyday lives leads to positive spin. Once the designers understand the way that they perceive the messages, they may link relevant benefits and incentives to the messages with various marketing and branding strategies and tactics.

Second, health campaign should be audience-driven by listening to group members to identify cultural norms and values counter to what they deliver in brands. If they do not understand what audiences want, message–audience nonfit may occur and lead to a boomerang or iatrogenic effect. Cultural adaptation is required to avoid this nonfit. We suggest that health message designers employ participatory and interactive research to reflect cultural norms and values embedded in each culture. By doing so, health messages can deliver the messages that resonate cultural identities and membership.

Third, health implementers should prepare for unintended effects. After the prevention program, the program should be evaluated to investigate if there are any unintended effects. The DRS research team measured the effectiveness of the culturally grounded prevention program at the immediate posttest as well as 14-month follow-up test (Hecht *et al.* 2006). The tests may increase the chances to detect unintended effects because these provide important information about the effect of the program on the rate and pattern of change in substance use over time (Hecht *et al.* 2003).

Finally, narratives can be an alternative to resolve challenges to branding approaches. As discussed above, a brand is not just images, but stories in public health context. If health implementers utilize the stories of the group members, they can effectively reflect the implicit assumptions of each culture. By doing so, these narratives can also provide 'good reasons' to justify their actions based upon the dominant stories within each group and do so with fidelity and in a coherent fashion.

Conclusion

The culturally grounded approach to branding is based upon an elaborated conceptualization of culture that considers cultural codes (system of meaning), conversations (way of interacting) and communities (membership). Cultural grounding starts with the experiences of group members and identifies their stories in order to capture these three features of culture. Traditionally, culturally adapted approaches just modified the universal messages; however, cultural grounding emphasizes messages that incorporate the deep structure of culture, such as values, norms and identity, while starting with the code, conversation and communities of a culture rather than adding these features later.

The *keepin' it REAL* curriculum is a culturally grounded approach to preventing adolescents' substance abuse and provides a template for branded health messages. Through formative research the Drug Resistance Strategies project has developed health messages that are grounded in group members' salient meanings, narratives and identities. The cultural narratives identified in this research led to highly salient health messages that provide 'good reasons' to justify actions as well as models for their behaviors. This multicultural curriculum, with its proven efficacy, provides a model of developing culturally grounded, branded health messages. There is, of course, much to learn in this area. *keepin' it REAL* is meant to be an exemplar of a method for developing health messages that provides a starting point for developing culturally grounded health brands. We believe that this approach can be productively applied to public service announcements and other different types of health messages utilizing branding strategies with cultural and social forces.

References

Aaker, D. (1996). *Building strong brands*, New York, NY: Simon and Schuster Inc.

Aaker, L. A., Benet-Martinez, V., and Garolera, J. (2001). Consumption symbols as carriers of culture: A study of Japanese and Spanish brand personality constructs. *Journal of Personality and Social Psychology* **81**:492–508.

Appiah, O. (2001). Black, White, Hispanic, and Asian American adolescents' responses to culturally embedded ads. *The Howard Journal of Communications* **12**:29–48.

Appiah, O. (2004). Effects of ethnic identification on web-browsers' attitudes toward navigational patterns on race-targeted sites. *Communication Research*. **31**:312–37.

Algesheimer, R., Dholakia, U. M., and Herrmann, A. (2005). The social influence of brand community: evidence from European car clubs. *Journal of Marketing* **69**:19–34.

Allen, M., Bruflat, R., Fucilla, R., Kramer, M., McKellips, S., Ryan, D. J., and Spiegelhoff, M. (2000). Testing the persuasiveness of evidence: Combining narrative and statistical forms. *Communication Research Reports* **17**:331–336.

Baldwin, J. R., Faulkner, S. L., Hecht, M. L., and Lindsley, S. L. (2006). *Redefining culture: perspectives across the disciplines*, Mahwah, NJ: Lawrence Erlbaum Associates.

Bandura, A. (1986). *Social foundations of thought and action: a social cognitive theory.* Englewood Cliffs, NJ: Prentice Hall.

Batra, R., Myers, J. G., and Aaker, D. (1996). *Advertising management* (5th edn). Upper Saddle River, NJ: Prentice Hall.

Campanelli, M. (1991). The African American market: community, growth, and change. *Sales and Marketing Management* **143**:75–81.

Castro, F. G., Barrera, M., and Martinez, C. R. (2004). The cultural adaptation of prevention interventions: Resolving tensions between fidelity and fit. *Prevention Science* **5**:41–5.

Cock, K. D., Mbori-Ngacha, D., and Marum, E. (2002). Shadow on the continent: public health and HIV/AIDS in Africa in the 21st century. *Lancet* **360**:67–72.

Dana, L. and Oldfield, B. M. (1999). Lublin Coca-Cola Bottles Ltd. *International Marketing Review* **16**:291–8.

DiFranza, J. R., Richards, J. W., Paulman, P. M., Wolf-Gillespie, N., Fletcher, C., Jaffer, R. D., and Murray, D. (1992). RJR Nabisco's cartoon camel promotes Camel cigarettes to children. *Journal of the American Medical Association* **266**:3149–53.

Elek, E., Miller-Day, M., and Hecht, M. L. (2006). Influences of personal, injunctive, and descriptive norms on early adolescent substance use. *Journal of Drug Issues* **36**:147–72.

Evans, D., Price, S., and Blahut, S. (2005). Evaluating the Truth® brand. *Journal of Health Communication* **10**:181–92.

Farrelly, M. C., Healton, C. G., Davis, K. C., Messeri, P., Hersey, J. C., and Haviland, M. L. (2002). Getting to the Truth®: Evaluating national tobacco counter-marketing campaigns. *American Journal of Public Health* **92**:901–7.

Fisher, W. R. (1987). Human communication as a narration: toward a philosophy of reason, value, and action. Columbia, SC: University of South Carolina Press.

Gosin, M. N., Dustman, P. A., Harthun, M. L., and Drapeau, A. E. (2003). Participatory action research: Creating an effective prevention curriculum for adolescents in the southwest. *Health Education Research: Theory and Practice* **18**:363–79.

Gosin, M., Marsiglia, F. F., and Hecht, M. L. (2003). *Keepin' it REAL*: A drug resistance curriculum tailored to the strengths and needs of pre-adolescents of the Southwest. *Journal of Drug Education* **33**:119–42.

Green, M. C. (2006). Narratives and cancer communication. *Journal of Communication* **56**:163–83.

Greene, K. and Brinn, L. S. (2003). Messages influencing college women's tanning bed use: Statistical versus narrative evidence format and a self-assessment to increase perceived susceptibility. *Journal of Health Communication* **8**:443–61.

Hammer, T. (1989). The increase in alcohol consumption among women: A phenomenon related to accessibility or stress: A general population study. *British Journal of Addiction* **84**:767–75.

Hecht, M. L. (1993). 2002 – A research odyssey: Toward the development of a communication theory of identity. *Communication Monographs*, **60**:76–82.

Hecht, M. L. and Krieger, J. L. (2006). The principle of cultural grounding in school-based substance abuse prevention: The Drug Resistance Strategies project. *Journal of Language and Social Psychology* **25**:301–19.

Hecht, M. L. and Miller-Day, M. (2007). The Drug Resistance Strategies project as transitional research. *Journal of Applied Communication Research* **35**:343–9.

Hecht, M. L. and Miller-Day, M. (in press). The Drug Resistance Strategies project: a communication approach to preventing adolescent drug use. In L. Frey and K. Cissna (eds.) *Handbook of Applied Communication*. London, UK: Taylor and Francis.

Hecht, M. L., Corman, S. R., and Miller-Rassulo, M. (1993). An evaluation of the drug resistance project: A comparison of film versus live performance media. *Health Communication* **5**:75–88.

Hecht, M. L., Marsiglia, F. F., Elek, E., Wagstaff, D. A., Kulis, S., Dustman, P., and Miller-Day, M. (2003). Culturally grounded substance use prevention: An evaluation of the *keepin' it REAL* curriculum. *Prevention Science* **4**:233–47.

Hecht, M. L., Warren, J., Jung, J., and Krieger, J. (2004). Communication theory of identity. In W. B. Gudykunst (ed.) *Theorizing about intercultural communication*. Newbury Park, CA: Sage, pp. 257–278.

Hecht, M. L., Graham, J. W., and Elek, E. (2006). The Drug Resistance Strategies intervention: program effects on substance use. *Health Communication* **20**:267–76.

Howard, G. S. (1991). Culture tales: a narrative approach to thinking, cross-cultural psychology, and psychotherapy. *American Psychologist* **46**:187–97.

Huesman, L. R., Eron-Klein, R., Brice, P., and Fischer, P. (1983). Mitigating the imitation of aggressive behaviors by changing children's attitudes about medical violence. *Journal of Personality and Psychology* **44**:899–10.

Keegan, W. J. and Green, M. C. (2005). *Global marketing*. Upper Saddle River, NJ: Pearson Prentice Hall, pp. 119–21.

Keller, K. L. (1998). Branding perspectives on social marketing. *Advances in Consumer Research* **25**:299–302.

Keller, K. L. (2007). *Strategic brand management: building, measuring, and managing brand equity.* Upper Saddle River, NJ: Pearson Prentice Hall.

Kishii T. (1988). Message vs. mood: A look at some of the differences between Japanese and Western television commercials. *Dentsu Japan Marketing/Advertising Year Book.* Tokyo, Japan: Dentsu, Inc. pp. 51–57.

Koss, L. A. and Vargas, J. D. (1992). *Working with culture: psychotherapeutic intervention with ethnic minority children and adolescents.* San Francisco, CA: Jossey-Bass.

Korzenny, F. and Korzenny, B. A. (2005). *Hispanic marketing: a cultural perspective.* Oxford: Elsevier-Butterworth-Heinemann.

Kotler, P. (2002). *Marketing management.* Upper Saddle River, NJ: Pearson Prentice Hall.

Kreuter, M. W., Lukwago, S. N., Buchholtz, D. C., Clark, E. M., and Sanders-Thompson, V. S. (2003). Achieving cultural appropriateness in health promotion programs: targeted and tailored approaches. *Health Education and Behavior* **30**:133–46.

Kulis, S., Nieri, T. Yabiku, S., Stromwall, L. K., and Marsiglia, F. F. (2007a). Promoting reduced and discontinued substance use among adolescent substance users: Effectiveness of a universal prevention program. *Prevention Science* **8**:35–49.

Kulis, S., Yabiku, S. P., Marsiglia, F. F., Nieri, T., and Crossman, A. (2007b). Differences by gender, ethnicity, and acculturation in the efficacy of the *keepin' it REAL* model prevention program. *Journal of Drug Education* **37**:123–44.

Lake, R. A. (1997). Argumentation and self: the enactment of identity in 'Dances with Wolves'. *Argumentation and Advocacy* **34**:66–89.

McGuire, W. (1984). Search for the self: going beyond self-esteem and the reactive self. In R. A. Zucker, J. Aronoff, and A. I. Rabin (eds.) *Personality and prediction of behavior.* New York: Academic Press, pp. 73–120.

Melewar, T. C., Meadows, M., Zheng W., and Rickards, R. (2004). The influence of culture on brand building in the Chinese market: a brief insight. *Journal of Brand Management* **11**:449–61.

Mooij, M. K. (1997). *Global marketing and advertising: understanding cultural paradoxes.* Thousand Oaks, CA: Sage.

Ono, Y. (1997). Japan warms to McDonald's doting dad ads. *Wall Street Journal*, pp. B1, B12.

Philipsen, G. (1992). *Speaking culturally: explorations in social communication.* Albany, NY: State University of New York Press.

Resnicow, K., Baranowski, T., Ahluwalia, J. S., and Braithwaite, R. L. (1999). Cultural sensitivity in public health: defined and demystified. *Ethnicity and Disease* **9**:10–21.

Richins, M. L. (1994). Valuing things: The private and public meanings of possessions. *Journal of Consumer Research* **21**:504–21.

Robin, S. S. and Johnson, E. O. (1996). Attitude and peer cross pressure: adolescent drug and alcohol use. *Journal of Drug Education* **26**:69–99.

Rothschild, M. and Andreasen, A. R. (1998). Considering social marketing from the perspective of several consumer research paradigms. *Advances in Consumer Research* **25**:295–8.

Schinke, S. P., Botvin, G. J., Orlandi, M. A., Schilling, R. F., and Gordon, A. N. (1990). African-American and Hispanic-American adolescents HIV infection and preventive intervention. *AIDS Education and Prevention* **2**:305–12.

Shavitt, S. (1990). The role of attitude objects in attitude functions. *Journal of Experimental Social Psychology* **26**:124–148.

Stevenson, T. H. and McIntyre, P. E. (1995). A comparison of the portrayal and frequency of Hispanics and whites in English language television advertising. *Journal of Current Issues and Research in Advertising* **17**:65–74.

Strasburger, V. C. (2000). Children, adolescents, drugs, and the media. In D. G. Singer and J. L. Singer (eds.) *Handbook of children and the media*. Thousand Oaks, CA: Sage, pp. 415–45.

Street, R. L. and Giles, H. (1982). Speech accommodation theory: A social cognitive approach to language and speech behavior. In M. Roloff and C. R. Berger (eds.) *Social cognition and communication*. Beverly Hills, CA: Sage, pp. 193–226.

US Department of Health and Human Services (US DHHS) and The Advertising Council. (2004). Healthy lifestyles and disease prevention media campaign: Take a small step to get healthy. Available from: http://www.smallstep.gov/pdf/obesity_whitepaperfinal_71205.pdf (accessed 7 November 2007).

Vaughan, P. W. and Rogers, E. M. (2000). A staged model of communication effects: Evidence from an entertainment-education radio soap opera in Tanzania. *Journal of Health Communication* 5:203–27.

Warren, J. R., Hecht, M. L., Wagstaff, D. A., Elek, E., Ndiaye, K., Dustman, P., and Marsiglia, F. F. (2006). Communicating prevention: The effects of the *keepin' it REAL* classroom videotapes and televised PSAs on middle-school students' substance use. *Journal of Applied Communication Research* 34:209–27.

Whittler, T. E. (1991). The effects of actors' race in commercial advertising: review and extension. *Journal of Advertising* 20:54–60.

Williams, J. D. and Tharp, M. C. (2001). African Americans: ethnic roots, cultural diversity. In M. C. Tharp (ed.) *Marketing and consumer identity in multicultural America*. Thousand Oaks, CA: Sage, pp. 206–7.

10

Public health branding Down Under

Robert J. Donovan and Tom E. Carroll

Summary

- Brand image or positioning refers to the associations people have when reminded of or when confronted with the brand's logo, products or services.
- All elements of an integrated marketing mix contribute to brand image, but the most visible are the brand's promotional activities (advertising, sponsorship, publicity, etc.).
- Public health brands have traditionally focused on increasing target audiences' awareness of various health issues (agenda setting) and increasing awareness and encouraging adoption of preventive behaviours to reduce disease and injury.
- Following lessons from commercial marketing, public health campaigns can be even more successful by developing brand positionings that go beyond being simply informative, and begin to establish relationships with their target audiences.
- Public health campaigns are far more limited in funding than commercial campaigns, and hence more restricted in opportunities available for establishing a desired brand positioning. However, using formative research with the target audience to guide creativity in developing the actual brand name and graphics can contribute substantially to establishing the desired brand image.

Introduction – defining 'brands' and 'branding'

In this chapter we note and accept Bennett's long-established definition of a brand in commercial marketing as: 'a name, term, sign, symbol, or design, or a combination of these intended to identify the goods or services of one seller or group of sellers and to differentiate them from those of their competitors' (Kotler 1980: 366). While the 'identify' perhaps signifies the literal branding that occurred on livestock, the key element of this definition in current competitive commercial marketing is the word 'differentiate'. The differentiation may be in terms of product attributes (such as a toothpaste that contains 'whitening ingredient X'), or in emotive or lifestyle positionings around the brand (such as a toothpaste for young, on-the-go professionals). The latter differentiation is the hallmark of today's consumer society, which is characterized by a surplus of parity products and services, and where differentiation within product lines is often on a quality or product attribute or features basis. Twitchell (2004) describes branding as applying a 'story' to a product or service, and that for parity products, such narratives are the only difference between alternative brands.

'Branding' is taken to mean the process by which a brand image, identity or positioning is developed. 'Brand positioning' ('what the brand stands for') refers to the thoughts, feelings and images the brand generates in the target consumer's mind – and particularly relative to other brands (Ries and Trout 1981). That is, the brand's positioning is competitively derived to appeal to particular target segments. Brand positionings are sometimes measured in terms of 'brand personality' – sets of attributes (e.g. strong or weak, modern or old-fashioned, bold or timid, dull or exciting, and so on), or aim for a single strong perception (e.g. Volvo and safety, Maytag and dependability, Nordstrom and service, Mercedes and prestige). Such attributes are often related to measures of 'brand equity'. Brand equity is variously defined, but for us is the set of evaluative beliefs and images held by target consumers about the brand. The more favourable these are, the higher the brand equity. Brand equity can be measured in dollar terms by comparing what a consumer does (or would) pay for the same product but differently branded. A good example of this occurred recently in Australia where a Melbourne art gallery painting thought to be a Van Gogh turned out not to be so. Although clearly a good painting for the mistake to have been made (it was not a forgery), the value of the painting plummeted from AU$50 million to less than $5 million in the absence of the Van Gogh 'brand' (Perkins 2007).

Following Bennett's definition, the *brand name* is the voiced part, while the *brand mark* is the non-voiced part. In commercial marketing, most brands begin as the manufacturer's or owner's name, with many still based on the manufacturer's name or names that mean little other than what the brand's positioning has created (e.g. Nike, Hertz, Kraft, Marlboro, Harley-Davidson and so on). For more recent brand names, apart from being easy to pronounce and easy to remember (e.g. Kodak), it is desirable (but not essential) for the brand name to indicate something about the brand's use, benefits or strengths (e.g. Snugglers, Weight Watchers, Toys 'R' Us, Mr Muscle, Diet Coke, Energiser). Noting the opportunity for charging higher prices for better quality, marijuana smuggler Alan Long separated his supplies on quality, branding his top grade crop 'Columbia *Gold*' and his lower grade 'Columbia *Red*' (Sabbag 2002). In a few cases, the brand name has attempted to describe the product's use (e.g. Shake 'n' Bake, Dial-a-Dinner, Post-It Notes).

A brand's logo is often a combination of the brand name and a graphic design, or simply a graphic design. Some brands have invested heavily in a graphic (e.g. Nike's swoosh; McDonald's arches; the Playboy bunny) or colour(s) (e.g. John Deere's green; Marlboro's red; Kodak's yellow) to aid recognition and differentiation.

There is also the issue of 'brands' and 'slogans' – statements attached to the brand (e.g. General Electric's 'We bring good things to life', dropped in 2003 after 24 years). Attaching slogans to brand names was one of the early attempts to create brand positionings around what were essentially manufacturer's names. Slogans can contribute very positively to brand image and reinforce the brand's positioning (although consumers do not always match slogans with the correct brand). Many Australian public health brands can be viewed as slogans about one or other aspects of a healthy lifestyle attached to a logo, where the slogan describes the desired behaviour and the graphics are used to communicate brand attributes and the target audience. For example, Colac Area Health's *Be Active Eat Well* project aimed to build the capacity of the Colac community to promote healthy eating and physical activity. The primary target audiences were children aged 2–12 years and their parents and carers. Their campaign brand/logo (Fig. 10.1) can be viewed as a slogan with accompanying graphics to appeal to its target audience of young children (incidentally accompanied by a further slogan: 'Making it easy').

Overall then, in commercial marketing, a brand is defined by multiple characteristics – the style and graphic design, font style, colours, etc., as well as by the messages delivered about the brand, and how and where these messages are delivered. This is the integration element of the marketing mix: packaging, pricing, distribution, advertising content and execution all contribute to and must be consistent with the brand image (e.g. an up-market perfume for elegant evening wear must be packaged in expensive looking materials, sold only through up-market stores and feature glamorous rather than sporting models). As emphasized in Chapter 1, branding encapsulates the relationship between individuals and the promoted product, and the added value in the exchange associated with using the product.

For our purposes, the branding of public health campaigns in Australia can be viewed as having operated primarily at three levels. At the basic level, branding is assumed to have occurred when the campaign has developed a specific brand and logo that, like the branding of livestock, has been placed on campaign materials to signify the campaign source, and where campaign materials follow a consistent graphical style. Recent examples include The National Tobacco Campaign and The National Alcohol Campaign brands. While these brands were accompanied with a tagline 'Every cigarette is doing you damage' and 'Drinking. Where are your choices taking you?' respectively, at this basic level there is far less concern for the 'brand image' than for ensuring people's understanding of the campaign's public health focus.

At a second level, a number of public health brands were developed around the specific behavioural message. Some early (and continuing) Australian brands that reflect this primary concern for the behaviour change message and lesser concern for brand attributes

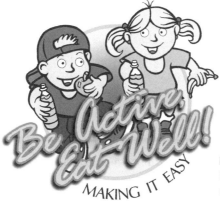

Fig. 10.1 *Be Active Eat Well* brand/logo. Reproduced with permission from *Be Active Eat Well*.

include *Slip, Slop, Slap* (sun protection), *2 Fruit 'n' 5 Veg* (now *Go for 2&5*) (nutrition), *Under 05 or Under Arrest* (drinking and driving), *Drink Safe* and *Alcohol. Go Easy* (alcohol), and *Be Active* and *Find 30* (physical activity).

At a third level, campaign originators are explicitly concerned with how their brand is perceived in the minds of the target audience. This type of public health branding, which seeks to establish a relationship with its target audience members in the same way as commercial marketers do, is illustrated later in this chapter through case studies of the *Freedom from Fear* domestic violence campaign and Mentally Healthy WA's *Act-Belong-Commit* campaign.

One example of how a brand has transformed over the years is in the area of sun protection. The *Slip, Slop, Slap* brand of the 1990s was used by a number of agencies to clearly signal the desired behavioural responses of *slipping* on a shirt, *slopping* on sunscreen and *slapping* on a hat. While these sun protection messages remain and have now been added to with *sliding* on sunglasses and *seeking* some shade, the *Slip, Slop, Slap* branding for sun protection campaigns has been replaced by *SunSmart*, representing 'what consumers are' when they adopt these sun protection behaviours. This *SunSmart* brand is now used effectively to market sun protection products and encompasses broader sun protection programmes and upstream policy initiatives.

As well as concern about the way a brand is perceived by the particular target audience with respect to its messages, a brand developed for government-sponsored campaigns will inevitably be developed with a view to how stakeholders will perceive its appropriateness for a publicly funded programme of activity (i.e. organizational branding). Similarly, non-government organizations will be concerned with perceived appropriateness of fit by funding agencies, supporters and stakeholders.

Some early public health brands in Australia

Quit and the Quitline

Quit is one of Australia's earliest and most recognized health brands. Use of the *Quit* brand dates back to the late 1970s when a quit smoking campaign was trialled as part of the North Coast Healthy Lifestyle Campaign in Australia's most populous state of New South Wales. This brand was initially developed as *Quit. For life*, signalling a health behaviour as well as a health goal and duration for the behaviour change. Based on the success of this trial (Egger *et al.* 1983), the *Quit. For life* campaign was extended throughout New South Wales in 1983. Tobacco control campaigns bearing the *Quit* brand (shortened from *Quit. For life*) soon emerged in other Australian states. The branding was followed through to the telephone counselling 'Quitline' and products such as the '5-day Quit Book', and in 1987, to sponsorship of a league football team. These campaigns focused on the objective of motivating and supporting smokers to quit smoking with little attention paid to how people viewed the campaign brand per se. However, although there were no explicit brand attribute objectives, it was implicitly desired that the *Quit* campaign was not seen to be 'telling' smokers what to do, but rather presenting them with information about the health consequences of smoking and letting them make up their own mind. In this sense, the concern was not about the word (brand) 'Quit' per se being seen as directive, but rather that advertising and other messages delivered by *Quit* should not be seen as directive.

Despite the fact that *Quit* campaigns operated at a state and territory jurisdictional level throughout Australia, sometimes operating within state governments and sometimes within Cancer Council non-government organizations, the *Quit* brand became nationally recognized as the graphics and style were adopted consistently across jurisdictions. This resulted in additional awareness for the brand throughout Australia when any national media reported on *Quit* campaign activity in any state, as well as facilitating sharing of resources across jurisdictions. This nationally consistent *Quit* branding also translated effectively to the establishment and promotion of a single Quitline telephone counselling and information service for advertising under Australia's successful National Tobacco Campaign (Hill and Carroll 2003), and, more recently, to the placement of a single Quitline number alongside graphic health warnings on tobacco products sold in Australia (Australian Government Department of Health and Ageing 2007). As *Quit* is a cessation message targeting smokers, sub-brands such as *Smoking. No way!* and *Smokefree* have been developed for prevention initiatives. While *Quit* could be categorized as a level two public health brand initially, primarily focused on a behavioural message, the brand would now reflect the characteristics of a level three brand, particularly with respect to its Quitline variant where significant effort is being directed into generating positive perceptions of a trusting relationship between potential callers and the Quitline counsellors.

The Drug Offensive

Another well-known Australian public health brand in the 1980s and 1990s was *The Drug Offensive*. In 1985 the Australian federal, state and territory governments came together for what was termed The Drug Summit. As a result of this meeting, a commitment was made to fund the National Campaign Against Drug Abuse (NCADA), involving initiatives in education, treatment, rehabilitation and research as well as increasing the commitment to controls and enforcement (NCADA 1985). Significantly, it was decided that the NCADA would focus on reducing problems associated with alcohol and tobacco use in addition to illegal drugs. While the total campaign was to be called the National Campaign Against Drug Abuse, a sub-brand was developed for its media and social marketing activities called *The Drug Offensive* (1986–1995). The following description of *The Drug Offensive* draws on Carroll (1996).

The Drug Offensive adopted a literal branding style, appearing as 'a stamp' featuring a map of Australia and the words 'The Drug Offensive' in bold uppercase, with a subscript 'A Federal and State initiative' to signal the collaborative arrangements between these levels of government (see Fig. 10.2).

The brand logo was designed to show a strong national commitment by Australia's governments to addressing the problems of drug abuse in Australia. However, as the brand came to be used for specific campaigns primarily addressing youth audiences, the perceptions of young people toward the brand as the source of campaign messages became an important consideration.

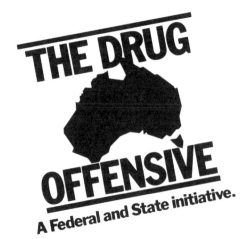

Fig. 10.2 The Drug Offensive logo.

For a decade, *The Drug Offensive* campaigns played a key role during the NCADA and the subsequent National Drug Strategy and were successful in reaching significant numbers of their respective target audiences and communicating effectively in line with designated communication objectives. After an initial public awareness campaign about drugs and the components of the NCADA in 1986, various drug-specific campaigns were staged from 1987 to 1995, beginning with heroin use, and covering teenage smoking, teenage and adult alcohol consumption, pharmaceutical drug misuse, tobacco smoking among young women, alcohol-related violence and amphetamine use. This was an example of how a single brand can be utilized to encompass a number of related health behaviours. Consistently branding messages about tobacco use and excessive alcohol consumption under *The Drug Offensive* along with messages about illegal drugs resulted in a reassessment of the public's perceptions of what constitutes a 'drug problem'. In other words, the branding increased perceptions of the harm associated with legal drugs (Makkai and McAllister 1998).

However, the major target audiences for *The Drug Offensive* campaigns were young people. Social marketing initiatives that provided continuity of engagement and communication with youth target audiences played an important role in building equity and positive attributes for the brand. Sponsorship marketing played a key role in positioning *The Drug Offensive* brand. For example, at the time of *The Drug Offensive* anti-amphetamine campaign, amphetamines were seen to fit with the dance party scene and dance music. Hence the central element of sponsorship was a series of *Drug Offensive*/Video Smash Hits Dance Parties, staged around the country in capital cities and regional areas in conjunction with the Seven Television Network's Video Smash Hits programme. The dance parties featured nine of Australia's then most popular young dance artists who endorsed *The Drug Offensive* campaign brand. In this way the campaign brand was taken to dance floors across the country by the stars of popular dance culture themselves. Importantly, endorsement of the campaign brand was not just coming from an individual celebrity but from a number of celebrities, thereby increasing the breadth of appeal to individual target audience members.

Through association over a number of years with youth music (e.g. weekly live concert broadcasts, artist endorsements and sponsorship of awards nights), sport events (e.g. surfing, basketball) and youth cultural events (The Rock Eisteddfod school student dance performance), *The Drug Offensive* brand came to be viewed by Australian youth as a credible message source for messages about both legal and illegal drugs. A brand perception study showed that while NACADA was seen to represent 'adults who wore suits and funded various government services', *The Drug Offensive* was perceived as being run by 'young people who wore jeans and spent a lot of time relating to teenagers'. While both brands were government 'owned', this stark contrast in brand perceptions reflected a strong degree of trust and credibility by young Australians in *The Drug Offensive* brand.

This brand equity led to the creative decision to open later campaign radio commercials with 'A message from *The Drug Offensive*' instead of the source being identified at the end of an advertisement. Research indicated that young people actually paid more attention to the radio advertisement's message when they were alerted to the fact that it was *The Drug Offensive* talking to them than when the source came later. It can be seen that the characteristics of *The Drug Offensive* brand transformed from what was described above as a basic-level branding to what would be viewed as a level three brand over the course of its use.

Case studies

We now present two case studies. The first concerns a relatively well established area (domestic violence) but where a new approach was being undertaken (targeting violent men to voluntarily seek help). In this case it was crucial that the overall branding be sensitive to the acceptance of this new approach in the established stakeholder groups. The second involves developing a brand in the relatively new and far broader area of mental health promotion, hence requiring far more thought to the specifics of the actual words and graphics used in the branding. Each of the case studies follows the same presentation format.

Case study 1: Targeting male perpetrators of intimate partner violence – the Freedom From Fear campaign

Overview

Western Australia's *Freedom From Fear* domestic violence campaign targets male perpetrators of intimate partner violence. Mass media advertising is used to create and maintain awareness of the 'Men's Domestic Violence Helpline' and to encourage violent and potentially violent men to call the helpline. The primary aim of the helpline counsellors is to refer as many as possible qualified callers into no-fee government-funded counselling programmes provided primarily by private sector organizations. The following description is drawn from publications by Donovan and colleagues (Donovan *et al.* 1999; Donovan *et al.* 2000; Donovan and Henley 2003).

Background

Violence against women by their partners is recognized as a major international public health problem, in both developed and developing countries. While intimate partner violence also involves female-to-male partner violence and same sex partner violence, male-to-female partner violence occurs more frequently and with far more serious consequences in terms of injury and death (Sorenson *et al.* 1996).

Intimate partner violence has major consequences for the physical and mental health of the women and for children and other family members (Gomel 1997). The victim-related economic cost of partner violence in the USA has been estimated to be in the vicinity of $67 billion (APS Observer 1997). The costs of such violence cannot be calculated simply in terms of emergency ward treatments, hospital bed nights, refugee home placements, lives lost in homicides and suicides, and so on. There also are enormous costs in terms of children's lost happiness and subsequent dysfunctional behaviours. Incarceration costs for convicted perpetrators also must be taken into account.

Most programmes aimed at the reduction of abuse have been based around the criminal justice system, targeting both police and the judiciary (Donovan and Vlais 2006). Where public education components have accompanied such campaigns, these have aimed at increasing the public's (and perpetrators') perception that domestic violence is a crime (Buchanan 1996). Such campaigns generally encourage women to report incidents, and, where necessary, to leave the family home and to take out civil protection (or 'restraining') orders against violent partners.

While the incarceration of violent men and the issuing of protection orders do alleviate some violence (Keilitz *et al.* 1998), they do not – and cannot – remove the fear women experience in terms of the man reappearing at some time in some place, often with tragic consequences (De Becker 1998). Furthermore, many women do not want to leave the relationship, nor do they want the man incarcerated; they simply want the violence to stop; in short, they literally want freedom from fear in their relationship.

The *Freedom From Fear* campaign

'*Freedom From Fear*' was originally designed as a ten-year community education programme complementing criminal justice and other community interventions. As far as we are aware, this campaign was a then unique initiative, being the first government-funded, mass media based, non-punitive campaign focusing primarily on male perpetrators of domestic violence, asking them to voluntarily seek help to change their violent ways.

The idea for this approach – targeting male perpetrators to voluntarily seek help – arose from a government task force established in 1995 to address the issue of family and domestic violence in Western Australia. However, directing resources towards male perpetrator programmes was generally viewed negatively by female victim support organizations. Hence it was crucial to gain women's organizations' and female victims' support for the programme in principle, and then ensure their continued support for the various programme materials as they were produced. It was required that this sector be reassured that targeting perpetrators and funding perpetrator programmes was consistent with the 'feminist' philosophy with respect to domestic violence prevention; that is, that victim safety is paramount and that directing services towards men must ultimately be about victim safety and freedom from fear.

After extensive consultations with all relevant stakeholders, especially women's advocacy groups, women's refuges and women themselves, and with the government promising extra funding for the campaign (i.e. no reduction in funds for women and children), sufficient tentative support was obtained for formative research to begin in 1996. After extensive pretesting against all stakeholders and target groups (Donovan *et al.* 2000), the campaign was launched toward the end of 1998.

Campaign goals and overall strategy

The overall goals of the campaign are the reduction of violence against women by male partners and, consequently, increased physical and mental health among victims. Fig. 10.3 summarizes the overall campaign strategy. Mass media advertising is used to motivate perpetrators and potential perpetrators of physical violence against their female partner to call a confidential helpline manned by trained counsellors. The goal of telephone counselling is to enrol men in a behaviour change programme.

Campaign target groups

While the primary beneficiaries of the campaign were the women and children of men who use violence, the primary target audiences for the campaign were male perpetrators

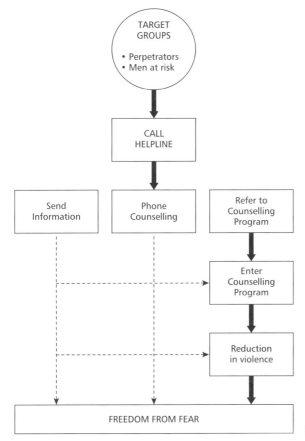

Fig. 10.3 Campaign overview.

and potential perpetrators in Prochaska's contemplation, ready for action or action stages (Prochaska and DiClemente 1984) with respect to doing something about their violence or potential violence. While these men may still minimize and deny (at some level or on some occasions) full responsibility for their behaviour, they are reachable through mass media because they do accept *some* responsibility for their behaviour. Hardcore perpetrators still in a strong state of denial (Eisikovits and Buchbinder 1997) were not part of the primary target audience for this campaign.

Potential perpetrators were defined as those subjecting their partner to non-physical forms of abuse (e.g. emotional abuse, financial deprivation, social isolation). Potential perpetrators also include men with undesirable attitudes towards partner abuse (e.g. believed violence by the male partner was justified or often provoked in certain situations).

Secondary target audiences consisted of 'all other 18–40 year old males' and those individuals who might encourage the primary target audiences to seek assistance: victims; family members, friends and professionals with whom they might come in contact (e.g. lawyers, doctors, nurses, police officers, counsellors). For example, police were encouraged to promote perpetrators' use of the telephone counselling service when called to 'domestics', and particularly where no charges could or would be laid. Finally, the campaign targeted all members of the community in terms of maintaining the salience of domestic violence as a community concern, and in terms of reinforcing men not engaged in violent behaviour. It was also important to create and reinforce positive community attitudes to the counselling of violent men as a legitimate domestic violence prevention strategy (complementary to police arrest and sentencing, and mandatory referral into counselling by courts), and hence worthy of government funding.

Communication and behavioural objectives

Among members of the primary and secondary target groups, the main communication objectives were to increase awareness that non-punitive, anonymous help was available and to stimulate motivations and intentions to seek help. The intermediate behavioural objective was that they should call the helpline for assistance, or seek assistance from some credible source. The final behavioural objectives, particularly following counselling, were a reduction in violent incidents – both physical and verbal – among perpetrators, and the prevention of violence among potentials.

For all audiences, the implicit communication objectives were that: (a) the perpetrator, not the victim, is responsible for the violence; and (b) that there are no circumstances in which violence is justified.

Campaign development and branding

Formative research was required to firstly 'get the right message' and then 'get the message right' (Egger *et al.* 1993). Getting the right message refers to establishing what message content would motivate violent men to seek help. Getting the message right refers to executing the message in a language and style that violent men would pay attention to, understand and find believable, yet not be seen to condemn nor condone their violence. Furthermore, the ads could not make victims of domestic violence feel responsible, guilty or more helpless.

A number of concepts were tested among groups of men who used violence and men in general. The testing showed that the damaging impact on children exposed to their violence was the most powerful motivator among perpetrators to take steps to stop their violence. All expressed strong feelings for their children, recalling that their children's reactions to specific instances of domestic violence had a very vivid impact on them, and many could relate to their own feelings when they were children. Thus, this theme had relevance whether or not they themselves had children. Furthermore, the damage to children theme was accepted by pre-contemplator perpetrators, and hence had potential to move this group towards contemplation. This theme was also considered to be effective by men in general and was selected as the key message strategy for the initial phase of the campaign.

Help being available was universally endorsed by contemplator perpetrators; it was seen as a positive message and contemplators were aware that they needed help but did not know how to go about getting it. This theme was also strongly endorsed by men in general and there was broad community support for a media campaign to publicize this assistance.

Overall then, the phase one formative research confirmed a potentially substantial number of violent and potentially violent men that could be reached by, and would respond to, a mass media campaign that offered formal assistance. The key to reaching this audience was to avoid being judgmental and to focus on the damaging effects on children of men's violence toward their partner as the motivator to take action.

It was crucial that the ads, although scheduled to be run only at 'adult times', did not trigger clinical stress symptoms in children, especially children of victims, and that children did not misunderstand the ads and think they were being asked to call the helpline or that they should ask their father to call the helpline. Hence groups of children at selected women's refuges were exposed to the advertising materials while a child psychologist observed and probed the children's reactions.

Three television commercials were aired in the first phase of the campaign:

- *'Nightmare'*: depicts a child tossing and turning in bed against a shadowy background and brief visuals and sound effects of a man abusing a woman. Subtitles state that 'this little boy is not having a nightmare, he is living one'.

- *'Horror Movie'*: two children are watching television against a similar background as above. The subtitles state that 'these children are not watching a horror movie, they are watching something far more frightening'.

- *'Back Seat'*: a child's view, from the back seat of a car, of a male verbally abusing a woman in the front seat. The child tosses to and fro covering her ears. The subtitles state: 'this 6 year old hates travelling by car … because the trip often ends with someone getting hurt'.

The ads end with spoken words such as 'Do something about it. Call the Men's Domestic Violence Helpline' and 'You can stop domestic violence. We can help you change'.

Branding the campaign

Given the diversity of interest groups in the domestic violence area and the initial reluctance among some to support this approach, an umbrella brand name was sought that would unite all of these groups under a common goal. Furthermore, although the campaign was targeting male perpetrators, the brand was required to reflect that the primary beneficiaries of the campaign were to be the women and children involved.

Freedom from fear is one of the four basic freedoms espoused by Franklin Roosevelt in his 1941 annual address to congress. Roosevelt used the term in relation to fear of physical acts of aggression by one country against another. The term is particularly apt in this area as it is the stress from constant fear of violence that is as debilitating, if not more so in many cases, as the actual violence. It directly reflects what women subject to violence actually want, and what is more likely to be delivered by a voluntary rather than mandatory commitment to counselling.

Overall, *Freedom From Fear* encapsulates the goal of all those working to stop violence against women and children's exposure to violence in the home, and explicitly states the underlying benefit promised by the campaign to women.

The name and graphics (see Fig. 10.4) are also positive in that the brand offers hope and is goal-directed. It is gender-free and can therefore unite all persons working against violence and can apply to same-sex partner violence as well as violence against men by a female intimate partner. Another major consideration was that the name could apply to all areas of violence – not just intimate partner violence and hence could eventually serve as a general umbrella brand against all forms of violence in the community.

The *Freedom From Fear* brand was initially directed primarily at professionals and others in the areas of family violence and violence against women and was present on all mass media and print materials, although where the materials targeted men, it was smaller than the sub-brand of the *Men's Domestic Violence Helpline* (see Fig. 10.5).

Sub-branding

The *Men's Domestic Violence Helpline* was a sub-brand of the campaign designed to have direct appeal to the primary target audiences (see Fig. 10.5). The message was succinct, the font was 'masculine', and the words 'Men's' and 'Helpline' dominated the branding, with the emphasis on 'Men's'.

The graphics depicted a telephone inside a man's head. Lines around the head depicted the 'pressure' men reported feeling when they used violence and afterwards. The colours

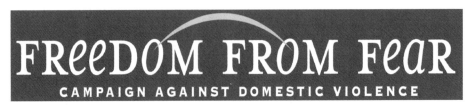

Fig. 10.4 *Freedom From Fear* brand/logo.

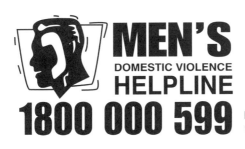

Fig. 10.5 *Mens' Domestic Violence Helpline brand/logo.*

(black and tan) and style were carried through to the self-help materials sent to men who called the helpline.

Both the *Men's Domestic Violence Helpline* sub-brand and the overall *Freedom From Fear* brand offered men a resolution to the anxiety, stress and remorse they felt as a result of their violence. The brands also offered them the promise of, and the way to achieve, a better relationship with their partners and children in exchange for their calling the helpline and enrolling in a counselling programme.

The marketing mix

The following is based on the '4 Ps' of tangible product marketing – product, price, promotion and place, in addition to the fifth 'P' (people) for services marketing (after Cowell 1984).

Product The 'core' product, that is, the value or end-benefit being offered by the brand to violent men in relationships, was the opportunity to keep their relationship and family intact by ending the violence towards their partner.

'Actual' products (services) were:

- Counselling (or 'behaviour change') programmes delivered by private service providers, subsidized by the government. Prior to this campaign there were few such programmes available (mostly attended by men under court orders), nor were counselling programmes promoted. Six new perpetrator and five new victim/children's counselling programmes were funded by the state government.

- The Men's Domestic Violence Helpline, staffed by trained counsellors who offered counselling over the phone and attempted to get violent callers into counselling programmes ('referrals'). Prior to this campaign there was no helpline specifically for perpetrators who voluntarily sought help.

- Self-help booklets and audio-cassettes (for men with literacy difficulties) that provided tips on how to control violence and how to contact service providers.

People The telephone counsellors were men who had considerable skills training and experience in dealing with men who used violence. These counsellors were able to gain the trust of men, 'listen' to their stories, assess level of denial and minimization, yet confront men with these aspects of their behaviour, undertake counselling and encourage them into programmes. If the caller could not be encouraged to accept referral – which required the caller to provide contact details for forwarding to the service provider – the telephone counsellors delivered counselling over the phone or attempted to engage the caller sufficiently so as to obtain permission to send, at no cost, educational self-help materials to an address nominated by the caller.

Promotion The primary medium for reaching violent and potentially violent men was television advertising (especially in sporting programmes), supported by radio advertising and posters. Extensive formative research was undertaken to ensure acceptance of the ad messages by the target group without negatively impacting victims/children and relevant stakeholders. It was necessary to avoid being judgmental so as to engage the attention and acceptance of members of the target audience. Simultaneously, it was essential – from victims' and other stakeholders' points of view – not to be seen to condone violence.

Extensive public relations activities were undertaken with relevant stakeholders, especially women's groups, police, counselling professions and other government departments. This involved repeated visits to these organizations and continually updating them on campaign developments.

Campaign information packs were distributed by mail to worksites with the assistance of a number of trade unions. The main aim in phase one was to distribute posters advertising the helpline to worksites and to alert the appropriate worksite professionals (usually the occupational health and safety officer or human resources manager) about the campaign.

Price With respect to dollar costs, although domestic violence occurs across all income levels, preliminary investigations and service-provider experience suggested that fees for courses and materials could serve as a barrier (or be rationalized as such) for many members of the primary target audience. Hence, all materials and most counselling programmes were provided at no cost to participants who were referred through the helpline. This pricing strategy also attempted to ensure that victims of low-income perpetrators would not be disadvantaged by their partner's limited income.

To minimize potential psychological and legal costs, the helpline assured anonymity and the counsellors were trained to deal with shame and embarrassment issues.

Place Where the caller accepted a referral, the counsellor took details from the caller and completed a referral form, which was faxed to the appropriate service provider the same day. Service providers were required to contact callers within two days to make an appointment for an assessment interview. Most callers were seen within one week. The referral process involved cooperation between two government departments and all (competing) service providers. This cooperation was gained only after extensive consultation and interpersonal networking.

Service providers were located throughout the metropolitan area and in six regional areas throughout the state. Programmes were scheduled to allow employed males access in non-working hours. However, access to programmes (but not to telephone counselling) was geographically limited outside major population centres. The telephone counselling and self-help booklets were especially useful for those not able to access a counselling programme. The decision to make a call requires some 'courage' on the part of the caller, with the act of calling often following a period of indecision. Hence, it was important that sufficient staff were always on hand to receive and act on calls. Putting callers on hold or asking them to call back can result in the caller losing motivation and cycling back one or more stages of change. That is, for some men, there is only a small 'window of opportunity' when the perpetrator actually makes the call, usually in the remorse phase of what is known as the 'cycle of abuse' (Roberts 1984).

Campaign results

By January 2005, the campaign had received over 21,000 calls, almost 13,000 of which were from the target group. Of these, 8,200 men identified themselves as perpetrators and 3,800 voluntarily entered counselling. Self-report evaluation instruments indicate that men who complete the programme say they are less likely to use physical violence and more likely to accept that they, and not their partners or their children, are responsible for the violence (Cant 2002).

Comment

This innovative campaign clearly demonstrated the feasibility of using social marketing principles to achieve voluntary behaviour change in an area where the emphasis has traditionally been – and continues to be – on criminal justice threats. This has been a significant breakthrough in the domestic violence area, where support for funds directed at perpetrators has not been readily forthcoming. These positive outcomes reflect that the investment in money, time and effort to ensure that the message strategy was right and that the ads were executed appropriately was a sound investment. This was particularly important for a campaign that would be subject to intense scrutiny because of its departure from traditional approaches and the scarcity of funds in this area.

The success of the campaign has been facilitated by the integration of all aspects of the campaign (price, promotion, people, place, and product); the extensive and sensitive use of research; the use of conceptual frameworks (i.e. stages of change, communication principles in message design); and the formation of partnerships with all relevant stakeholders across the public and private sectors in a highly political and socially sensitive area.

The strong, positive *Freedom From Fear* branding of the campaign facilitated the job of regional domestic violence coordinators and provided a focus for all working in the area of family and domestic violence. A major benefit was that the strong branding via the television advertising – and the name itself – made it much easier to gain access to worksites and other institutions. Domestic violence workers reported that calling and introducing themselves as from the *Freedom From Fear* campaign received a much more friendly response than did 'I'm the regional domestic violence coordinator', and far more acceptance of a visit by the worker to talk about domestic violence.

The sub-branding of the *Men's Domestic Violence Helpline* provided a clear indication to men who used violence that this telephone service was specifically for them, that the individuals on the other end of the helpline would understand their feelings, and that the helpline would offer confidentiality and 'real' help.

More information is available from the campaign website (www.freedomfrom fear.wa.gov.au).

Case study 2: Promoting positive mental health – *Mentally Healthy WA*

Overview

The *Mentally Healthy WA* campaign is conducted by a research group within the Faculty of Health Sciences at Curtin University in Western Australia (WA). The campaign targets individuals to be proactive about their mental health and wellbeing, and simultaneously targets organizations that provide mentally healthy activities to promote their activities under the *Act-Belong-Commit* banner. The campaign provides a simple framework to assist mental health promotion professionals communicate with and gain the cooperation of potential partners and stakeholders for mental health promotion programmes. This description draws on Donovan *et al.* (2003, 2006a, 2007).

Background

Using measures of disability-adjusted life years, Murray and Lopez (1996) have shown that mental health disorders emerge as a highly significant component of global disease burden when disability, as well as death, is taken into account. Their projections show that mental health conditions could increase their share of the total global burden by almost half, from 10.5 per cent of the total burden to almost 15 per cent by 2020.

The growth of mental health problems and consequent demand for treatment services have led to growing international interest in promotion, prevention and early intervention for mental health. However, interventions to date have been largely directed towards those suffering mental health problems, early identification of at-risk individuals or de-stigmatization of the mentally ill (e.g. Morrow *et al.* 2002; European Commission 2004; Davis and Tsiantis 2005; Janè-Llopis *et al.* 2005; Saxena *et al.* 2005). While there are a number of school and worksite interventions aimed at building positive mental health (Durlak and Wells 1997; Stewart *et al.* 2004), other than the Victorian Health Promotion Foundation's (VicHealth) current *Together we do better* campaign (Walker *et al.* 2004) and California's 1982 *Friends can be good medicine* campaign (Hersey *et al.* 1984; Taylor *et al.* 1984), we could find no published literature on population-wide mental health promotion campaigns that targeted people to be proactive about maintaining and building their own (and others') mental health. For example, the World Health Organization and World Federation for Mental Health joint publication, *Mental health promotion: case studies from countries* (Saxena and Garrison 2004) describes 35 programmes from around the world, none of which is a comprehensive community-wide positive mental health promotion campaign.

The *Mentally Healthy WA* campaign

Given the increasing awareness of the need for positive mental health promotion, the Western Australian Health Promotion Foundation (Healthway) commissioned qualitative research with people in general as well as mental health professionals to inform a mental health promotion campaign in Western Australia (Donovan *et al.* 2003).

The researchers suggested two possible starting points for a mental health promotion campaign in Western Australia: one targeting individuals in general to be more proactive about their own mental health; and one targeting individuals in authority over others to be more aware of their impact on their charges' mental health. The former would encourage individuals to engage in activities that would enhance their mental health (e.g. social, arts and sporting organization membership; community involvement; physical and mental activities; family socializing; hobbies; etc.), and would simultaneously encourage the numerous community organizations offering such activities to promote their activities under a mental health benefit message. The latter would focus on interactions between those in authority and those under their charge or care (i.e. supervisors and their workers; parents and their children; teachers and their students; coaches and their trainees; service personnel and customers), with the aim of replacing coercive, negative styles with encouraging, positive styles.

It was decided in the first phase of the campaign to focus on the individual/community organization focus. After a six-month feasibility study to recruit intervention sites and personnel, and to develop and pretest communication materials, the campaign was piloted and evaluated in six towns in regional Western Australia. It was launched in the six towns progressively through October and November 2005 for a two-year period.

Campaign goals and overall strategy

Given that people rarely consider what they could or should be doing for their mental health (in contrast to the salience and proactive intentions about their physical health), a primary objective was to reframe people's perceptions of mental health away from the absence of mental illness, to the belief that people can (and should) act proactively to protect and strengthen their mental health.

The campaign objectives were to increase individuals' awareness of things they can (and should) do to enhance or improve their own mental health and to increase individuals' participation in individual and community activities that increase mental health and reduce vulnerability to mental health problems.

Broader goals were to build cohesion in communities by fostering links between organizations around a unifying theme of positive mental health and building links between those in the community dealing with mental health problems and those in the community with the capacity to strengthen positive mental health.

In essence, the campaign aims to increase individual and community wellbeing by increasing and strengthening connections between community members via their participation in family and community events and organizations, as well as increasing collaborations between community organizations that offer activities conducive to good mental health and wellbeing. This is depicted in Figs 10.6 and 10.7, where people are shown on the right-hand side and organizations on the left-hand side. Lines show people's participation in organizations and connections between organizations. Towns with high social capital will already have many strong connections between people and organizations. In Fig. 10.7, the *Mentally Healthy WA* project officer

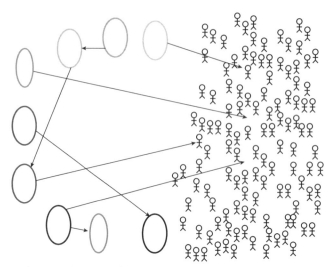

Fig. 10.6 Community Organization and community members prior to *Act-Belong-Commit* unconnected or weakly connected

'parachutes into town' with the task of building these connections: getting people participating in community organizations' activities and getting the organizations to collaborate more – hence increasing and strengthening connections between and among people and organizations in the town.

Campaign target groups

Our two primary target groups were individual community members and office holders or owners of community organizations or businesses that offered activities conducive to good mental health (e.g. libraries, sporting and recreational clubs, tourism operators, volunteer associations, walking groups, educational institutions, eco-environmental groups, arts and craft groups, etc.). In a sense, these constituted respectively, 'end-consumers' and 'retailers' (partners). These organizations provided both a channel through which to deliver messages (e.g. posters and banners at events) as well as the 'products' (behaviours) for end-consumers to 'purchase' (i.e. adopt or participate in).

Communication and behavioural objectives

The communication objectives for individuals in general were to increase their awareness of what they could and should do to increase or maintain good mental health and to motivate intentions to act proactively for their mental health. Communication objectives for community organization office-holders were to increase their awareness that the activities they provided were good for participants' mental health and to motivate intentions to join in the campaign and promote their activities under the (additional) benefit of contributing to good mental health.

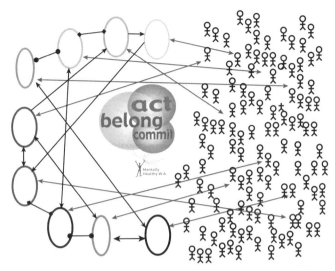

Fig. 10.7 Community Organization and community members after to *Act-Belong-Commit more connections, more strongly connected*

The advertising, publicity and sponsorship were designed to sensitize people to local organizations' promotion of their activities, and, in conjunction with these promotions, to get people to participate in specific events or become more active in organizations of which they were already a member. For organizations, the behavioural objectives were to undertake activities to increase attendance, participation, membership and volunteerism in their organizations, and to form partnerships with other organizations to achieve these aims.

Campaign development and branding

The formative research delineated a number of factors that people perceived to affect positive mental health, ranging from economic and sociocultural factors to individual personality and lifestyle factors. There was near universal support for the concepts that remaining active (physically, socially and mentally), having good friends, being a member of various groups in the community, and feeling in control of one's circumstances were necessary for good mental health. There was also widespread agreement that having opportunities for achievable challenges – at home, school or work, or in hobbies, sports or the arts – are important for a good sense of self. Helping others (including volunteering, coaching and mentoring) was frequently mentioned as a great source of satisfaction, as well as providing a source of activity and involvement with others.

These findings were used to develop the campaign to target individuals and community organizations, as noted above. However, we first required an overall brand under which different mental health promotion campaigns could be launched.

The *Mentally Healthy WA* brand

Formative research with a broad variety of individuals about their understanding of mental health indicated that people rarely thought proactively about their mental health and that the term 'mental health' primarily had connotations of mental *illness* (e.g. schizophrenia, psychiatry, manic-depression, depression, etc.).

On the other hand, the term 'mental*ly* healthy' had primarily positive connotations (e.g. alert, happy, able to cope, socially adept, emotionally stable, etc.). The researchers suggested a mental health promotion campaign use the term 'mentally healthy' as often as possible in conjunction with the term 'mental health' to neutralize the negative connotations and build positive connotations to the term 'mental health'. We therefore decided to brand the overall campaign as the *Mentally Healthy WA* campaign.

Other features of this umbrella brand name were:

◆ Inclusion of the state as part of the brand to engage a sense of community participation and ownership (Western Australians have a reputation for being parochial – probably because of the sheer physical separation from the rest of the Australian states). Hence the inclusion of the state initials, as people commonly refer to the state via the letters 'W' and 'A', and rarely use the full words 'Western Australia'. (None of the other states' populations refer to their state in this way).

◆ Mindful that other jurisdictions could be interested in adopting the campaign, and to aid diffusion, another desired feature was that individual towns, or other states or countries could easily adapt the brand format (e.g. 'Mentally Healthy USA'). The Mental Health Council of Australia (the peak body for organizations dealing with mental illness) now uses 'Mentally Healthy Oz' (and the *Act-Belong-Commit* logo) in its national campaign around world mental health week.

Sub-branding the phase one campaign: *Act-Belong-Commit*

Our first requirement was that the sub-brand go beyond slogans or belief statements such as 'together we do better' and 'friends are good medicine' and connect directly to the actions we wanted people to take (in the same way that other health promotion/injury prevention campaigns include their basic desired behaviour in their branding or logo (e.g. *Quit, Belt Up, DrinkSafe, 2 Fruit 'n' 5 Veg, Eat less fat*, etc.). We therefore looked to the formative research findings and to the literature for the basic behaviours that contributed to good mental health.

Given the potential complexity of the mental health/illness area, we also imposed the requirement that acting on the campaign's primary messages be 'as simple as ABC'. This resulted in searching for behaviours beginning with the letters 'A', 'B' and 'C' that reflected the formative research and literature.

We chose the verbs 'act', 'belong' and 'commit' as they not only provide the opportunity to tell people that maintaining good mental health 'is as easy as A-B-C', but they also represent the three major domains of factors that both the literature and people in general consider contribute to good mental health (Donovan *et al.* 2003, 2005; Donovan 2004; Ross and Blackwell 2004; Rychetnik and Todd 2004; Shah and Marks 2004).

Act means that individuals should strive to keep themselves physically, socially and cognitively active. Being active is a fundamental requirement for mental health: there is substantial evidence from a variety of sources that individuals with higher levels of physical, cognitive and/or social activity have higher levels of wellbeing and mental health, and that such activities can alleviate mental problems such as anxiety and depression. At the basic physical and cognitive levels, individuals can act alone: take a walk, read a book, do a crossword puzzle, garden, take a correspondence course, visit a museum, and so on. At a basic social level, individuals can interact with salespeople while shopping, talk to their neighbours and maintain contact with family and friends.

Belong refers to being a member of a group or organization (whether or not face-to-face), such that an individual's connectedness with the community and sense of identity are strengthened. Groups can be formal or informal. Many activities can be done alone or as a member of a group (e.g. read a book versus join a book club; go for a walk alone or join a walking group; play solitaire or bridge games). In some cases there are synergistic effects: belonging to a book club not only adds a connectedness dimension but is likely to expand the cognitive activity involved; joining a walking group is likely to expand the physical activity while adding a social connection. Regular involvement in social activities, whether via hobby groups, professional interest groups, or family and friends is likely to result in a strong personal support group, one of the most important factors for maintaining mental (and physical) health. Involvement in local community activities and organizations also builds social cohesion (or social capital), which is important for individuals' mental health. Overall, the more an individual is active within the context of connectedness, the greater contribution to mental health, and the greater the availability of assistance in coping with the vicissitudes of life and threats to mental health. The California-based *Friends are good medicine* and VicHealth's *Together we do better* campaigns are examples of campaigns that focus on the 'belong' domain.

Commit refers to the extent to which an individual becomes involved with (or commits to) some activity or organization. Commitment provides a sense of purpose and meaning in people's lives. Commitment can be to a cause or organization that benefits the group or wider community, or can be to the achievement of some personal goal. For example, one can be a spectator member of the local theatre group or sport club, or one can be an active participant, or one can volunteer to be treasurer or go on a recruiting drive or in some other way make a deeper commitment to the organization. Meeting challenges provides a sense of accomplishment, feelings of efficacy and a stronger sense of self (Csikszentmihalyi 1990). There is widespread agreement in the general population that volunteering and activities undertaken to benefit the community at large, especially where these involve the disadvantaged, have special returns for feeling good about oneself, and indeed have mental health benefits, particularly in the retired elderly. Volunteering and greater participation in community activities and organizations have substantial implications for community cohesion and social capital, and hence quality of life (ESRC 2004).

In short, positive mental health relies on people keeping physically, socially and mentally active, participating in group activities, keeping up social interactions, getting involved in community activities and taking up causes or setting goals and achieving them.

These three domains may be viewed as a hierarchy of increasing contribution to an individual's sense of self and mental health. For example, a person could *act* by reading a book; *belong* by joining a book club; *commit* by becoming the secretary/organizer for the book club, or by occasionally reading challenging books rather than just 'pulp fiction'. Similarly a person could *act* by going for a walk alone; *belong* by joining a walking group; *commit* by becoming the secretary/organizer for the walking group, or by increasing the difficulty or challenge of the walk (e.g. uphill, orienteering aspects, etc.).

The visual brand

The *Act-Belong-Commit* brand logo was required to reframe good mental health as more than the absence of illness. It was required to reflect people's positive connotations to the term 'mentally healthy'. Hence we chose balloons as signifying 'lightness', sociability and generally positive affect and energy.

A single non-gender character was chosen to have non-specific appeal. This also has the advantage of being adapted in other promotional areas (e.g. a TV ad), and because this could be further elaborated by other partners (the Mental Health Council of Australia sought permission to add a child figure, which blended with their own logo of a similar adult character shown in a protective pose with a child figure).

Several variations were tested to ensure that the brand was seen as 'friendly' and was generally 'liked'. We also ensured that the logo achieved high ratings on 'easy to read' and 'easy to remember'.

Another reason for choosing to base the logo on balloons was that the three balloons could be easily displayed at sponsored/branded events. Project officers were provided with a good supply of 'act', 'belong', and 'commit', balloons in the appropriate colours, in addition to anchors and a gas cylinder. Trios of balloons were displayed at events – not only reinforcing brand recognition, but clearly branding the event as an *Act-Belong-Commit* event as well as adding to the sociability/fun atmosphere of the event. The balloons proved popular with children who asked for the balloons – thus serving to bring their parent or carer into contact with the brand.

The marketing mix

Product The 'core' product or value offered to individuals was 'good mental health' and feelings of wellbeing in exchange for their taking up activities suggested in the Act-Belong-Commit messages. The value offered to organization operators was facilitation in reaching their own organizational goals in exchange for promoting their activities under or in conjunction with the Act-Belong-Commit brand.

'Actual' products offered to individuals were all the activities offered by organizations that promoted their activities under or alongside the *Act-Belong-Commit* banner. 'Actual' products offered to organizations were the skills of the A-B-C project officers, who helped organize events and obtain sponsorship funding and publicity for organizations and their activities, along with merchandising items (described below). All of these served to establish and maintain a good relationship with partners.

People The project officers in each town were required to have health promotion expertise and good interpersonal skills. The campaign benefited greatly from the enthusiasm and the ability of the project officers to engage with people in the towns. Our project officers also offered expertise in assisting community organizations apply for funding from grant bodies (e.g. government and charity arts and sports funding bodies) in return for their partnership cooperation.

A small management group (6–10 persons) was set up in each town, consisting of representatives of the main partner organizations in each town. This group served to support the project officer as well as provide links to other organizations in each town.

Promotion A media advertising and publicity campaign was developed to inform and encourage individuals to engage in activities that would enhance their mental health, while a direct approach to potential partners simultaneously encouraged community organizations offering such activities to promote their activities under a mental health benefit message. In exchange for partners ('retailers') promoting their activities under our banner, we offered merchandise resources (T-shirts, water bottles, stickers, hats, etc.), paid advertising support, and promotional expertise that many community organizations did not have.

A set of four press ads was developed (Figs 10.8–10.12) for the launch and first six months of the campaign. The ads were designed to appear on consecutive right-hand pages for maximal impact. Donovan *et al.*'s (2003) summary of people's understanding of mental health suggested that people in Western Australia would be responsive to mental health promotion messages if delivered in everyday language. Hence the ad content was deliberately designed to avoid technical jargon and the notion that mental health concepts were complex. The copy refers to people already knowing what's good for their mental health, with 'health experts' now confirming that knowledge.

The ads are supplemented by publicity and press releases for local events. The campaign expected – and generally received – good use of press releases and coverage of local events held under the *Act-Belong-Commit* brand. Other mutually beneficial

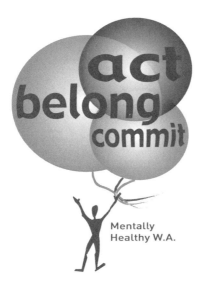

Fig. 10.8 *Act-Belong-Commit* Brand/logo

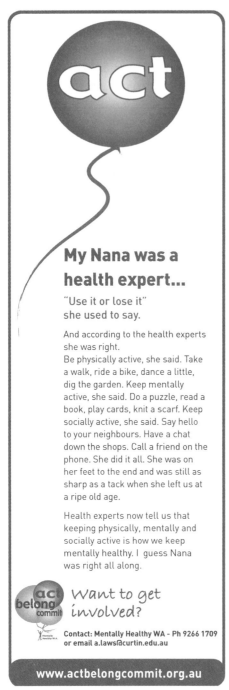

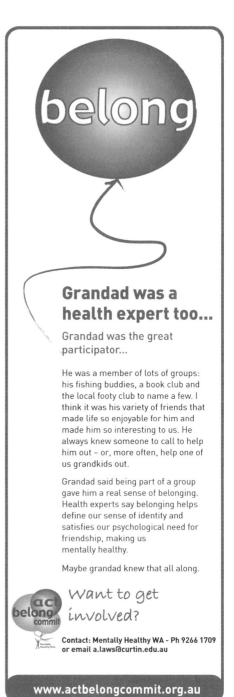

Fig. 10.9 *Act* press advertisement.

Fig. 10.10 *Belong* press advertisement.

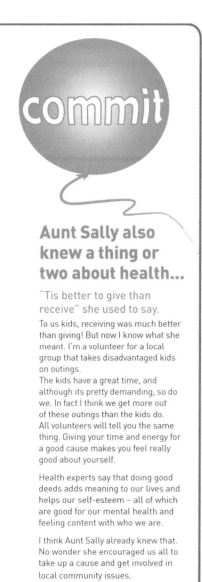

Fig. 10.11 *Commit* press advertisement.

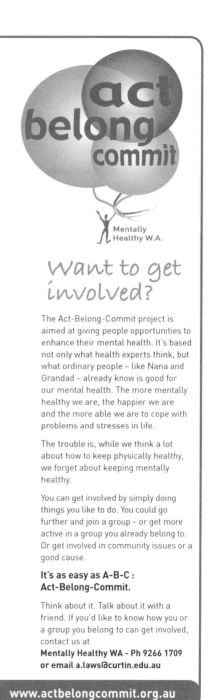

Fig. 10.12 *Get Involved* press advertisement.

newspaper features have been negotiated in some towns (e.g. one town's newspaper features a 'club of the month', describing the club's activities and contact details, along with the *Act-Belong-Commit* logo and message). A monthly newsletter is circulated, mainly among collaborating organizations, with the aim of keeping people informed and maintaining individuals' interest by recounting personalized, local stories about the campaign's implementation.

Price While participation in some events and activities has required a monetary outlay, most of the co-branded events to date have not. Instead, what they have required are psychological costs such as time (primarily), effort, overcoming shyness or dealing with potential social embarrassment (e.g. in attending an intergenerational concert and meeting, greeting and conversing with strangers).

Place There are two levels of place. First, campaign project officers were physically located in each town. In a commercial sense these were our 'sales offices' in each town.

As a first step, we visited the six participating regional towns and invited community organizations to a community forum to discuss the project and to generate ideas on what they might do and how they might cooperate. Ideas and partnerships mooted at these forums have been incorporated in the planning for each town. Organizations willing to participate are asked to 'sign on' to the campaign. These collaborating organizations are encouraged and assisted to promote participation in their activities under the *Act-Belong-Commit* banner. These organizations (e.g. local government organizations, businesses, libraries, tertiary and technical education services, sporting and arts clubs/groups, professional associations, schools, worksites, recreational groups, including indigenous and other ethnic groups, and so on) become a second level of place, in that their premises (or use of public spaces) are where the 'behaviours' are engaged in.

ABC guide to promoting mental health via targeting individuals in authority

A tentative ABC guide for targeting individuals in authority over others has been developed for the second phase of the *Mentally Healthy WA* campaign: *Actively involve* (those in your care) – *Build* (their) skills – *Celebrate* (their) achievements. This guide suggests three major ways that individuals in charge can enhance the mental health of those in their care. The fundamental notions are that each and every individual in their care should be given the opportunity to actively participate in the group or organization's activities and relevant decisions, be provided with challenges that increase their skills and sense of self-efficacy, and have their achievements recognized. These three concepts are based on individuals' beliefs about factors influencing one's mental health or vulnerability to illness (Donovan *et al.* 2003; Donovan *et al.* 2006b), and are consistent with the literature (Csikszentmihalyi 1990; Warr 1994; Stewart *et al.* 2004; Oxenstierna *et al.* 2005), particularly Hawkins *et al.*'s (1992) concept of bonding, and concepts of control and reward imbalance (Vezina *et al.* 2004).

Campaign results

For the first 12 months of the campaign, the emphasis was on establishing partnerships in the towns and building brand awareness and knowledge among potential partners.

Use of media to reach the general community was limited to advertising and publicity in each town's local newspaper. In the first 12 months, 59 key partnerships were established, 115 co-branded community events and activities were held, and the campaign generated a total of 124 campaign-related press articles in the local newspapers (27,538 cm^2).

Benchmark and two 12-month follow-up telephone surveys (random selection) of the intervention town residents ($n = 200$ per town) have been undertaken and results in the intervention sites will be compared with telephone surveys of metropolitan residents and non-intervention rural town residents ($n = 1,000$). The final survey was undertaken in October 2007. Campaign awareness after the first 12 months of limited local newspaper advertising varied from 20 per cent to 30 per cent in the various towns. Those exposed to the campaign reported greater participation in mentally healthy activities than those not exposed. A television ad was developed and launched in February 2007 in an attempt to increase population awareness in the second year of the campaign. Preliminary results show that even with a limited budget ($60,000 for the whole state excluding the metropolitan area), campaign awareness increased to approximately 65 per cent across all intervention sites.

Organization partners were also surveyed after 12 months. Among other questions, respondents were asked to provide an overall rating on a ten-point scale, of how beneficial they considered their collaboration with the campaign to have been and whether 'In the future, would you be willing to collaborate with the *Act-Belong-Commit* campaign in running events or activities?' The overall mean beneficial rating was almost eight out of ten, and 100 per cent stated they would be willing to collaborate with the campaign in the future.

The intervention has had an upstream impact on the health system in that the Western Australian Country Health Services has agreed to continue to deliver the *Act-Belong-Commit* mental health promotion in all country areas. We will also measure the extent to which mental health promotion becomes a major activity of the Division of Mental Health within the Health Department of Western Australia.

The intervention activities are designed to be self-sustaining. At the end of the two-year intervention, we hope to leave a network of collaborating organizations in each town who have the capacity to obtain sufficient funding to maintain their activities under the *Act-Belong-Commit* brand, with the support of not just the Department of Health but other government sectors (such as Sport and Recreation, Conservation and Land Management, Education, Office of Seniors Interest, etc.) and a variety of local community organizations and businesses.

Comment

A major positive for the campaign has been the readiness with which people from all walks of life and backgrounds readily relate to the simplicity and relevance of the *Act-Belong-Commit* branding. This has facilitated partnerships with a broad variety of organizations as these organizations readily understand how their activities contribute to individual and community mental health.

Another major positive of the campaign's brand positioning is that by engaging community organizations of all sorts – arts, crafts, theatre, sporting groups, libraries, educational groups, etc – mental health is removed form a 'health department'/'hospital' context, and placed in an everyday, community responsibility context; which is where it should be.

More information is available on the campaign website (www.actbelongcommit.org.au).

Conclusion

Because the actual brand names and graphics in both of these cases were based on formative research with target audiences, they contributed significantly to establishing these brands' values to their target audiences and inviting participation in the exchanges being offered. Both *Freedom From Fear* and *Mentally Healthy WA* were positive if not aspirational, offering improved wellbeing in return for adopting their respective recommended behaviours encapsulated in their respective sub-brands, the *Men's Domestic Violence Helpline* and *Act-Belong-Commit*. Probably far more than for commercial brands – where the recommended behaviour is usually obvious, and where there are significantly greater budgets for developing brand values and relationships external to the actual name and graphics – public health brands are best served by ensuring that their names and graphics incorporate both the recommended behaviours as well as the values promised in exchange.

Acknowledgments

The Mentally Healthy WA intervention is funded largely by Healthway, supported by WA Country Health Services, Lotterywest, The Office of Mental Health and Pilbara Iron Ltd. The Centre for Behavioural Research in Cancer Control is part funded by the Cancer Council of Western Australia. The Australian Drug Offensive Campaigns were developed and implemented by the Campaigns Unit in the then Commonwealth Department of Health and Family Services.

References

APS Observer Special Issue. (1997). *Human capital initiative – reducing violence: a behavioral science research plan for violence*. Washington, DC: American Psychological Society.

Australian Government Department of Health and Ageing. (2007). Graphic Health Warnings – labelling of tobacco products. Available at: http://www.quitnow. info. au/internet/quitnow/publishing.nsf/Content/warnings-lp (accessed 8 June 2007).

Buchanan, F. (1996). Zero tolerance in South Australia: a statewide community initiative. *Australian Journal of Primary Health-Interchange* 2:107–12.

Cant, R., Downie, R., Fisher, C., Henry, P., and Froyland, I. (2002). *Evaluation of perpetrator programs for mandated and voluntary participants in Western Australia*. Perth: Centre for Research on Women, Family and Domestic Violence Unit.

Carroll, T. (1996). *The role of social marketing campaigns within Australia's National Drug Strategy*. Sydney: Commonwealth Department of Health and Family Services. A submission to the National Drug Strategy Evaluation. Drug Info Clearinghouse no. JE60 CAR.

Cowell, D. W. (1984). *The marketing of services*. Institute of Marketing and the CAM Foundation, London Heineman Professional Publishing.

Csikszentmihalyi, M. (1990). *Flow: the psychology of optimal experience*. New York: Harper Perennial.

Davis, H. and Tsiantis, J. (2005). Promoting children's mental health: the European Early Promotion Project (EEPP). *International Journal of Mental Health Promotion* **7**:4–16.

De Becker, G. (1998). *A gift of fear: survival signals that protect us from violence*. New York: Dell Publishing.

Donovan, R. J. (2004). North Queenslanders' beliefs about mental health and mental health promotion. Townsville: Tropical Public Health Unit, Queensland Health.

Donovan, R. and Henley, N. (2003). *Social Marketing: Principles and Practice*. Melbourne: IP Communications.

Donovan, R. J. and Vlais, R. (2006). A review of communication components of anti- racism and prodiversity social marketing/public education campaigns (Paper 1). Melbourne: VicHealth.

Donovan, R. J., Paterson, D., and Francas, M. (1999). Targeting male perpetrators of intimate partner violence: Western Australia's 'Freedom from Fear' campaign. *Social Marketing Quarterly* **5**:127–43.

Donovan, R. J., Francas, M., Paterson, D., and Zappelli, R. (2000). Formative research for mass media-based campaigns: Western Australia's 'Freedom From Fear' campaign targeting male perpetrators of intimate partner violence. *Health Promotion Journal of Australia* **10**:78–83.

Donovan, R. J., Watson, N., and Henley, N., James, R., Zubrick, S., Sillburn, S. *et al.* (2003). *Report to Healthway: Mental Health Promotion Scoping Project*. Perth: Curtin University, Centre for Developmental Health.

Donovan, R. J., Henley, N., Watson, N., Zubrick, S., Silburn, S., and Williams, A. (2005) People's beliefs about factors contributing to mental health: implications for mental health promotion. *Health Promotion Journal of Australia* **18**:50–6.

Donovan, R. J., James, R., Jalleh, G., and Sidebottom, C. (2006a). Implementing mental health promotion in Western Australia. *International Journal of Mental Health Promotion* **8**:29–38.

Donovan, R. J., Henley, N., Watson, N., Zubrick, S., Silburn, S., and William, A. (2006b). The impact on mental health in others of those in a position of authority: a perspective of parents, teachers, trainers and supervisors. *Australian e-Journal for the Advancement of Mental Health* **5**(1). Available at: http://www.auseinet.com/journal/vol5iss1/donovan.pdf.

Donovan R. J., Henley N., Watson N., Zubrick S., Silburn S., and Williams, A. (2007). People's beliefs about factors contributing to mental health: implications for mental health promotion. *Health Promotion Journal of Australia* **18**:50–6.

Durlak, J. A. and Wells, A. M. (1997). Primary prevention mental health programs for children and adolescents: a meta-analytic review. *American Journal of Community Psychology* **25**:115–52.

Economic Research Council (ESRC) (2004). *The art of happiness … is volunteering the blueprint for bliss?* Press Release. Available at: http://www.esrc.ac.uk/esrccontent/news/september04-2.asp.

Egger, G., Fitzgerald, W., Frape, G., Monaem, A., Rubenstein, P., Tyler, C., and Mackay, B. (1983). Results of a large-scale media anti-smoking campaign in Australia: The North Coast Healthy Lifestyle Program. *British Medical Journal* **287**:1125–287.

Egger, G., Donovan, R. J., and Spark, R. (1993). *Health and the media: principles and practice for health promotion*. Sydney: McGraw-Hill.

Eisikovits, Z. and Buchbinder, E. (1997). Talking violent: a phenomenological study of metaphors battering men use. *Violence Against Women* **3**:482–98.

European Commission (2004). *Actions against depression: improving mental and well-being by combating the adverse health, social and economic consequences of depression*. Luxembourg: Health and Consumer Protection Directorate-General.

Gomel, M. (1997). *A focus on women*. Geneva: Nations for Mental Health, World Health Organization.

Hawkins, J. D., Catalano, R. F., and Miller, J. Y. (1992). Risk and protective factors for alcohol and other drug problems in adolescence and early adulthood: Implications for substance abuse prevention. *Psychological Bulletin* **112**:64–105.

Hersey, J. C., Klibanoff, L. S., Lam, D. J., and Taylor, R. L. (1984). Promoting social support: the impact of California's 'Friends can be good medicine' campaign. *Health Education Quarterly* **11**:293–311.

Hill, D. and Carroll, T. (2003). Australia's National Tobacco Campaign. *Tobacco Control* **12**(S2): ii9–14.

Janè-Llopis, E., Barry, M., Hosman, C., and Patel, V. (2005). Mental health promotion works: a review. *Promotion and Education*, S2:9–25.

Keilitz, S. L., Davis, C., Efkeman, H. S., Flango, C., and Hannaford, P. L. (1998). *Civil protection orders: victims' views on effectiveness*. National Institute of Justice.

Kotler, P. (1980). *Principles of marketing*. Englewood Cliffs, NJ: Prentice-Hall.

Makkai, T. and McAllister, I. (1998). *Public opinions towards drug policies in Australia 1985–95*. Canberra, ACT: Commonwealth of Australia.

Morrow, L., Verins, I., and Willis, E. (Eds) (2002). *Mental health and work: issues and perspectives*. Adelaide: Aussinet: The Australian Network for Promotion, Prevention and Early Intervention for Mental Health.

Murray, C. J. L. and Lopez, A. D. (1996) *The Global Burden of Disease*. Cambridge, MA: WHO.

National Campaign Against Drug Abuse (NCADA). (1985) Campaign document issued following the Special Premiers' Conference, Canberra, 2 April. Canberra: Australian Government Publishing Service.

Oxenstierna, G., Ferrie, J., Hyde, M., Westerlund, H., and Theorell, T. (2005). Dual source support and control at work in relation to poor health. *Scandinavian Journal of Public Health* **33**:455–63.

Perkins, C. (2007) Great head, pity it's no Van Gogh. *The Australian*. Available at: http://www.theaustralian.news.com.au/story/0,25197,22186222-5013571,00.html (accessed August 8, 2007).

Prochaska, J. O. and DiClemente, C. C. (1984). *The transtheoretical approach: crossing the traditional boundaries of therapy*. Irwin, IL: Dow-Jones Research Center.

Ries, A. and Trout, J. (1981) *Positioning, the battle for your mind*. New York: Warner Books, McGraw-Hill.

Roberts, A. R. (ed.) (1984). *Battered women and their families: intervention strategies and treatment programs*. New York: Springer.

Roosevelt, F. (1941). Annual address to congress – the 'four freedoms'. Available at: http://www.fdrlibrary.marist.edu/od4frees.html (accessed 17 July 2007).

Ross, R. and Blackwell, A. G. (2004). *The influence of community factors on health: annotated bibliography*. New York: PolickLink and The California Endowment.

Rychetnik, L. and Todd, A. (2004). *VicHealth mental health promotion evidence review: a literature review focusing on the VicHealth 1999–2002 Mental Health Promotion Framework*. New South Wales: University of Sydney.

Sabbag, R. (2002). *Smoke screen: a true adventure*. Edinburgh: Canongate.

Saxena, S., Ommeren, M. V., Tang, K. C., and Armstrong, T. P. (2005). Mental health benefits of physical activity. *Journal of Mental Health* **14**:445–51.

Saxena, S. and Garrison, P. J. (2004). *Mental health promotion: case studies from countries*. World Health Organization and World Federation for Mental Health. Geneva: WHO.

Shah, H. and Marks, N. (2004) *A well-being manifesto for a flourishing society*. London, UK: New Economics Foundation.

Sorenson, S. B., Upchurch, D. M., and Shen, H. (1996). Violence and injury in marital arguments: risk patterns and gender differences. *American Journal of Public Health* **86**:35–40.

Stewart, D., Sun, J., Patterson, C., Lamerle, K., and Hardie, M. (2004). Promoting and building resilience in primary school communities: evidence from a comprehensive 'health promoting school' approach. *International Journal of Mental Health Promotion* **6**:26–33.

Taylor, R. L., Lam, D. J., Roppel, C. E., and Barter, J. T. (1984). Friends can be good medicine: an excursion into mental health promotion. *Community Mental Health Journal* **20**:294–303.

Twitchell, J. (2004). *Branded nation: the marketing of Megachurch, College Inc., and Museum World.* New York: Simon and Schuster.

Vezina, M., Bourbonnais, R., Brisson, C., and Trudel, L. (2004). Workplace prevention and promotion strategies. *Healthcare Papers* **5**:32–44.

Walker, L., Moodie, R., and Herrman, H. (2004). Promoting mental health and wellbeing. In R. Moodie and A. Hulme (eds) *Hands on health promotion*. Melbourne: IP Communications. pp. 238–248.

Warr, P. (1994). A conceptual framework for the study of work and mental health. *Work and Stress* **8**:84–97.

Part III

Practice and applications of public health branding

11

Public health brands in the developing world

W. Douglas Evans and Muhiuddin Haider

Summary

- Public health brands are a rapidly growing social marketing strategy in the developing world.
- There are parallels between public health brands in the developed and developing worlds in terms of health issues addressed and the difference in terms of channels used and social context.
- Care studies from HIV/AIDS, malaria prevention, and reproductive health illustrate public health branding in the developing world.
- There are important research questions concerning the marketing mix and effects of social context in brand equity.

Introduction

Social marketing has been a staple of international efforts to change health behavior (UNAIDS 2002). In recent years, branding strategies have increasingly been incorporated into social marketing efforts funded by major donors such as the US Agency for International Development, the World Health Organization (WHO), and large foundations with global focus, such as Gates and Rockefeller. Branded health campaigns have tremendous potential to reach audiences and change modifiable behaviors related to HIV/AIDS, reproductive health, environmental risk factors, and chronic disease risks through mass media, community outreach and other strategies in the developing world. As with branded health messages delivered in Europe, the USA, Oceania and other developed countries, such brands seek to create positive associations with healthy lifestyles and act as powerful mediators to increase uptake of health-promoting and disease-preventing behaviors such as use of condoms, quitting or not initiating smoking, or improved sanitation practices.

In this chapter, we argue that branding in the developed and developing worlds are similar in many ways, but there are important social, cultural, economic and technological differences that condition the development of public health brands, and present important challenges and lessons for social marketers. The developing world is in some ways a more difficult environment in which to deploy public health brands, but there are important underlying similarities with the developed world that are reflected in case studies we will examine later in the chapter. For example, there are the same issues of diversity (e.g. the last UK census recorded no fewer than 112 languages being spoken in one London borough, just as there is tremendous linguistic diversity in Indonesia or South Africa), and inequality (e.g. health disparities in chronic and infectious diseases between recent immigrants, and African-Americans, as compared with European-Americans, just as there is tremendous health inequality in Africa and South Asia). There are also issues about the changing environment of channels based on new media (e.g. the proliferation of cell phones and wireless internet access, which is burgeoning in both the developed and developing world) and their effect on the marketing mix.

There is much public health can learn from examining branding in the developing world, and the similarities and differences between the two contexts provide valuable lessons for future brand development. We illustrate these points of comparison by examining the background of global public health brands, and then turning to individual case studies of social marketing in several African and South Asian countries.

Parallels between public health brands in the developed and developing world

There are both parallels and differences in the context and challenges facing branded health messaging in the developing world, as compared with the developed world. In general, public health brands share many common characteristics in terms of purposes, outcomes and strategies across population, community and country settings. They are about establishing a positive reputation for a healthy lifestyle, or an organization promoting healthy lifestyles. In other words, the purposes of public health brands are the same regardless of setting.

Public health brands are also universally about achieving better health outcomes. In other words, a branded campaign to promote condom use in the USA, such as the *Know HIV/AIDS* campaign sponsored by the Kaiser Family Foundation (www.knowhivaids.org), and the African *loveLife* campaign (Stadler and Hlongwa 2002), are both about promoting increased condom use and not about selling condoms or promoting any other commercial interest. Thus the outcomes of public health campaigns are the same in the developed and developing world.

Specifically, there are three main parallels. First, public health brands are more than just *communication*. Public health brands in all contexts seek to position a lifestyle as the preferred alternative to unhealthy behaviors, and accomplish this through many communication strategies such as mass media, community outreach and mobilization, and policy and organizational change. For example, both *Know HIV/AIDS* and *loveLife* have used multiple strategies, including advertising promotions, event sponsorship, community outreach, policy advocacy and policy change promotion, as part of a concerted branding strategy (Rideout 2004; Stadler and Hlongwa 2002).

Second, and related to the first parallel, public health brands in developing countries are both about affecting upstream environmental factors, such as community actors, aid donors and non-governmental organizations (NGOs), and about affecting individual-level behavior and promoting behavior change. For example, the *Zuia Mbu* (Prevent Mosquitoes) brand in Tanzania addressed factors affecting adoption of treated mosquito netting along organizational/workplace dimensions (e.g. hospitals, development projects and employers), and by marketing directly to villagers using multiple outreach and media strategies.

Third, public health brands are affected by, and in turn seek to change, the social environments in which they are developed and delivered. Public health branding in any context is ultimately a broad-based marketing strategy that models techniques from commercial branding but differs importantly in purposes and outcomes. Public health brands in developing countries use persuasive mechanisms that make the brand appealing and therefore an effective marketing tool. Such mechanisms include: aspiration to appealing external ideals; modeling of socially desirable behaviors or other goods; and association with appealing imagery (e.g. forming beliefs, engaging in behaviors that associate the individual with the appealing imagery).

Differences in context between the developed and developing world

There are also important differences in opportunities to build public health brands in areas such as Europe, Oceania and North America, and developing contexts such as Africa and parts of Asia. Access, availability and use of media channels differ in many important respects, and thus the promotional strategies for public health brands must differ, at least for the near future. For example, in the USA, television penetrates over 99 per cent of households and it has been estimated that the average US consumer is exposed to over 40,000 television advertisements per year (Calvert 2008). If social marketing can capture even a small percentage of those exposures through paid advertisements or public service announcement (PSA), it represents a tremendous opportunity to promote a public health brand as part of an integrated promotional strategy that may include many other components such as partnerships, community outreach, and other upstream and downstream strategies.

Television penetration and use, as well as that of other 'new' media such as the internet, are sharply lower in developing countries. For example, while penetration is increasing, in 2001 television only penetrated approximately 7 per cent of Indian homes, or about 79 million households out of a population of 1.13 billion (Government of India Census, NRS-2001). In China, one of the most advanced of the so-called developing nations, in 2001 there were televisions in about 21 per cent of homes, or 269 million out of a population of 1.278 billion.

Rates of television penetration in Africa vary widely, and are somewhat higher in many English-speaking countries. In Kenya, some estimate there are televisions in approximately 60 per cent of households (Internet World Stats 2007).

Overall, however, there are far fewer opportunities to reach the population with health or consumer brand messages through mass media in the developing world than in

Europe, Oceania and the USA. This is even more of an issue with respect to so-called 'new' media such as computers, the internet and handheld devices

In the developed world, the use of new media has greatly expanded opportunities to promote all forms of brands. In the 27 European Union countries, internet penetration has been estimated at over 51 per cent, or 252 million out of a population of some 493 million (Internet World Stats 2007). In the USA, nearly 70 per cent of the population has internet access, or over 210 million out of 301 million (Internet World Stats 2007).

However, penetration of new media in developing countries is far lower, with fewer opportunities for public health and commercial brands to extend their reach through mass media. In India, internet penetration is 3.7 per cent, or about 42 million users out of some 1.13 billion population. In Africa, the overall rate of internet usage is comparable, at 3.6 per cent (Internet World Stats 2006), but there are substantial differences between countries. In South Africa, approximately 10.3 per cent of the population has internet access, or over 5 million out of a population of nearly 50 million. By contrast, in Kenya, internet penetration was approximately 3 per cent in 2005 (Internet World Stats 2006) or just over 1 million people out of a total population of 35 million. In the poorest African nations, there is much less access (and exposure) to mass media. For example, in the Democratic Republic of Congo, it is estimated that only 0.2 per cent of the population are internet users, or just 140,000 out of over 60 million (Internet World Stats 2006).

As a result of these differences in media patterns, the future opportunities and past history of social marketing efforts to promote public health brands differ in some respects. While televised mass media campaigns are used (e.g. *loveLife*, reported in Stadler and Hlongwa 2002) and present an important channel, they have far less reach than in say, the UK, and are only one tool that social marketers need to utilize to reach developing world audiences. Other mass media, such as radio and popular print magazines, may be more useful. The choice of channel is especially context-sensitive in light of the low literacy rates present in some developing countries.

For example, in developing a nutrition promotion campaign in South Africa, Evans *et al.* (forthcoming) found that small wattage local radio and magazines available in townships were the preferred media channels to receive health information. Formative research with parents living in townships, urban and rural areas demonstrated consistent utilization of these channels, but differed in extent of television and new media usage. Low technology options bypass issues of media access and the 'digital divide' and take advantage of culturally-relevant and population-specific channels used in local communities.

One important exception to these media use patterns may be cell phones, and the increasing opportunities they represent to deliver branded health and other messages through broadband connections. For example, many people in Kenya, Tanzania and other sub-Saharan African countries do not have fixed phone lines, and yet there is relatively high, and growing, cell phone penetration. From 1999 through 2004, the number of mobile subscribers in Africa jumped to 76.8 million, from 7.5 million, an average annual increase of 58 per cent. South Africa accounted for approximately 20 per cent of that growth (LaFraniere 2005). The number of mobile subscribers in Asia increased by 34 per cent during this same period. Cell phones are a relatively inexpensive, highly portable means of accessing digital information. As broadband cellular access increases, a growing number of people in developing countries who otherwise lack access to television, internet (through computers), and other media channels will have access to a wealth of digital information through their cell phones. This represents an important opportunity in these countries for social marketers to deliver branded health messages to individuals otherwise deprived of health information.

Case studies of five branded health campaigns from Africa and Asia

In this chapter, we explore these posited parallels and differences, and thereby identify the challenges and opportunities for branded health messaging in developing world contexts. We discuss the brand characteristics, promotional strategies and evidence of effectiveness of five campaigns in the developing world identified in a systematic review of published literature (Evans *et al.*, forthcoming). This study, described in Evans and Hastings in Chapter 1 of this volume, identified a total of 37 publications on branded health campaigns that met a set of relatively strict review criteria (i.e. their sole outcome objective was the improvement of health outcomes and not promotion or distribution of commercial products). These campaigns covered the domains of HIV/AIDS, reproductive health (men's involvement in their pregnant wives' health) and malaria control. Table 11.1 summarizes these five published campaigns.

Although growing in number, published research and reports on public health brands are relatively rare in the peer-reviewed literature. But there are numerous examples of 'gray' (non-peer reviewed reports or brief summaries) that can also provide useful information. Organizations such as Population Services International (PSI) (www.psi.org), the Academy for Educational Development (www.aed.org), and other major social marketing organizations working in the developing world routinely produce programmatic and research reports on their projects.

For example, in June 2006, PSI reported on the *Nimechill* campaign, Kenya's first large-scale abstinence program (PSI 2006a). This report describes the concept underlying

Table 11.1 Overview of branded health campaigns from the developing world.

Topic area	Citation	Public health campaign	Research design	Location
HIV/Aids prevention	Agha (2003)	*Trust* (condom campaign)	Observational	Kenya
HIV/Aids prevention	Eloundou-Enyegue *et al.* (2005)	*Salama*	Observational	Tanzania
HIV/Aids prevention	Stadler and Hlongwa (2002)	*loveLife*	Observational	South Africa
Malaria control	Armstrong Schellenberg *et al.* (1999)	*Zuia Mbu* (Prevent Mosquitos)	Observational	Tanzania
Reproductive health	Shefner-Rogers (2004)	*Suami SIAGA* (I'm an Alert Husband)	Observational	Indonesia

Nimechill, meaning 'I have chilled' or 'I am abstaining', and development of a brand around the social desirability of abstinence, exemplified by a logo of a yellow hand giving a 'V' or a 'peace' sign to brand the campaign.

Clearly, there have been numerous other branded social marketing campaigns in the developing world. To illustrate the range of public health brand strategies, we will focus on the five published brands.

Trust (HIV/AIDS prevention in Kenya)

As a result of rising public awareness and interest in fighting HIV/AIDS in the late 1990s (Eriksson *et al.* 1997), the government of Kenya worked with PSI Kenya to develop the *Trust* campaign. The objective of the campaign was to promote the Trust condom as a positive lifestyle choice. The Trust condom advertising strategy reinforced condom efficacy and encouraged users to always be prepared. The government provided free airtime for HIV prevention broadcasts to PSI Kenya. This airtime was used to supplement an ongoing branded social marketing campaign being implemented by PSI Kenya.

PSI Kenya used formative research to develop branded and generic mass media campaigns. As a result, PSI Kenya developed a brand strategy around *Trust* as a 'cool' and contemporary choice that distinguished the user from the crowd. For example, in one radio spot, a man repeatedly calls a woman to ask for a date. The woman refuses to speak with him on several occasions. When she does agree to listen to him, the man describes the lengths that he has gone to organize the date, including getting transport to and from the movie. He finally manages to get her attention when he mentions his intention of bringing 20 packets of Trust condoms for her birthday party. This prompts her to say that he is cool and to agree to go out with him.

In addition to the branded mass media campaign promoted both openness with a partner and openness about condoms in order to develop a new image of condoms that associated condoms with trusting one's partner. Similar lifestyle-oriented approaches have been successful in other social marketing interventions in sub-Saharan Africa (Agha *et al.* 2001). The visual presence of Trust condoms was enhanced by the use of outdoor advertising, including a wall branding (mural) campaign. Various other special events such as concerts were also part of the brand advertising activities.

In addition to the branded campaign, there was a generic campaign that used fear appeal messages. To avoid *Trust* losing brand equity through a potentially confusing or seemingly contradictory message to its branded 'social desirability' message, a separate generic campaign was developed to induce uncertainty/fear about the consequences of not using condoms consistently. In one of these generic advertisements, several men and women introduce themselves by saying 'Hi, I'm Fred', 'Hi, I'm Mary', etc. The listener is asked to guess which of these persons has HIV. The message behind the advertisement is that it is not possible to guess if someone has AIDS and that condoms should be used whenever one has sexual relations.

Agha (2003) reports findings from an evaluation of the *Trust* campaign. The objective of this study was to determine whether an AIDS prevention mass media campaign influenced risk perception, self-efficacy and other behavioral predictors. Using house-hold survey data collected from 2213 sexually experienced male and female Kenyans aged 15–39. Respondents were administered a questionnaire asking them about their exposure to the branded *Trust* and generic mass media messages concerning HIV/AIDS and condom use. They were asked questions concerning their personal risk perception, self-efficacy, condom effectiveness, condom availability, and their embarrassment in obtaining condoms. Logistic regression analysis revealed that those exposed to branded advertising messages were significantly more likely to consider themselves at higher risk of acquiring HIV and to believe in the severity of AIDS. Exposure to branded messages was also associated with a higher level of personal self-efficacy, a greater belief in the efficacy of condoms, a lower level of perceived difficulty in obtaining condoms, and reduced embarrassment in purchasing condoms. There was also a dose–response relationship: a higher intensity of exposure to advertising was associated with more posi-tive outcomes. Exposure to generic advertising messages was less frequently associated with positive health beliefs and these relationships were also weaker. Agha (2003) concludes that branded mass media campaigns that promote condom use as an attractive lifestyle choice are likely to contribute to the development of perceptions that are conducive to the adoption of condom use.

What is distinctive about *Trust* is its focus on the condom – not as a commercial product – but as a symbol of a lifestyle choice. Based on the Evans *et al.* (forthcoming) criteria that a public health brand's objective must be solely health promotion and not product promotion for commercial purposes, *Trust* was aimed at making the choice to always use condoms socially desirable. The condom was an instrument to effect the choice of personal responsibility and control as mechanisms of social acceptability. The condom also represented a call to action for the brand – always be prepared with a Trust condom. *Trust* represents a distinctive strategy in that it sought to build a social norm of condom use through an object, a product, not as a commercial end in itself, but as the focus of a healthy lifestyle choice.

Salama (HIV/AIDS prevention in Tanzania)

The *Salama* campaign represents a different approach to branding condom use. Also developed and implemented by PSI, *Salama* targeted high-risk groups, primarily young people aged 15–24 as well as other target groups, in its campaign against spread of HIV/AIDS. While vulnerable, the campaign also operated on the principle that young people are more susceptible to behavior change communication messages. *Salama* also targeted high-risk groups, including key transmitters of HIV/AIDS such as commercial sex workers, truck drivers and other transient groups, as well as the rural Tanzanian population, which suffers from lack of information on HIV/AIDS.

PSI used a balance of behavioral prevention and condom use promotion strategies to reach these targeted high-risk groups. Strategies included: abstinence and delayed sexual debut to young people who are not yet sexually active; mutual fidelity and condom use for those active but in stable relationships; and condoms and partner reduction for high-risk groups (e.g. truck drivers) and the general population exhibiting high-risk behavior (PSI 2006b). *Salama* used a wide variety of channels, and relied heavily on community outreach such as roadshows, cultural shows, mobile video units, promotion events, concerts, sport tournaments and the *Amua* newsletter which is distributed in schools. There was also a mass media campaign that included paid and government-sponsored local and national television and radio advertising and billboards.

In addition to these largely individual-level strategies, *Salama* also worked upstream in workplaces, schools and other NGOs. For example, PSI promoted workplace health policies and using workplaces to deliver the strategies highlighted above.

The stigma surrounding HIV/AIDS, and surrounding prevention strategies, was a major focus of *Salama*. For example, PSI developed messages targeting the 'trusted partner syndrome', in which partners who have regular sexual relations and develop a level of trust choose not to use condoms. *Salama* also targeted stigma among the 15–24-year-old target group associated with buying or getting condoms (PSI 2006b).

Eloundou-Eneygue *et al.* (2005) show that *Salama* also offers distinctive lessons about public health brand evaluation. The authors conducted retrospective event-history analysis covering a four-year period to examine the timing of exposure to HIV/AIDS education and social marketing condom promotion campaigns, relative to the timing of changes in sexual risk behavior in Tanzania. This analysis showed that the process of exposure to AIDS education messages and exposure to brand advertising for Salama brand condoms was very different. While exposure to AIDS education was early and gradual, exposure to Salama brand condoms started later, but was much more rapid. After one year of advertising, over half of the 15–24-year-old population had been reached by the *Salama* advertising campaign, mostly through newspapers, radio and television. During the study period, condom use increased from 15 per cent at the beginning of 1993 to 42 per cent at the end of 1996. Increases in condom use were driven both by males who became sexually active, and by males who were not yet protected, or not fully protected. This study also found that once males adopted condom use, they were unlikely to return to more risky behavior, suggesting the potential for long-term behavior maintenance.

Salama highlights the multifaceted nature of sexual risk behavior related to HIV/AIDS, and the differences in target groups engaging in and affected by these diverse behaviors. As much or more than other health risk behaviors, HIV/AIDS calls for multiple branded messages and promotion strategies. Abstinence is an important option for young people, especially those who have not yet become sexually active, but condom use and partner reduction is needed for older, sexually active, and/or transient audiences. In Tanzania, issues of stigma and lack of access to mass media channels such as television and internet for most of the target population further heighten the need to use multiple channels to achieve the broadest possible reach and exposure.

loveLife (HIV/AIDS prevention in South Africa)

The South African *loveLife* brand represents the third, and most comprehensive, approach to public health branding of HIV/AIDS prevention. The *loveLife* brand is the largest effort ever launched in South Africa to change adolescent sexual behavior, with the aim of reducing the rate of HIV infection among 15–20-year-olds by 50 per cent, reducing other sexually transmitted infections, and reducing the incidence of teenage pregnancy. The brand promotion campaign was launched in September 1999, by a consortium of leading South African public health organizations in partnership with a coalition of more than 100 community-based organizations, the South African government, major South African media groups and the Kaiser Family Foundation.

The *loveLife* brand is based on promoting a holistic lifestyle choice that values abstinence, delayed initiation of sexual activity, reduction of sexual partners among already sexually active teenagers, and condom usage. Branded behaviors and supporting values include more open communication about HIV/AIDS, sex and relationships; gender relations based on informed choice; shared responsibility for sexual decisions; and healthy lifestyle and aspirations. Brand promotion combines a highly-visible, long-term multimedia HIV education and awareness campaign with nationwide adolescent-centered reproductive health services in government clinics and a network of youth outreach and support (Kaiser Family Foundation 2007).

The *loveLife* brand builds on the optimism of young South Africans – especially those under 16 years of age – who have not had sex and are not HIV positive. The brands calls young people to action – to 'maintain an AIDS-free lifestyle and to achieve your dreams and aspirations through self-motivation and leadership'.

The major campaign strategies include: (1) a sustained *loveLife* brand promotion and HIV/AIDS awareness campaign – including television, radio, outdoor media and print – aimed at educating young people about HIV and promoting dialogue about sexual health issues; (2) educational entertainment programming including two *loveLife* television series – *JikaJika*, and *S'camto*; (3) the National Adolescent-Friendly Clinic Initiative, a major drive to establish adolescent health services in South Africa's 5000 public clinics; (4) a national network of 16 multipurpose youth facilities, known as 'Y-Centres', providing recreation and skills training, as well as sexual health education and care in non-clinical settings; (5) a countrywide program of community-level outreach and support to young people (including 3500 schools) led by a national volunteer corps of more than 1500 18–25-year-olds known as *loveLife groundbreakers*; (6) a nationally accessible toll-free telephone helpline for young people providing specialized sexual health information, counseling and referrals averaging 300 000 calls per month; and (7) *loveLife Games*, the largest school sports competition in South Africa, promoting healthy living, self-motivation and personal achievement to more than 400 000 school students annually (Stadler and Hlongwa 2002; Kaiser Family Foundation 2007).

The *loveLife* brand has been evaluated following a five-year research and evaluation plan including a multiyear comprehensive observational study, tracking of brand equity and formation of branded associations; message recall and receptivity; and change in a range of behavioral indicators and in sexual health outcomes. Stadler and Hlongwa (2002) report that from 1999 to 2001 *loveLife* reached more than 4 million South African youth. Sixty-two per cent of youth and 59 per cent of their parents/guardians recognized the brand, while the vast majority of parents (97 per cent) and youth (89 per cent) exposed to *loveLife* identified *loveLife* as being positive. A subsequent evaluation sponsored by the Kaiser Family Foundation found that by 2004 nearly 85 per cent of South African youth reported confirmed awareness of *loveLife*; more than two-thirds had been exposed to at least three *loveLife* advertisements, programs or products; significant correlation (in cross-sectional survey data) between brand exposure and abstinence, waiting to have sex, and condom use among those sexually active; and significantly lower odds of HIV-positive status after brand exposure.

The *loveLife* brand is distinctive first in its comprehensive scope and ability to deploy and sustain significant financial, media, community, government and NGO sector resources to the epidemic of HIV/AIDS. Its sheer scale and sustained effort is a model that few other public health brands in the developing or developed world have achieved. But *loveLife* is also distinctive in using innovative strategies, such as educational entertainment programming, that enhance the brand's integration into the audience's daily lives and provide opportunities to elaborate on messages and arguments for behavior change (Petty and Cacioppo 1986). Finally, the campaign's resources and context in a more advanced developing country such as South Africa have enabled it to use methodologies utilized in many developed-world branded campaigns. For example, the brand promoted young adults as social role models (*loveLife groundbreakers*), which has been successfully used in promotion for the *truth* tobacco countermarketing brand in the USA (Holden *et al.* 2005). It has also used sports participation to build brand equity and promote team sports as an alternative to health risk behaviors, much as the *VERB* campaign has promoted sports as an alternative to sedentary behavior (Huhman *et al.* 2005). Figure 11.1 captures the community outreach component of *loveLife*.

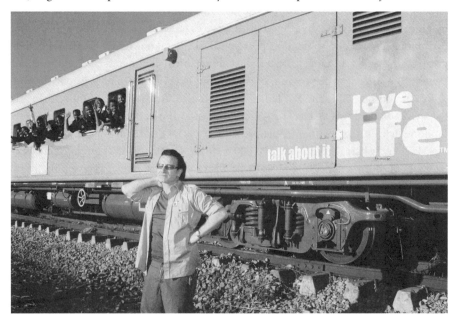

Fig. 11.1 *loveLife* brand imagery. Reproduced with permission from the Henry J. Kaiser Family Foundation.

Zuia Mbu (Malaria prevention in Tanzania)

The *Zuia Mbu* (Kiswahili for 'prevent mosquitoes') brand utilized indigenous knowledge and communication practices to promote insecticide-treated nets (ITNs) to prevent and control malaria infection in the Kilombero Valley region of Southern Tanzania. The *Zuia Mbu* brand was developed through the Kilombero Treated Net (KINET) Project, funded by the US Agency for International Development (Armstrong Schellenberg *et al.* 2001; IHRDC 2001). The project developed *Zuia Mbu* as part of a social marketing strategy to distribute and promote utilization of ITNs and insecticide to a rural population of 480 000 people living in the Kilombero Valley (Armstrong Schellenberg *et al.* 1999; Abdulla *et al.* 2001). The KINET project operated from July 1996 to June 2000.

The idea behind *Zuia Mbu* was to build on existing interpersonal communication channels and knowledge to build a relationship between the brand and villagers. The conceptual basis of *Zuia Mbu* derives from work by Mundy and Compton (1995) in which they call attention to the interface of exogenous and indigenous knowledge and communication and the importance of this interface for the development process. They suggest a conceptual model that contrasts exogenous (e.g. for the Kilombero residents, mass communication strategies) and indigenous types of knowledge and communication, and identifies opportunities to communicate indigenous knowledge through exogenous channels.

As discussed earlier in this chapter, brand promotion efforts in all cultural and country settings utilize mass media of various kinds to communicate behavior change messages. The alternative, indigenous approach emphasizes locally organized channels and folk media like local theatre groups staging plays to disseminate knowledge about a variety of health and community issues, such as family planning programs in Indonesia (Mundy and Compton 1995: 121). Little has been published on indigenous knowledge that has been taken up and spread through exogenous channels, although this type of information flow carries great potential (Minja and Obrist 2005).

Armstrong Schellenberg *et al.* (1999) describe the *Zuia Mbu* brand promotion campaign to promote ITN adoption and use. Formative and market research were conducted in order to understand community perceptions, knowledge, attitudes and practice with respect to the products to be socially marketed. *Zuiu Mbu* was used as the brand name for both ITNs and single-dose insecticide treatment sachets. Brand promotion included a mix of public and private channels. The first step was identification of local agents (village leaders, shop owners, priests and health workers) to promote ITN use in Kilombero and communicate indigenous knowledge about mosquito prevention. For single-dose treatment, young people were appointed in the same villages and trained as agents. Other institutions in Kilombero such as hospitals, development projects and employers were also involved in distribution. Promotion for both products used a variety of channels, including posters and a leaflet, informed by formative research and drawn by a local artist and pilot-tested; billboards posted along main roads and a local bus with the *Zuia Mbu* logo; and a discount system to reduce further the cost of a net for mothers of young children and pregnant women, developed for use through health clinics.

Armstrong Schellenberg *et al.* (1999) report that a total of 22 410 nets and 8072 treatments were sold during the first year: 18 months after launching, 46 per cent of 312 families with children aged under five years reported that they were sleeping under treated nets.

The *Zuia Mbu* brand represents an innovative conceptual model to reaching rural, indigenous populations in the developing world that are not closely connected to the mass media channels used for most public health brand promotion. The use of indigenous knowledge and communication channels, use of cost reductions as a component of a branded social marketing promotion, and use of indigenous actors as channels for health information are all distinctive components of this malaria prevention brand.

Suami SIAGA (Reproductive health in Indonesia)

Shefner-Rogers and Sood (2004) describe the branded *Suami SIAGA* (Kiswahilli for: I'm an Alert Husband) campaign in Indonesia, which was promoted through a multimedia campaign that also utilized entertainment education, and targeted husbands with messages about birth preparedness. Shared responsibility was at the heart of the brand strategy to reduce potentially fatal delays in treatment before, during and after the birthing process. As delays can occur at different times and places, preparedness and readiness must therefore occur at different places and involve a variety of people and places. Under the *Suami SIAGA* initiative, the core behaviors and intervention steps promoted for husbands were recognizing danger signs and preparing for childbirth by saving funds, arranging for transportation to a health facility if necessary, and identifying a skilled provider and birthing place.

Evaluation of the *Suami SIAGA* (alert husband) in 2000 and baseline assessment in six West Java districts in 2000–2001 provided insights and recommendations for the development of the subsequent *Warga SIAGA* (alert citizen) and *Bidan SIAGA* (alert midwife) campaigns (Shefner-Rogers and Sood 2004). Each phase of the *SIAGA* campaign shared a common brand identity, but had distinctive goals and approaches. Popular Indonesian singer Iis Dahlia served as the spokesperson through each *SIAGA* campaign. Launched in 2001, *Warga SIAGA* encouraged individual citizens to be alert and prepared for delivery by doing their part in arranging for transport, funds, a blood donor, and recognizing danger signs. Launched in 2002, *Bidan SIAGA* promoted the midwife as a skilled and friendly provider prepared to help throughout the pregnancy. As a result, *SIAGA* became the brand name for safe motherhood in Indonesia (Johns Hopkins University, Center for Communication Programs 1998).

Shefner-Rogers and Sood (2004) found that when husbands were directly exposed to the messages from the *Suami SIAGA* campaign, there was knowledge gain about birth preparedness activities. However, the interaction of direct exposure to the campaign and the interpersonal communication stimulated by the campaign about *Suami SIAGA* was an even stronger predictor of knowledge gain and taking birth preparedness actions. As this was a post-only evaluation, findings should be treated with caution as there was no control for baseline differences in potential confounding variables (e.g. previous related knowledge, attitudes, beliefs and practices) that may have affected the interaction. However, the *SIAGA* brands achieved high levels of awareness and appear to have changed social norms about shared parental and community responsibility for birth preparedness and action.

The *SIAGA* brands are distinctive in that they took a multilevel approach, seeking to change the social norms of multiple levels of influence on the health behavior (interpersonal, community) that has been adopted as best practice in health promotion (Green and Kreuter 1999). The campaign also sought to change behaviors not directly related to the individual's health, but to the health of loved ones, appealing to shared responsibility as an interpersonal and community commitment, and branding overall community wellbeing as opposed to individual health benefit. This approach may have potential for other social issues such as environmental protection (i.e. the individual contributing to a larger social benefit) in which immediate returns on effort invested accrue to others, or society as a whole.

Challenges facing public health brand promotion in developing countries

Channels

Some of the biggest challenges facing public health brand promotion were suggested in the earlier discussion of media use patterns. Low penetration of media channels into rural and low-income populations poses a significant promotional challenge, but one that the campaigns discussed earlier, and others, have overcome or worked around. The solution has naturally been to do formative research on what channels target audiences use, and then use appropriate channels, including highly localized channels such as the *Zuia Mbu* approach of using indigenous knowledge and communication, or in the case of well-funded efforts, to use a very wide diversity of channels at multiple levels, such as in *loveLife*.

But another major challenge is local media capability and resources to develop materials and access existing media channels. For example, in Kenya there appears to be growth in the number of locally-owned media production firms. This change is apparently a result of the increasing popularity of the Kenyan film industry and also the increasing attraction of Kenya as a shooting location for international film companies. The film producers' 2005 directory listed 40 locally-owned and 13 international or foreign-owned independent television/film production companies in Kenya (Africa Film and TV 2007).

Data on advertising agency growth are not readily available, but there has definitely been an increase in market research, with Steadman Research and Consumer Insight being the leaders in collecting media market data. There are currently around 70 advertising agencies, 13 market research agencies and 22 marketing consultants in Kenya. Some of the leading international advertising agencies, including Ogilvy & Mather, McCann-Erickson and Young & Rubicam, have local offices or affiliates.

Several other challenges emerged from, or are suggested by, the case studies that should be considered:

- *Reaching diverse audience segments.* Many developing countries, such as South Africa and Indonesia, have extreme racial, ethnic, linguistic, religious and other cultural diversities. These factors are all well known to affect message reactions and receptivity (Petty and Cacioppo 1986; Evans *et al.* 2005), and combined with limitations in terms of media usage and the need to use multiple or non-traditional channels (at least by developed world standards) create a very complex communication and media environment. Public health brand promotion in these contexts needs to consider strategies such as development of a core brand with a common purpose, outcome and reputation, which can be decomposed into sub-brands, such as in the case of *SIAGA*, with a common look and feel. In highly diverse developing country settings, public health brand promoters should consider developing parent brand and then implementation of sub-brands as time, resources, audience reactions and mental energy permit.

- *Health and general literacy.* Health literacy is critical to message development, delivery, and reactions and receptivity (Bernhardt *et al.*, 2003). The Indonesian husbands receiving *SIAGA* messages initially had low health literacy about birth preparedness, and the campaign was thus in part educational and in part motivational to promote preparedness and action. In *Salama*, the target audiences lacked knowledge of HIV/AIDS risk factors and needed this foundation in order to acquire motivational elements of brand equity (e.g. brand loyalty, awareness). At the same time, general literacy levels vary greatly across the developing world, with low levels in poorer nations such as Tanzania, and great diversity within regions and populations in more prosperous countries such as South Africa. Logo development, channel selection, promotional messages, and most other brand development components hinge on these elements, and this adds another layer of complexity to brand strategy.

- *Credibility of media sources.* Media source credibility is central to message receptivity and reactions (Evans *et al.* forthcoming). Developing contexts calls for careful formative research on media sources, and consideration of trade-offs between reach (mass level often better) and potential reactions (local level often better). The work by Mundy and Compton (1995) shows the potential for more refined levels of cultural targeting and small population tailoring of messages and channels, especially in situations where the population is deprived of health information, such as in rural developing country settings.

Conclusions and implications for public health branding and social marketing

This brief review of public health brands in the developing world suggests a few overarching conclusions, future directions for brand development and research, and some general conclusions for social marketing. First, the behavior change communication theory and mix of theoretical assumptions underlying developing world public health brands may differ.

What constitutes an idealized external image or a credible source obviously differs between many audience segmentation factors, as noted above. But what is less obvious, and brands such as *SIAGA* and *Zuia Mbu* make clear, is that these differences can be fundamental, as there is in many cases a near absence of shared cultural experience between populations highly exposed to modern mass media (e.g. in Dar es Salaam) and those sheltered from substantial portions of that 24/7 onslaught (e.g. residents of the Kilombero Valley).

Second, there may be differences in what behaviors we can realistically hope to affect in developing world contexts as compared with the developed world. Some behaviors, such as promoting abstinence in adolescents, have proven intractable in the USA, or at least the available evidence suggests that intervention strategies to date have been ineffective (Trenholm *et al.* 2007). Yet exposure to brands such as *Salama* and *loveLife* was associated with abstinence in this same population in Tanzania and South Africa. The myriad of cultural and sociodemographic factors, such as the relative cost–benefit of abstinence in two societies – say the USA and Tanzania – with widely differing average personal income and future earning potential, may help to explain these differences in outcomes. But this review at least suggests the potential for differing behavior change 'gradients' – the degree of difficulty and ultimate tractability – for different health behaviors between the developed and developing world contexts.

Third, there may be differences in optimal marketing mixes and execution strategies stemming from these differences, and from the issues of cultural differences in message receptivity and reaction. We saw similar marketing mixes in terms of promotional, placement and product strategies in *Trust* and *Salama* in two relatively similar country contexts. Meanwhile, on the same topic but in a somewhat wealthier country and more diverse population context, with *loveLife* we found a wider variety of product (e.g. using educational entertainment programming) and promotional strategies. Granted, *loveLife* was blessed with greater financial and other resources, but the marketing mixes were also largely a function of audience and available channels (e.g. television penetration for the *loveLife* programming). The marketing mix clearly varied among the five case studies, and there may be more effective marketing mixes that future public health brands can utilize in specific developing contexts.

This review raises some questions to be answered by future brand development and research activities, including:

- To what extent are branding evidence and strategies from the developed world applicable to developing world contexts?
- What models can be articulated for the marketing mix in developing country contexts?
  - Is there an optimal mix of price, promotion, placement and product strategies depending on local conditions and factors such as media use patterns, health literacy and sociodemographics?
- How can we expand and improve the evaluation methods used in, and quality of evidence derived from, branding evaluations? Are randomized experimental designs, or close alternatives such as delayed intervention designs (such as planned in Evans *et al.*, forthcoming) desirable, feasible and ethical?

◆ What are the ethical implications of branded messages in low literacy (and low media access and health literacy) populations? What special obligations do brand developers have in terms of limiting the use of behavior change messages to populations that have limited ability to critically examine the implications of those messages for themselves, their families and communities?

Finally, the strategies being used by commercial marketers in developing countries may also suggest future directions for public health branding. While much recent trade has flowed from large developing countries such as India and China to the West, Western multinationals have also had success with brand promotion. With large populations of young people in developing countries, many Western companies have targeted the younger audience with brand promotions. In China, for example, Marlboro was the most popular cigarette brand even when it was officially banned and illegal in the 1990s, and was something of a black market phenomenon among younger consumers. In India, where there are estimated to be more than 150 million middle class consumers, Western-style shopping malls with offerings from McDonald's to Nike are expanding rapidly.

Western brands have capitalized on a new, typically young, urban, upwardly mobile population that has reaped benefits of globalization. For example, marketers are developing sophisticated strategies to reach the young Indian middle class, which has grown with the development of information technology-related industries in the country (MarketingSherpa 2007). At the same time, the young people targeted by these brands also disproportionately use new media and are increasingly exposed to online advertising, including through web-enabled handheld devices which, as discussed in this chapter, are in widespread and growing use.

In short, young people are an access point for brands of all kinds into developing markets. These same young people are also often at greatest health risk for behaviors such as tobacco use and unprotected sex, and are natural targets for protective messages from social marketing campaigns. The confluence of media use patterns, success in commercial brand promotion, and socioeconomic development enabled by globalization present new opportunities for public health branding in the developing world.

References

Abdulla, S., Armstrong Schellenberg, J. R. M., Nathan, R., Mukasa, O., Marchant, T., Smith, T., *et al.* (2001). Impact on malaria morbidity of a programme supplying insecticide treated nets in children aged under 2 years in Tanzania: community cross-sectional study. *British Medical Journal* **322**:270–3.

Africa Film and TV. (2007). Available at: http://www.afridigital.net/ (accessed 22 October 2007).

Agha, S. (2003). The impact of a mass media campaign on personal risk perception, perceived self-efficacy and on other behavioral predictors. *Aids Care* **15**:749–62.

Agha, S., Karlyn, A., and Meekers, D. (2001). The promotion of condom use in non-regular sexual partnerships in urban Mozambique. *Health Policy and Planning* **16**:144–51.

Armstrong Schellenberg, J. R. M., Abdulla, S., Minja, H., Nathan, R., Mukasa, O., Marchant, T., *et al* (1999). KINET: A social marketing programme of treated nets and net treatment for malaria control in Tanzania, with evaluation of child health and long-term survival. *Transactions of the Royal Society of Tropical Medicine and Hygiene* **93**:225–31.

Armstrong Schellenberg, J. R. M., Abdulla, S., Nathan, R., Mukasa, O., Marchant, T., Kikumbih, N., *et al.* (2001) Effect of large-scale social marketing of insecticide-treated nets on child survival in rural Tanzania. *Lancet* **357**:1241–47.

Bernhardt, J.M. and Cameron, K.A. (2003). Accessrly, understanding, and Applying Health Communicative Messages: The Challenge of Health Literary. In T.L.Thamson, A.M. Dassey, K.I. Miller, and R. Parrott (eds.). Handbook of Health Communication Mahwah, NJ: Lawrence Erlbaum Associates, p. 583–605.

Calvert, S. (2008). Using media to sell: marketing to children and media campaigns. *Future of Children: Children, Media, and Technology* 18(1):205–34.

Eloundou-Enyegue, P. M., Meekers, D., and Calves, A. E. (2005) 'From awareness to adoption: the effect of AIDS education and condom social marketing on condom use in Tanzania (1993–1996)', *Journal of Biosocial Science* **37**:257–68.

Eriksson, T., Sonesson, A., and Isacsson, A. (1997). HIV/AIDS information and knowledge: a comparative study of Kenyan and Swedish teenagers. *Scandinavian Journal of Social Medicine* **25**:111–18.

Evans, W. D., Blitstein, J., Lynch, C., de Villiers, A., Steyn, N., Draper, C. Lambert, V. (forthcoming). Childhood obesity prevention in South Africa: developing a family-centered social marketing intervention. *Social Marketing Quarterly.*

Evans, W.D., S. Price, and S. Blahut (2005). Evaluating the truth® brand. *Journal of Health Communication* **10**:181–92.

Government of India Census, NRS-2001. (2007). Available at: http://www.exchange4media.com/e4m/viewpoint/viewpoint_211002.asp (accessed 22 October 2007).

Green, L. W. and Kreuter, M. W. (1999). *Health promotion planning: An educational and ecological approach* (3rd edn). Mountain View, CA: Mayfield Publishing.

Holden, D., Evans, W. D., Hinnant, L., and Messeri, P. (2005). Modeling psychological empowerment among youth involved in local tobacco control efforts. *Health Education and Behavior* **32**:264–78.

Huhman, M., Potter, L., Wong, F., Banspach, S., Duke, J., and Heitzler, C. (2005). Effects of a mass media campaign to increase physical activity among children: year-1 results of the VERB campaign. *Pediatrics* **116**:e247–e254.

Kaiser Family Foundation. (2007). KNOW HIV/AIDS: Learn about the campaign. Available at: http://www.kff.org/about/lovelife.cfm (accessed 10 August 2007).

Ifakaora Health Research and Development Centre (IHRDC) (2001). The Kinet Project. An overview. Ifakara: Ifakara Health Research and Development Centre.

Internet World Stats. (2006). Available at: http://www.internetworldstats.com/africa.htm (accessed 22 October 2007).

Internet World Stats. (2007). Available at: http://www.internetworldstats.com/america.htm (accessed 22 October 2007).

Johns Hopkins University, Center for Communication Programs. (1998). *Safe motherhood: a partnership and family approach, IEC strategy and implementation plan.* Baltimore, MD: Johns Hopkins University, Center for Communication Programs.

LaFraniere, S. (2005). Cellphones catapult rural Africa to 21st century. *New York Times*, 24 August. 1–2

MarketingSherpa. (2007). How to market to India online. Available at: https://www.marketingsherpa.com/barrier.php?ident=29656 (accessed 23 October 2007).

Minja, H. and Obrist, B. (2005). Integrating local and biomedical knowledge and communication: experiences from KINET Project in Southern Tanzania. *Human Organization* **64**:157–65.

Mundy, P. A. and Compton, J. L. (1995). Indigenous communication and indigenous knowledge. In D. M. Warren, L. J. Slikkerveer, and D. Brokensha (eds.) *The cultural dimension of development: indigenous knowledge systems.* London: Intermediate Technology Publications. pp. 157–65.

Petty, R. E. and Cacioppo, J. T. (1986). *Communication and persuasion: central and peripheral routes to attitude change*. New York: Springer-Verlag.

Population Services International (PSI). (2006a). Kenya. Available at: www.psi.org/where_we_work/kenya.html (accessed 3 March 2008).

Population Services International (PSI). (2006b). Tanzania. Available at: http://www.psi.org/where_we_work/tanzania.html (accessed 3 March 2008).

Rideout, V. (2004). *Assessing public education programming on HIV/AIDS: a national survey of African Americans*. Washington, DC: Kaiser Family Foundation.

Shefner-Rogers, C.L., and Sood, S. (2004). Involving husbands in safe motherhood: effects of the SUAMI SIAGA campaign in Indonesia. *Journal of Health Communication* **9**:233–58.

Stadler J, Hlongwa L. (2002). Monitoring and evaluation of loveLife's AIDS prevention and advocacy activities in South Africa 1999–2001. *Evaluation and Program Planning* **25**:365–76.

Trenholm, C., Devaney, B., Fortson, K., Quay, L., Wheeler, J., and Clark, M. Impacts of Four Title V, Section 510 Abstinence Education Programs. Final Report submitted to USDHHS, Assistant Secretary for Planning and Evaluation. Available at: http://aspe.hhs.gov/hsp/abstinence07/ (accessed 22 October 2007).

UNAIDS. (2002). *Report on the global HIV/AIDS epidemic 2002*. Geneva: Joint United Nations Program on HIV/AIDS.

12

Branding of international public health organizations
Applying commercial marketing to global public health

Muhiuddin Haider and Michelle J. Lee

Summary

- Organizational brands in public health transcend products and services and seek to develop a relationship and a sense of trust with the target audience.
- Organizational branding is both about transforming the internal culture of an organization's environment through people and process-related change and about projecting the vision, goals and focus of the organization into its products and services for the goal of behavior change.
- There is no single approach to organizational branding in public health. However, the most effective approaches are achieved by organizations whose products and services reflect the core mission and values of the organization itself
- In public health, organizational branding still has much to learn and to apply from corporate branding. Organizational branding as an approach to behavior change often lacks clarity. Adequate documentation of successes is needed.

Introduction

Businesses of all types have long tailored their products and services to reach their target audiences in greater numbers. While the emergence of international markets has consistently added a wrinkle to traditional marketing and branding conceptions, corporations have responded to that challenge by pursuing cross-cultural relevance or culturally-specific resonance. The ability of corporate brands to transcend geographical and cultural barriers to similarly evoke the same emotions, desires and consumption patterns is indicative of the power of brands. The history of international health initiatives reflects a similar search for the optimal provision of goods and services. However, it is the focus on behavioral change rather than merely consumption and optimization of profits that warrants a different approach and application of branding principles. The attempt to address complex social problems by bringing about changes in social attitudes and behaviors affords a much more challenging front. Concepts such as social marketing have made efforts to address these challenges through the application and active use of commercial marketing strategies to induce change in behavior and societal conditions and policies.

This chapter, a primer on international organizational health branding, attempts to demonstrate a branding practice beyond that of products and services that addresses the movement of social marketing in international health. Acknowledging the numerous actors in the international health scene, we further explore different organizational approaches to branding in international health initiatives. As a patchwork of public, private and religious outreach, international health has gained a following of donors, practitioners and advocates that have influenced the course of action in addressing international health issues. Hailing from the various fields of psychology, marketing, medicine, economics and politics, the actors in international public health bring an amalgam of specialized knowledge and skills to strategic public health responses to reducing the worldwide burden of disease and improving health status. The gathering of these complex and sustained stratagems across disciplines into a brand can be a potent advantage.

When organizations are brands in and of themselves, the products and services they offer automatically fall within that brand. Branding therefore involves strategically and effectively crafting all elements of the audience's interactions with the organization and its products and services so that they evoke the right emotions and support the right image, namely behavior change. The challenge for public health institutions, particularly at an international level, is to understand how to efficiently and effectively utilize the principles of branding strategy in the institutional context, while realizing that these efforts result in the communication of core values to their target audience. While clear recognition of the brand by target audiences is invariably central to successful branding, how institutions communicate their promise and deliver on that promise are also crucial ingredients for success as described in the introductory chapter of this book. This chapter examines some principles inherent to the practice of organizational branding and how this translates across sectors.

Types of branding: the products, services and organization continuum

In the corporate world, branding can happen at three different levels: the corporate, the product business and the product. As we are concerned with behavior change and not just product movement, all three become necessary elements of health branding. Brands are a means for public health organizations to achieve their goals in promoting behavior change. In this way, the branding of an organization cannot be distanced from the branding of its products and services. Branding must operate at all levels of the product, service and organization. Due to the inclusion of a chapter on international health branding of products and services, we focus here on organizational branding which incorporates but is not wholly defined by products and services. However, because organizational branding cannot be understood without the basic framework of the product and service concepts, we very briefly revisit them here.

Product branding is familiar and abundantly recognized in society. Products are branded by differentiating them with a name and/or symbol such as a logo, trademark or package design. This is often intended to identify the goods of an organization and to create a unique position in the mind of the consumer or other stakeholders. Likewise, services are branded to be differentiated. Services bring the audience and organization or program representatives and providers in closer and more meaningful interaction. These services may include educational sessions or even actual provision of clinical services, such as giving contraceptive injections. Through these interpersonal interactions, the service provided directly reflects upon the organization's performance.

In each instance, the identity of a brand represents what the organization stands for. Whereas visibility and recognition are key elements that determine the success of the brand, a brand is much more than just the product itself, or the visuals created to promote the product. Beyond recognition, the brand is how the audience connects with what you are promoting at an emotional level. In this sense, it is a combination of how the product is marketed, and how the audience experiences it. It further implies a promise to the public from the organization's members (Aaker 1996: 68). It can be viewed as a contract between the organization and audience regarding the value delivered by the product or service in support of the behavior change (Kotler and Armstrong 2005). Certainly, the successful narrative of products and services has been about finding areas neglected and needs not addressed by established markets. There is an increasingly recognized market for health products and services in developing countries (expanding with identification, access and transmission, while shrinking only with effective and curative health response) which is and will continue to be addressed, met, and sometimes exploited for profit. What concerns us in international health branding is not simply the provision of products for profits, but also the promotion of sustainable behavior change. Such a change does often coincide with products – condoms coupled with healthy sexual behavior, for example – though this is not always the case. Here, the promise of branding in international health is the delivery of full knowledge of lifestyle, prevention and treatment into a recognizable and culturally appropriate package.

The delivery of the brand to its target audience plays an important role in its acceptance and success. Together, with recognition and promise, the delivery of brands communicates a message. This message carries the values of the organization the brand represents as well as of the product or service it may be promoting. Numerous organizations have utilized health programs and campaigns as a bridge to bring essential health messages, products and services to targeted audiences. However, the question remains whether or not organizations are harnessing all aspects of these mechanisms in a manner suitable to reaching overall goals in health promotion and behavior change.

Organizational branding in the public health context

Branding is a central component of business strategy, and it stands to reason that public health organizations would be concerned with how their brand helps them distinguish themselves and how it conveys their personality, values, principles, vision, purpose and mission (Sargeant and Ford 2007). Although the stake in health markets is more pressing, branding still involves shaping how the organization contributes, supports and enhances relationships with the public, including the targeted audiences as well as donors and stakeholders. The strengthening of these relationships through branding is accomplished via managing brand equity, brand quality, brand loyalty and brand associations, concepts explored in earlier chapters.

A dearth of literature exists regarding the role of organizational branding in the public health context. Much of the research centers on corporate strategies and for-profit settings, but has unique contributions and applications in the abstraction of the strategies and principles in public health. Aaker (1996) proposes the 'brand-as-organization' concept, which relates to the strength of the organization's image as a brand. This perspective focuses on much of the internal aspects as well as external aspects of brand management within an organization, such as the institution's personnel, culture, values and external programs. The importance and contribution of each of these facets of brand management are discussed in more detail throughout the chapter.

Implementing branding strategies in international public health organizations and successfully incorporating these strategies at an operational level for dissemination both internally and externally helps to establish a connection between the brand and the cause in both employee and consumer minds (Evans *et al.* 2005). Brands demonstrate a value in a public health organization's efforts to bring about social influence (Andreasen 2006). The value of a brand is not in the recognition of the name so much as it is in the trust people have in the organization and its products and services (Grunig *et al.* 2002). When organizations act with integrity; demonstrate credibility and consistency in their provision of products and services; are accessible and responsive; and communicate their level of commitment to the public, they are strengthening their brand (Duncan and Moriarty 1997) while building and strengthening relationships with their public. The trust established through these relationships is more likely to readily translate into changed behaviors and increased awareness.

Relationship building is an essential part of successful marketing. Much like commercial marketing, marketing in public health (also known as social marketing) attempts to go beyond a one-time transaction. Even more than a campaign or program that targets behavior change by itself, the focus should be on building relationships with the audiences whose behavior we want to change. The utilization of programs and campaigns in public health to reach these means have been observed, particularly through the health promotion and disease prevention efforts of social marketing. Because social marketing often addresses behaviors that need long-term efforts and high involvement to change, and in fact, may require lifestyle change, strategic relationship marketing as opposed to traditional transactional thinking is more likely to encourage behavior change (Hastings 2003; Siegel and Lotenberg 2007).

The power of an organization in actively building relationships with its target audience is inherent in its every aspect – physical spaces, communications, products, services and employees (Siegel and Lotenbnerg 2006). An organization's brand may act as the driver of the relationship as it communicates the values the organization stands for and represents the benefits, whether psychological or functional, that are being offered (Roman *et al.* 2003: 13).

> Public health institutions have brand identities, whether or not they want to, and unfamiliarity with brand management can lead to mistakes and missed opportunities. Every public health institution has an identity in the mind of funding agencies, potential partners, the media, and target audiences. The identity may be fuzzy or clear, positive, neutral or negative; but it exists.
>
> (Siegel and Lotenberg 2007: 226).

The importance of building, managing and sustaining brands and their relationships, internally as well as externally, cannot be understated. External brand management 'involves understanding the needs, wants, and desires of consumers to create marketing programs for brands that fulfill and even surpass consumer expectations' (Keller 2000: 134). Organizations accomplish this through their collective processes of formative research, including audience segmentation.

> With these [external brand management] marketing programs, consumers would have a clear picture of what the brand represents and why it is special. Consumers would then view the brand as a 'trusted friend' and value its dependability and superiority. With external brand management, marketers engage in dialogue with consumers, listening to their product joys and frustrations, and establishing a rapport and relationship that would transcend mere commercial exchanges. Marketers would develop a deep understanding of what makes their brand successful, retaining enduring core elements while modifying peripheral elements that fail to add value.
>
> (Keller 2000: 134)

It is easy to maintain an outward public focus when working with the development of public health brands. After all, societal interests are at hand. However, as key players in the branding strategy, organizational employees and partners must also 'appreciate and understand basic branding notions, and how they can impact, help, or hurt the equity of brands' (Keller 2000: 134). This facet of internal brand management requires that the brand be implemented in a consistent manner across all branded materials and messages that are distributed to strategic publics. Thus, proper internal brand management helps to ensure that the brand is consistently and effectively managed externally. There should be a lack of dissonance between the messages projected by the organization and the experience of the target audience.

Thus, internal brand management can be considered an upstream level of branding that branding helps to unify and express the established vision, values and goals of the organization at an organizational and policy level. Communication and delivery of the vision, values and goals for the downstream-level behavior change of individuals is often mediated through the different kinds of organizational branding, including social marketing and corporate social responsibility. Numerous organizations have utilized such branding strategies as a bridge to bring essential messages, products and services to targeted audiences to inspire change at an individual level.

Branding of organizations

Ultimately, however, brands are much more than just a label, logo or a service concept. One of the objectives of the brand in public health is to influence the values and behaviors of consumers (McFarland 2007). This influence will in part stem from the consumer's perception of the organization just as much as their perception of the product or service provided to them. So then, branding must start from the organizational core (Sargeant and Ford 2007). The branding framework for an organization includes the organization's vision, mission, purpose, values, actions, principles and personalities; it is, therefore, an amalgam of everything the organization is, says and does (Sargeant and Ford 2007). This core is integrated throughout the organization and establishes the direction, leadership, clarity of purpose, and energy for the organization's brand. Good and effective organizational brands start with a clear understanding of the organization itself. It is from this that the communications and visual elements such as logos flow.

As part of the organizational core, brands must convey an attractive personality as well as a distinctive one (Andreasen 2006). As Grunig (1993) rightly warns, symbolic relationships alone are not enough. They must be used in conjunction with behavioral relationships that are formed with the public through organizational branding. What makes an organization distinctive is its values, the actions it takes, and the manner in which these actions are undertaken (Sargeant and Ford 2007). Strong brands help organizations improve their effectiveness by raising their visibility among their target audience and also by helping them develop deeper relationships with their stakeholders (Sargeant 2007).

A powerful example of successful organizational branding in the corporate world is embodied by Apple. In spite of its continuous releases of innovative products, marketing experts view Apple's brand, not its products, as its key to survival (Gobe 2001). Apple has successfully launched a brand that people connect to at an emotional level as opposed to a purely consumer-oriented level of product purchasing. The power of Apple's brand in connecting to target audiences on a personal level is reflected in three respects (Gobe 2001). First, the company projects a humanistic corporate culture through its long commitment and partnership with educational institutions. It also evokes a strong corporate ethic that resonates with people in bringing power to people through technology. Second, the company has established a recognizable visual and verbal vocabulary that is clearly represented in its product design and advertising. The monochromatic apple symbol and the streamlined and colorful visual elements of Apple's products set it apart from all others. Third, the company has learned to resonate with its consumers through the building of trust, loyalty and a sense of community. Indeed, many a Mac user will feel a certain kinship with a complete stranger just by having identified that person as a fellow Mac user. The company has built a relationship with the user that is beyond transactional, but gives the user a sense that they belong to a special community, one that they are loyal to and that they value. It is this power of the brand alongside its innovative products and designs that drives people to buy into the community, despite its monetary price tag.

International health organizations must completely harness this demonstrated power of brands to create a sense of community and value in the target audiences' minds about demonstrated behavior change. What do public health organizations gain by developing a strong brand, and how does this aid them in achieving their goals for behavior change? Sargeant and Ford (2007) adeptly describes four ways in which brands contribute to the strengthening of the organization. First, brands enhance learning by functioning as the point of reference that makes people aware of the organization and its products and services. Second, brands reduce risk for the organization. One of the ways to reassure the public, including donors and stakeholders, that the organization is committed to delivering quality goods and services is to develop a brand identity that communicates this value (Chajet and Shachtman 1991). Third, brands provide insurance. This insurance is, in a manner of speaking, a type of insurance to protect an organization's reputation. This 'reputation insurance' is the ability of the organization to weather any bad circumstances that might temporarily bring about damage. Depending on how well established the brand is, the organization may be able to withstand short-term damage (Sargeant and Ford 2007). Finally, organizations gain loyalty through the building of their brands. The public is drawn to organizations that they perceive as having a 'personality' similar to their own. This similarity in personality may signify the acceptance of values that they already hold, or ones they aspire to adopt (Aaker 1996). The supporters of the brand in the community form an important core outside of the organization that works to further the organization's brand and mission.

Adoption and acceptance of the organization's brand identity by its target audience is a step in helping to facilitate behavior change. When the audience is ready for the message offered by the public health organization, but they find they are still unable to adopt the new behavior, social marketing campaigns provide the means through which the organization can establish a relationship with the targeted audience and work to influence their behavior (Pirani and Reizes 2005: 132). In this sense, social marketing provides a framework for the use of branding in addressing public health goals of voluntary behavior change, particularly through product and/or service consumption and the reduction or removal of the barriers that formerly inhibited the behavior (Keller 1998; Andreason 2002).

The use of branding in social marketing

The rise of social marketing has proven an enormous asset to the construction of health initiatives as organizations have adapted their practices and others have specialized in providing such services. Social marketing campaigns are a means through which an organization seeks to establish its relationship with the public; and through the products and/or services it offers, influence behavior change in the target audience. The proper utilization of branding, and the presence of a strong brand identity and image contribute to the effectiveness of the program (Engelberg and Kirby 2001).

A branded social marketing campaign is focused. It follows that the consistent use of brand symbols and logos throughout the campaign helps to maintain the focus in the messages, products and services. The target audience must trust that the organization branding the health issue or behavior is credible and truthful about the health issue, the risks encountered by partaking in the unhealthy behavior, and the benefits of changing their behavior to reduce those risks. Trust is therefore a key factor in organizational branding.

Depending upon the public health organization, the approach to branding might differ. However, what remains constant is the establishment of bonds between the target audience and the brand. Current efforts in social marketing campaigns themselves have been criticized where social marketers have not been sufficiently concerned with developing brands or relationships, but have been more concerned with telling people how to behave (Rothschild 2001: 37). However, the relevance, significance and potential of brands in public health social marketing campaigns cannot be undermined, and need to be further examined and appropriately incorporated.

> Branding may provide an important function in social marketing programs by helping individuals to communicate and signal to themselves as well as others that they are engaging in desirable behaviors so that [they] are better able to realize more immediate benefits and receive positive reinforcement … In other words, branding personally and/or socially desirable behaviors could help individuals receive more immediate awards from the public approval and recognition of others as well as from the benefits of self-expression and personal approval and recognition.
>
> (Keller 1998: 299, author's emphasis)

Examining the approaches to organizational branding of international public health institutions

As previously discussed, the most effective and sustainable health advances require coordination between products and services – a state that can be efficiently achieved by an organization whose products and services reflect the core mission and performance of the organization itself. It should be no surprise that many organizations concerned with health follow the money trail as nearly as businesses do. While their aims are not profit-driven in nature, health organizations seek (and make themselves attractive) to donor countries and organizations in order to ensure a reliable source of funding to cover their operating expenses and, if wanted, to expand their coverage or range of products and services. International health organizations work in the trenches of a market failure, and the movement of targeted business marketing practices into the non-profit and public health world provides an interesting study of how market practices will address what has historically been neglected.

The social marketing approach

Population Services International (PSI) is a prime example of a firm that has incorporated tested commercial practices into a non-profit mission in order to achieve measurable health outcomes more effectively. Founded in 1970 with a focus on employing market strategies to improve reproductive health, PSI follows the social marketing organization construct rather than the manufacturer's model which fuels the general market of goods and services and results in the legions of unhealthy persons and neglected diseases overlooked by the market. To accomplish its mission, which has expanded beyond family planning to include oral rehydration therapy, HIV and malarial prevention, PSI often relies upon certain products as essential tools (e.g. mosquito nets, condoms, filtering systems). However, because behavior change is the essential goal beyond product provision, PSI uses these tools as only part of sustained health campaigns. To this end, condom promotion – a prime example of product branding and product-based intervention – matures to condom social marketing programs, where the product is but a piece of a intended branded message of safe sexual practices, gender equity, and the building of relationship trust through communication and mutual respect. Data collection goes beyond product movement to focus on measurable behavior change and demonstrated adoption of healthy practices. Such a concept is not particularly dynamic unless one understands the culture of international aid and the difficulty or reticence of data collection relevant for project evaluation.

International NGOs such as PSI must walk the line between being responsive not only to their targeted population (product and service end-users) but also their donors (who, in this case, are also consumers). Branding in such a case necessitates not only being both universally recognized for sound business practices, financial accountability and tangible results; it also requires cultural competence and local sensitivity of the type achieved by working with indigenous populations to maximize project effectiveness and brand 'stickiness'. Such an organization has the ability to brand products and services at the local level while operating under the organizational brand gained through its results. We profile PSI continually here because, invariably, when one looks at international health branding, there is one name that resurfaces. Two examples of such branding will be profiled later in the chapter.

The private sector approach

We try to maintain a distinction here between public health organizations and their programs and services devised around a product whose profitable distribution is the centerpiece of the initiative. The movement of some public health campaigns to focused cost recovery (e.g. SOMARC) begins to blur this distinction. Furthermore, a comprehensive discussion of organizational branding, which, we have repeatedly made clear, cannot be wholly separated from the products and services (themselves branded) that it provides, must touch upon the activities of the pharmaceutical industry.

Almost every major pharmaceutical company has some institutional involvement in an international health campaign. Some of them are self-financed and orchestrated, some are simply drug donations and supply, but many more are public–private partnerships with governments, foundations and NGOs to provide the goods at reduced or no cost to populations in critical demand. Treatments already exist for many diseases, such as schistosomiasis, onchocerciasis and lymphatic filariasis, which have long been combated by drugs donated free by corporations such as Merck and GlaxoSmithKline Beecham.

Other pharmaceutical companies are engaged in various partnerships, which they showcase in terms of public duty and corporate responsibility. At a time when hotly contested international intellectual property rights agreements could either extend their hold over medicinal patents or allow for the development of cheaper generics, pharmaceutical companies are certainly exhibiting their philanthropic side. And for a company with deep pockets, public–private partnerships can be win-win situations as they gloss the corporation's public image while developing important political contacts and laying the groundwork for expanded markets for their products. Much could be said about the branding lessons of pharmaceutical companies and the partnerships in which they take part, but as our focus is social health, it is enough to show these partnerships as serious actors in international health that have essential goods. Their agenda may not mirror the scores of international health NGOs, but it is not necessarily incompatible with meeting the needs of the underserved.

The public–private partnership approach

Public–private partnerships continue to assert themselves on the global stage in public health. The meteoric rise of the Bill and Melinda Gates Foundation and its attention to neglected diseases has reinvigorated the global health climate with purpose and funding. The successful negotiation of anti-retroviral (ARV) prices between the Clinton Foundation and pharmaceutical companies provides a further standard of corporate accountability in addressing modern global health crises of disease and lack of access. As much as the pharmaceutical industry is demonized for profiteering and ignoring the needs of millions suffering from easily curable or preventable diseases but characterized by the lack of ability to pay, some pharmaceutical companies have maintained longstanding programs (largely product-based initiatives) that have provided medicines, either through outright donation or significantly subsidized cost to areas characterized by previously inefficient demand. The ethics and effectiveness of such provision need to be monitored and underscore the goals of effective public health intervention and comprehensive branding. The emergence of multidrug-resistant tuberculosis has revealed the limits of the foresight of the World Health Organization (WHO) DOTS program – a brand that gained traction in developing nations as well as nearly religious (and slow to adjust) fervor among its supporters. ARV treatment, its expansion to developing nations a welcome although tardy event, is not an undiluted good if drug provision is the only end. The HIV/AIDS epidemic will long provide an opportunity and great challenge for sustained behavioral change. Creative, culturally adept and responsive branding in this arena is the hallmark of successful social marketing products. 'Use a condom' messages coupled with distribution, while they certainly can translate into hard statistics of access, do little to address the underlying behavior change with which public health centrally concerns itself.

The faith-based approach

Faith-based organizations (FBOs), while they have reemerged on the international circuit due to the debate over increased public funding by the US government, have long been on the frontlines of public health in both developing and developed nations.

Traditionally, religious organizations operated in the margin where they provided medical care (often with a proselytizing bent) – free or greatly subsidized – in villages in developing nations as often as in needy neighborhoods of major industrialized cities. To talk of organizational branding without mentioning FBOs and religious institutions themselves is to ignore one of the most sustained organizations to carry the organizational branding of commitment to the poor and underserved, while operating from the considerable brand of the church itself.

Encouraged by the familiar discourse persons of faith share with the institutions and representatives of that faith, health messages can be conveniently couched in the religious mileu where behavioral change theory finds an old hand at the same game.

Older and more laden with brand meaning than the modern pillars of corporate branding (Coca-Cola, Nike, etc.), religious institutions have the refinement (or confusion) of centuries and the lessons of canonical text distilled into their referent. Moreover, an unspoken trust and expectation often exists between the church and community members, regardless of belief. Beyond the established relationship between the institution and its adherents, the religious brand opens doors for funding through the parent organization, tithing, and the considerable financing mechanisms of the faithful; furthermore, the positive philanthropic associations with religious groups can be a powerful impetus for cooperation and behavioral change in many cases. Some of the largest NGOs (e.g. World Vision) continue to be FBOs, and of those, a large number work in the public health arena. The HIV/AIDS epidemic has become an especially busy challenge for religious institutions and organizations as hundreds of FBOs have swelled the ranks of aid organizations and the official religious institutions working against the disease.

As FBOs and religious institutions have taken a more active role in international health, their methods and effectiveness have begun to be more closely observed and studied. This is especially true due to the public funding of FBOs through the US PEPFAR program which prompted a great deal of debate about the legitimacy of using public funds to support religious organizations. As a result, their programs have endured greater scrutiny; however, the research on the strengths and weaknesses of religious organizational approaches to public health is still nascent. Some of the strengths, mentioned above, seem to play out in a variety of environments, but the approach is not without justified criticism. An organization operating with a religious brand benefits from the established network and positive associations of that brand; however, religious affiliation can have serious drawbacks in the realm of public health. Opposition to condom·use by the Catholic Church is one of the most intractable examples. For an organization to ally itself with the church and take advantage of the brand comes at the cost of not being sanctioned to employ one of the most effective barriers to HIV infection available. In a reversal, the same can be said of the promotion circumcision on religious grounds as being supported by recent medical science. While the quantifiable comparable effectiveness of organizations operating under a religious brand with the religion's restrictions requires some further study, the active role of the institution of the church in international health cannot be overlooked. A February WHO report found that between 30–70 per cent of health infrastructure in Africa is owned by faith-based organizations and their involvement is critical to finding lasting solutions to entrenched international health problems.

SOMARC: a case study from the social marketing approach

The Social Marketing for Change project (SOMARC) provides a case study through which to analyze the conceptual framework of organizational branding in international public health, and understand how its application or lack thereof contributed to the experience of the project. We will examine the utilization of branding at each of the levels of products, services and organization within SOMARC's strategy.

SOMARC was funded by the US Agency for International Development and was directed by Constella Futures (formerly known as The Futures Group International) in each of the three consecutive SOMARC contracts: SOMARC I, SOMARC II and SOMARC III, the totality of the program having lasted a period of 17 years. Since its inception in 1981, SOMARC applied traditional marketing tools, including branding principles, to the reproductive health and family planning issues in developing countries. SOMARC's use of social marketing in its family planning campaigns has been driven by the goal of influencing couples in developing countries to take responsibility with their reproductive choices. We will examine the role of branding in these efforts (Heilig 1998).

Product branding in SOMARC

SOMARC traditionally concentrated its efforts on the marketing of products, including condoms, oral contraceptives and intrauterine devices, injectables and other long-term family planning methods. At the product level, brand-specific approaches were found to help in promoting products and in motivating behavior change. The lesson learned was that such personalized strategies help move consumers through a product adoption continuum. For example, having taken into account the needs, cultural and religious values, and readiness of a society, the Protector condom was a success in multiple markets. This success was due in part to having taken advantage of the opportunity to create a brand based upon consumer profiling, so that the product was uniquely oriented and directed towards the target population. Intensive and involved research allowed SOMARC to identify a number of similarities in consumer preferences for condoms. This was the case in regards to product names, logo designs, packaging and promotional slogans. The name 'Protector' and the general theme of protection was widely and universally supported by consumers. This brand served to promote the self-expressive benefits of behavior change (i.e. using a condom) to the target audience. The meaning of and identification with protection struck a cultural chord and subsequent relationship with target groups.

Service branding in SOMARC

SOMARC then expanded its activities to include the marketing of reproductive health services as well. It found that effective products alone were not enough. For increased success, programs must also offer quality services. Behavioral change is a step-by-step, interactive process, and products alone do not generate the motivation needed to change behaviors. Therefore, education and counseling in using products is necessary to create an atmosphere conducive to change.

In ensuring increased quality of products and services provided, SOMARC additionally expanded the development of training programs. These programs shared information and instruction in regards to the growing broad spectrum of programs, products and services in and across countries and cultures. Such training can ensure the continuity of brand messages across the spectrum, and take advantage of the opportunity to impart instruction in strategic marketing management, market research techniques and the integration of marketing communications – all essential elements of successful brand management.

Organizational branding in SOMARC

Once the organization is able to build and sustain relationships with its target audience through its products and services, building partnering agreements with NGOs and/or private sector firms is essential to the long-term success of the initiatives. SOMARC was able to act as a broker between the public and private sectors, integrating the contributions each brings to the work at hand. In fact, in building alliances with the private and public sectors, SOMARC strived for a way to institutionalize programs over the long term, and thus 'graduate' programs and products into full self-sufficiency where they have the ability to support all of their own costs.

The example of SOMARC's work in Turkey provides a study of the movement from individual contraceptive products to a network of services and the role of SOMARC branding throughout. In 1991, Turkey was struggling to provide adequate family planning and reproductive health services to a rapidly growing and urbanized population. Although free healthcare was available, the public sector was not able to keep up with the demand. The preference for private sector services abounded, but was limited largely due to high costs as well as an unawareness of the availability of family planning services in the private sector. SOMARC utilized its strategies towards two main outcomes in Turkey.

First, SOMARC's role in brokering a relationship with the commercial pharmaceutical firm Eczacibasi Ilac and the Turkish Family Health and Planning Foundation resulted in the launch of the Okey condom campaign. This relationship with major stakeholders in both public and private sectors led to a leading brand of condom, the Okey condom, and the graduation to self-sufficiency within two years. Similarly, an oral contraceptive was marketed in collaboration with leading manufacturers, Wyeth, Schering and Organon. Working in tandem with SOMARC in marketing their product under a branded umbrella campaign resulted in a reduction in the fears of Turkish women regarding oral contraceptives, as well as a leading market product. The product marketed by the SOMARC team graduated into self-sufficiency within three years.

The success of the SOMARC initiatives in Turkey led to a collaboration in family planning and reproductive health on a grander scale. The private sector showed great potential in the provision of needed services in the form of practitioners, hospitals, clinics and general infrastructure. Furthermore, despite a growing private infrastructure that was serving the low-middle and low-income communities, the major obstacle was still the higher costs of services to be paid for by the consumers. The provision of and emphasis on family planning services among private practitioners was low, and misperceptions of family planning products ran high. SOMARC's solution produced a private network of providers in the area of family planning and reproductive health care. The network, Kadin Sagligi ve Aile Planlamasi Hizmet Sistemi (KAPS), translates to Women's Health and Family Planning Service System. The network has improved the delivery of services and has increased the awareness of women visiting these facilities that such services were available.

SOMARC integrated its own branding strategy into the standards set for delivering the services in such a network. As little regulation previously existed in the private sector, measures such as assessments were developed to assure the delivery of high-quality care, lest membership of the network be denied. Moreover, SOMARC developed a training program for staff and providers to ensure a standard level of care across the network. Care was taken to make sure the information provided was up to date and provided in a family planning context. In order to raise the network's visibility among its target audience, women were initially trained to talk personally with women about KAPS and to distribute brochures. As the network and visibility increased, the branded network found public recognition in mass media campaigns including television, radio, newspapers, women's magazines, and finally, a telephone hotline.

Along similar lines of striving for cost-recovery, leveraged support and sustainability while maintaining focus on the consumer, an initiative known as Commercial Market Strategies (CMS) joins the private and commercial sectors in the realm of healthcare to expand choices and opportunities for family planning and other healthcare products and services in developing countries. A central aspect of CMS is the building of demand for products and services in part by integrating services through packages provided at health centers. The innovative strategy CMS was able to bring to the developing country market was to make options more accessible by acting like a clearinghouse where social marketing programs are accessible; partnerships and relationships are facilitated with pharmaceutical companies to offer quality, low-cost products to consumers and public sector agencies; and technical assistance is provided as needed to support activities. Much of this was reflected in SOMARC III, though not on the same level of delivery. The progression towards organizational branding is reflected in these initiatives.

Ethics and challenges

As a social good and subject, public health is meant to benefit the masses. This means working to ensure equity and access, realizing particularly that the most disease-burdened countries are those where such important contributions to wellbeing are out of reach. Though meant to target disadvantaged populations where access is limited and inequity has driven the disparity in health, the reality remains that the poorest of the poor are the ones who are often most ill and are not being adequately reached through social marketing programs and the like.

This being said, many might view the approaches of social marketing programs and organizational initiatives as somewhat unethical, given that financial or geographic barriers may prevent the clientele most in need from accessing the relevant products or services, irrespective of successful branding. Part of the effectiveness of the organization and the campaign lies in the approach to social marketing. The tension between cost-recovery health interventions and realizing the 'social' aspect of social marketing plays itself out in the balance between starving off donor dependence (as in the case of SOMARC III) and having to maintain donor funding indefinitely if the poor and vulnerable are to be reached.

In addition, given the increasing role of public–private partnerships, it is easy to be skeptical regarding organizations that seek to profit from these populations despite their good intentions and practice of corporate social responsibility. The challenge remains in encouraging the active participation of the private sector in public health matters with increased access, equity and sustainability. As such, a battleground in public health continues over how to maintain programs while reaching those most in need of assistance.

A continuing challenge is often the lack of clarity of what organizational branding means in public health. Whereas much has been learned and applied from corporate organizational branding, there is still inadequate documentation regarding specific implementation of organizational branding within public health institutions. There is much to be garnered and learned from the processes of success and failure.

Looking forward: optimizing the future of organizational branding

The feverish, although sometimes cosmetic, adoption of corporate structure and practice as well as marketing functions and language have prodded some health organizations to realign themselves and their services in a more efficient and effective way. Addressing health provision inefficiencies through market solutions requires the diffusion of learned best practices and the replication of model campaigns and programs. Not surprisingly, this has led to moves towards franchising. When certain programs and their services or messages gain appreciable traction among the wider public, the organization can extend that brand by opening other offices or extending it to other health service models. It follows that an organizational brand representing quality care, reliable access and tangible results can take advantage of client knowledge and consumer confidence to buoy the attractiveness and stickiness of its products and services.

Exploring franchising in public health

Both NGOs and corporations are getting into the franchising game with successful replication of model clinics and services. PSI, through the New Start and ProFam networks, has expanded voluntary counseling and testing services as well as reproductive health throughout a number of countries. The New Start VCT social marketing program was initiated in Zimbabwe in 1999 and has since expanded throughout Zimbabwe and into 20 countries in total. The program's statistics show a precipitous increase in testing numbers as coverage and name recognition have widened access as well as demonstrated demand (Joseph 2006). A 2004 US AID report characterized the success of the New Start brand as follows:

> PSI/Z has also made a significant contribution to creating awareness and demand for VCT. The New Start 'brand' is well known in Zimbabwe ... New Start centres have set the standard for high quality services, with confidential and rapid testing provided by well-trained counsellors. The centres also have quality assurance and supervision measures in place to ensure consistent quality at direct and indirect sites. PSI/Z training for partners managing indirect centres, and the development of training and operational manuals, have played an important role in setting and maintaining standards. Other countries in the region have used the New Start approach as a basic model.
>
> (Population Services International 2006)

The remainder of the report is more critical of the program, citing examples where lack of a refined strategic approach has led to gaffes such as VCT awareness campaigns beginning in regions where VCT services had not yet been implemented. Other coordination problems continue to hamper New Start as it expands to cover more underserved populations. Nonetheless, the fact of its continued expansion and its testing of over 10 per cent of the Zimbabwean population reaffirm the traction that the brand has achieved and suggests the possibility of an even greater market share (Hales 2004). Quality, cost-effectiveness and cultural appropriateness remain the recognizable tenets of the network and account for its popularity. The impact of the Zimbabwe government's support of routine HIV testing should prove an interesting element to the program's relative success in the coming years.

Capitalizing on successful precedents: the Green Star Network

The potential of proper organizational branding in expanding relationships with target audiences and reaching the wide range of peoples with products, services and changed behaviors is great. The harnessing of such potential has been revealed in the Green Star Network of Pakistan. Green Star has shown the capacity to bring together the skills and offerings of private sector family planning providers throughout urban Pakistan to complement the rural sector family planning strategies of the national government by filling in where these services were falling short. Two public health organizations, PSI and its local affiliate, Social Marketing Pakistan, worked together to design the Green Star Network.

A major part of branding is in reaching as much of the target population as possible. This is where current family planning services were failing, and where the strength of organizational branding and the ensuing strength of relationships capable of being built between audiences, stakeholders and partners come in. The aim of Green Star was to encourage increased use of contraception by making high-quality family planning products and services more widely available to low-income people throughout urban Pakistan at prices they could afford.

The ultimate strategy for delivery of services followed a franchise model. Social franchising, much like social marketing, applies the principles of a commercial mechanism to initiatives that are designed to bring about social change rather than generate profit. A critical component that needs to be in place before an organization can engage in social franchising is the brand. This brand links a specific service delivery point with the franchise, and in addition to communicating a certain quality to the consumer, it must deliver what it claims to deliver, and by extension, envelop the personalities, visions and values of the participating organizations.

Social franchising ensures the establishment of a tested, trusted, culturally sensitive and recognizable brand that is registered as a trademark to prevent its misuse by providers outside the network who may not bring quality, standard care. By rolling out branded products under the umbrella brand of Green Star to franchisees within the network, a greater population is able to access a credible high-quality product and service, encouraging them in the use of contraception. To be kept in mind is the possible accommodation of new health categories and an increasing vision and goals for brand development. However, the core values and principles of the organization must be maintained.

Conclusion

Organizational branding is a central tenet in the context of international public health. By using organizational structures, processes and an understanding of local cultures and behaviors, strong branding has the ability to create global synergies and long-lasting relationships both between institutions and individuals, as well as between organizations themselves. These relationships and the trust on which they are built are integral to achieving the goals and missions of effecting behavior change.

Conceptually speaking, understanding and applying organizational branding principles is desirable as it has the potential to have a tremendous impact on public health and the greater visions of sustained behavior change. Individual components of different programs have been successful in exemplifying important elements of branding. For example, in SOMARC, the Protector brand of condoms resonated with its specific audience, an element necessary in the continuum towards behavior change. Likewise, the Green Star Network shows the potential of key partnerships, particularly when capitalizing upon the specific strengths and advantages offered by both the public and private sectors. The various elements necessary for organizational branding in international public health have been demonstrated in individual capacities. In an overall sense, however, these elements have suffered a lack of successful and focused coordination in respect to behavior change.

In order to be truly successful, organizational branding requires major policy changes within the developing world. By leveraging its ability to encourage health literacy, as seen with SOMARC and the Green Star Network's work with health providers, and its ability to promote health behavior change, we can hope to improve access and equity in health services. However, advances in organizational branding in the international public health realm demands substantial market research with a greater emphasis on consumer needs, service equality and organizational intelligence. We urge organizations to take a step back and holistically determine how their policies, visions and actions determine their brands and how these strategies align with the needs of their target audience, how they relate with their audience, and how these effect downstream behavioral change at the individual level.

References

Aaker, D. A. (1996). *Building strong brands*. New York: The Free Press.

African Religious Health Assets Programme (October 2006). 'Appreciating assets: the contribution of Religion to Universal Access in Africa', Report for the World Health Organization, Cape Town: ARHAP.

Andreasen, A. R. (2002). Marketing social marketing in the social change marketplace. *Journal of Public Policy and Marketing* **21**:3–13.

Andreasen, A. R. (2006). *Social marketing in the 21st century.* Thousand Oaks, CA: Sage.

Chajet, C. and Shachtman, T. (1991). *Image by design: from corporate vision to business reality.* Reading, MA: Addison-Wesley.

Duncan, T. and Moriarty, S. (1997). *Driving brand value: Using integrated marketing to manage profitable stakeholder relationships.* New York: McGraw-Hill.

Engelberg, M. and Kirby, S. D. (2001). Identity building in social marketing. *Social Marketing Quarterly* **7**:8–15.

Evans, W. D., Price, S., and Blahut, S. (2005). Evaluating the truth® brand. *Journal of Health Communication* **10**:181–93.

Gobe, M. (2001). *Emotional branding: the new paradigm for connecting brands to people.* New York: Allworth Press.

Grunig, J. E. (1993). Image and substance: from symbolic to behavioral relationships. *Public Relations Review* **19**:121–39.

Grunig, L. A., Grunig, J. E., Dozier, D. M. (2002). *Excellent public relations and effective organizations: a study of communication management in three countries.* Mahwah, NJ: Lawrence Erlbaum.

Hales, D., Attawel, K., Hayman, J., and Khan, N. (September 2004). PSI Zimbabwe Assessement Report. Prepared for USAID/Zimbabwe and DFID.

Heilig, G. (1998). *National building, one family at a time: the story of SOMARC.* Washington, DC: The Futures Group International.

Joseph, D. ed. (November 2006). VCT in Focus. **1** issue 4.

Keller, K. L. (1998). Branding perspectives on social marketing. *Advances in Consumer Research* **25**:299–302.

Keller, K. L. (2000). Building and managing corporate brand equity. In M. Schultz, M. J. Hatch, and M. H. Larsen (eds.) *The expressive organization: linking identity, reputation, and the corporate brand.* New York: Oxford University Press, pp. 115–37.

Kotler, P. and Armstrong, G. (2005). *Priciples of Marketing,* (10th edn). Upper Saddle River, NJ: Pearson Education. p. 293.

McFarland, D. (2007). Using concept mapping to develop advertising messages and identify brand attributes of breast cancer with African American women. In J. Biberman and A. Alkharaji (eds.) *Business research yearbook: global business perspectives,* Vol. XIV. Beltsville, MD: Interntional Academy of Business Disciplines and International Graphics.

Pirani, S. and Reizes, T. (2005). The turning point social marketing national excellence collaborative: integrating social marketing into routine public health practice. *Journal of Public Health Management Practice* **11**:131–8.

Population Services International (August 2006). Marketing HIV counselling and testing: Zimbabwe Program Expanded to 20 countries. Social marketing and communications for health: PSI.

Roman, K., Maas, J., and Nisenholtz, M. (2003). *How to advertise,* (3rd edn). New York: St. Martin's Press.

Rothschild, M. L. (2001). Building strong brands – review of the book *Building strong brands. Social Marketing Quarterly* **7**:36–40.

Sargeant, A. and Ford, J. B. (2007). The power of brands. *Stanford Social Innovation Review,* Winter, 41–7. Stanford, CA.

Siegel, M. and Lotenberg, L. D. (2007). *Marketing public health: strategies to promote social change.* Sudbury, MA: Jones and Bartlett.

13

The intersection between tailored health communication and branding for health promotion

Megan A. Lewis and Lauren A. McCormack

Summary

- Branding and tailoring are health communication strategies with roots in commercial marketing perspectives.
- Despite their apparent dissimilarities in scope, with branding focusing on populations and tailoring focusing on individuals, these two health communication strategies are relevant to each other.
- Branding could add value to tailored health messages by enhancing their visual nature, source credibility, or helping to build stronger relationships with consumers.
- Tailored health messages could add value to branding by enhancing brand equity assets.
- Research is needed to examine the value added by integrating branding and tailoring as health communication strategies.

Introduction

The goal of this chapter is to explore the connection between tailoring messages and the process of building brands and brand equity as a strategy for health promotion and health behavior change. At first blush, branding and tailored messaging might seem to have little in common. Tailored messages are narrow and individually focused while branded messages are broad and population focused, which begs the question, what can these communication strategies do for each other? Because this volume is focused on branding as a promising strategy for health promotion, we focus both on how tailored health messages can add value to branding, specifically by helping to build brand equity, and on how branding could add value to tailored messaging interventions. In this chapter we focus solely on 'downstream' branding as discussed in Chapter 1 of this volume, that is, we consider brands in respect to changing individual behavior as opposed to changing macro organizational or social determinants.

We begin by illustrating why despite their dissimilarities in scope we believe an integration of branding and tailoring is fruitful. We then describe the process of tailoring in more detail and distinguish it from other customized forms of communication. We do this to dispel the frequent misconceptions about what tailored communications entail and how they are developed. Here we highlight how branding could add value to tailored communications. We also review evidence showing the effectiveness of tailored messaging and hypothesize how branding could have been used in successful tailored interventions. We then discuss how tailoring could add value to branding specifically by building brand equity, and then conclude by describing how the integration of these two communication strategies could be evaluated.

As defined in earlier chapters, branding is the process of building associations and visual imagery to create brands that motivate attitudinal or behavioral change (Evans et al. 2002, 2005). The goal in the branding process is to create a brand, that is, a symbol, logo or slogan that has widespread influence and increases affinity for a particular product or, in the case of health promotion, a particular health-promoting idea or behavior. An important goal of the brand is to develop a long-term relationship with the consumer. Commercial marketers want people to keep coming back for more of the same or similar product. Therefore, in terms of population reach, branding is characterized in terms of breadth and generality.

In contrast, tailored messaging is a health communication strategy used to change behavior that is characterized as having great depth, specificity and individual focus. Tailored messaging is defined as 'any combination of strategies and information intended to reach one specific person, based on characteristics that are unique to that person, related to the outcome of interest, and derived from an individual assessment' (Kreuter et al. 1999). This method of informing and motivating individuals is different from the breadth associated with a brand. One of the themes of this chapter is how this apparent conceptual and practical distinction between breadth and generality, on the one hand, and depth and specificity on the other can be reconciled and integrated when it comes to branding and tailoring health messages for health promotion.

Why integrate branding and tailoring as strategies for health promotion?

Despite their apparent dissimilarities, we view the integration of these two communication strategies as an important goal for many reasons. First, consumers are increasingly exposed to more information, including health information, from a larger variety and number of channels that are sophisticated in information delivery style. This 'information overload' requires public health practitioners to be increasingly sophisticated in the development and delivery of health messages. Tailoring health messages as discussed below, and branding as discussed in this edited volume, are two ways that public health has begun to address this issue. We propose that the integration of these communication strategies may further strengthen public health intervention effectiveness and reach.

Second, brands are based on competition between products, services or behavior (Aaker 1991). The goal of the brand is to make the product, service or behavior more desirable, with the goal of outperforming the competing brand. Public health brands have to compete with a variety of commercial products that are unhealthy, including food that is not nutritious, products that promote sedentary lifestyles, and lifestyles that are health-threatening such as smoking, drinking to excess and drug use. As tailoring could target individual motivational determinants of behavior, it could help give brands, especially those focused on health promotion, a competitive edge against brands that promote unhealthy behavior, products or lifestyles.

Third, because of increasing interactivity in technology, marketing in the commercial world may become, if it has not already, increasingly individualized. For example, digital television allows for interactive TV advertising and will continue to develop so that branding and tailoring may both eventually encompass both breadth *and* depth. Advertisers will be able to collect information from consumers via digital TV, and use this information to personalize and tailor commercially branded messages. Marketers see interactive advertising as a way to head off advertising losses. Digital TV allows for 'personal' TV, video on demand, and digital video recording, all which allow consumers to skip through commercials. Interactive advertising allows consumers to get more information about a product or topic in various formats and lengths, and is seen as a counter to digital formats that allow consumers to skip commercials. To keep pace with changes in technology and how commercial marketers will deliver advertising of potentially unhealthy products, public health branding and tailoring will need to capitalize on these same technological advances. These advances could support the integration and synergy of tailoring and branding of health-promoting ideas and behaviors, by increasing both breadth and depth of the messages delivered.

Fourth, the integration of branding and tailoring may help support efforts in media literacy. In public health, the most vulnerable populations are typically thought to be children and older adults for a variety of developmental, social and biological reasons. These groups may be the most vulnerable when it comes to commercial marketing due to lower media literacy and/or health literacy (NAAL 2007). Interactive technology and sophisticated marketing techniques will make digital television, and have already made the internet, very influential and powerful media for selling unhealthy products. For example, websites that promote sugary breakfast cereals do so via 'electronic playgrounds' that looks nothing like the typical commercial. For older adults who have less experience with digital and internet media, media and health literacy may be lower and trust may be higher, making them more vulnerable to the promotion of harmful health messages and products. The integration of branding and tailoring in public health may help counteract the powerful influence internet and digital media may have in the promotion of unhealthy products and lifestyles for those who are potentially more vulnerable.

What are tailored health messages?

Like social marketing and branding, tailoring health messages came from the growing recognition that a great deal of variability exists in target audiences and that communication science and other fields, such as marketing, could be used to create more persuasive health messages (Rimer and Kreuter 2006). To address this variability and to make the message more persuasive, the idea is to make the message more personally relevant to the target audience member. On the continuum of personalization in communication, tailoring is more specific than other communication strategies used in public health and marketing, such as personalized messages, targeted messages or generic standard messages or even branded messages. *Personalized messages* and educational materials are generic in nature and reference the message recipient by name. *Targeted messages* are typically designed for a specific group of people, older adults, women or Latinos, for example. *Tailored messages* are designed specifically for an individual based on information supplied by, or about, that individual.

Rimer and Kreuter (2006) describe the emergence of tailored messaging as arising from the convergence of several innovations. First, there was a growing recognition that marketing approaches could be used to inform mass audiences about health promotion and disease prevention (Slater and Flora 1991). Second, theoretical advances, such as the transtheoretical model suggested that people changed behavior based on stages of change and that health messages would be more effective if they were matched to a target individual's particular stage of change (Prochaska *et al.* 1993). Third, advances in computing and information technology allowed storage and analysis of large data structures that could be used to develop tailored materials. The integration of marketing practices, theoretical innovations, and advances in information and computing technology helped support not only the personalization of health communication, but the capacity to individualize health communication. Tailored messaging strategies are a prime example of how interdisciplinary collaboration leads to innovation in health communication. Branding for public health promotion is another good example.

In public health research, tailored messages have been most commonly delivered via print, although are increasingly being delivered via the internet (Stretcher *et al.* 2007), telecounseling (Stretcher *et al.* 2002) or other venues that include electronic channels, such as kiosks. To understand the individual's attitudes, motivation and behavior, either some kind of preexisting information about the individual is used, or there is an initial assessment survey in which the individual answers closed-ended questions. Many times these questions or information concern determinants of a problem, such as behavioral history, barriers, or opportunities or health behavior constructs derived from health behavior theories, such as self-efficacy, perceived susceptibility, or social support perceptions. These are sometimes referred to as behavioral construct determinants (Kreuter *et al.* 2003). Answers to these kinds of questions are linked to health messages that have been developed in previous and extensive formative work. The match between individually endorsed determinants or information, and health messages is done via computer-based algorithms, and then the tailored messages are inserted into the delivery or channel modality. In addition to tailored messages, tailoring algorithms can insert graphics, pictures or other images that have been tailored to the individual. Table 13.1 provides a summary of how a tailored messaging library is built. Once the library is built it can be used, along with an assessment tool or preexisting data, to implement tailored health message interventions.

Table 13.1 Overview of objectives, methods and outcomes for developing a tailored message library.

	Step 1	Step 2	Step 3	Step 4
Objective	Identify determinants and refine conceptual framework of the problem	Develop assessment tool to identify prevalence of determinants	Develop and test message concepts and full-length messages	Write tailoring algorithms that link message libraries with assessment tools
Method	Systematic literature review, secondary data analysis, pilot data collection	Self-administered survey or interview, pre-existing data sets of individual-level data	Pretest messages	Programming
Outcome	Refined set of determinants to include in Step 2 assessment tool	Ranking of determinants that informs message development for Step 3	Final set of messages to include in message library for Step 4	Tailored message library and algorithms that have been tested and are ready for implementation

How can branding contribute to tailored messaging interventions?

Because tailored messaging interventions utilize graphics and other symbols in materials delivered via print, or electronically, there are several ways in which branding could contribute to tailored messages. First, brands could help enhance the visual nature of tailored messaging materials. A recent meta-analysis of tailored print interventions found that pamphlets, newsletters and magazines were more effective print modalities than were letters, manuals or booklets (Noar *et al.* 2007). These authors hypothesize that one reason certain types of printed materials may be more effective is because they include more pictures and graphics, and a better layout than those that were inferior at promoting behavior change. Brands could enhance the visual presentation of printed and electronic media that contain tailored messages.

Second, brands could contribute to source credibility. This may be especially true for internet sites that contain assessment protocols and tailored message libraries. If these sites were sponsored or branded by partners such as healthcare providers, well-known insurers and government agencies, the credibility of the site could be enhanced. For example, through its partnership program with non-profit, private and other government organizations, the National Cancer Institute's Cancer Information Service helps to reach people across the USA with cancer-related messages (Squiers *et al.* 2005), and has served as a tool for evaluating health communication, including tailored health communication. However, one study found very limited awareness of the Cancer Information Service, but higher awareness of the National Cancer Institute, suggesting the need to associate the Cancer Information Service and the National Cancer Institute 'brand' to enhance credibility and trust in the messenger (Squiers *et al.* 2006). Another example where this kind of association has already taken place is the US Department of Veterans Affairs' *Move!* weight management program that is delivered via the internet. The *Move!* program contains assessment tools and generates tailored communication to support better nutrition and physical activity among veterans.

Third, brands can help build stronger relationships with the target population. One way to build a stronger relationship is through a personal connection. The National Heart, Lung, and Blood Institute is sponsoring a national campaign called *The Heart Truth* with the goal of making women more aware of the danger of heart disease. Formative research showed 'a strong emotional link between a woman's focus on her outer self (appearance) and the need to focus on her inner self (health in general and heart health, in particular' (Ogilvy 2007). The campaign uses emotionally evocative stories about real women who have experienced heart disease and what it has meant to them, and a national symbol or brand – the Red Dress – to help deliver the message about heart-related health. The campaign employs Oglivy's Brand Stewardship® approach, which involves identifying and reaching all of the target audience's influencers in a systematic way. With this approach, the message, the spokespeople (e.g. Laura Bush), the media, and the partners, which include healthcare organizations (e.g. American Hospital Association), have a consistent theme and message to convey and influence women from multiple angles. The campaign might go one step further by allowing women to enter personal health risk information onto a website, so that tailored messages could be created, along with encouragement to speak to a healthcare provider.

What is the evidence supporting tailored messaging intervention, and how could branding increase effectiveness?

In this section we briefly review several examples of successful tailored health interventions and hypothesize how branding could have helped enhance the delivery of the intervention, by enhancing visual imagery, source credibility or the relationship with the target audience member. These hypotheses are derived based on our knowledge of branding and the information presented in the published literature. In fact, some tailored interventions may be already capitalizing on branded messages, but not describing or even understanding the independent effect such messages are having on the outcome of the intervention.

Tailoring health messages as a strategy for enhancing health behavior change have been applied to a variety of behaviors including smoking cessation (Strecher 1999; Stretcher *et al.* 2007), increasing fruits and vegetable consumption (Campbell *et al.* 1999; M. Campbell *et al.* 2002), increasing physical activity (Bull *et al.* 2000), and screening behaviors (Lipkus *et al.* 2000; Rimer *et al.* 2001). These examples are just illustrations of many other studies that could have been included. Tailored health messaging interventions have been used to change most of the behaviors linked to the leading causes of disability and death.

Tailored health messages are more effective than standard self-help or educational materials at changing health behaviors. For example, a Cochrane review of randomized trials that tested the effectiveness of tailored print materials for smoking cessation showed they were more effective in reducing smoking compared with standard self-help materials (Lancaster and Stead 2005). In addition, a review of tailored print communication concluded that tailored messages decreased fat intake, increased fruit and vegetable consumption, and increased mammography screening (Rimer and Glassman 1999). The most systematic and comprehensive review to date of printed tailored health communications was conducted by Noar and colleagues (2007). This meta-analysis included all tailored print communication interventions that measured a behavior change outcome, and supports the conclusion of earlier theoretical or narrative reviews.

Many early tailoring studies compared tailored messages based on transtheoretical model variables (Prochaska *et al.* 1993) to standard self-help or educational materials. Studies have become increasingly more sophisticated, using multicomponent interventions (Kristal *et al.* 2000) or focusing on multiple behavior changes (Rimer *et al.* 1999). They are also expanding beyond tailoring on traditional health behavior theories, such as the transtheoretical or health belief models, to include tailoring on cultural variables (Kreuter *et al.* 2005), social support (Campbell *et al.* 2002) and concepts such as the teachable moment (Fish 2006). These increasingly complicated and sophisticated studies continue to support the idea that tailoring is effective at changing important health behavior, and that increasing intensity of tailored communications is more effective than less intensive tailoring. For example, in a randomized trial of 1,227 lower-income African-American women recruited from health centers, women receiving print communication tailored on both behavioral constructs and cultural variables were more like to get a mammogram, and had greater increase in daily servings of fruits and vegetables compared with either behavioral or cultural tailoring alone or usual care conditions (Kreuter *et al.* 2005). Table 13.2 summarizes the main components of this study.

Table 13.2 Cultural tailoring for cancer prevention among low-income African-American women.

Problem Focus: To enhance mammography screening, and fruits and vegetable consumption for cancer prevention.

Theoretical Foundation: Health behavior change theories and culturally relevant concepts.

Target Population: 1227 low-income African-American women aged 18–65 from public health centers.

Study Design: Randomized trial comparing behavioral construct tailoring vs. culturally relevant tailoring and no treatment control.

Tailored Messages: 1) Behavioral tailored magazines based on knowledge, self-efficacy, interest, preferences, readiness to change, past behavior and family history. 2) Culturally tailored magazines focusing on two of four cultural variables including religiosity, racial pride, time orientation or collectivism. 3) Magazines that were both behaviorally and culturally tailored.

Findings: Women who received magazines that were tailored both culturally and with constructs from health behavior theory were more likely than those receiving only one type of tailoring or a control group to get a mammogram, and increase consumption of fruits and vegetables.

Source: Kreuter *et al.* (2005)

This innovative and successful tailored intervention demonstrated that cultural variables were as important as commonly used behavioral theory constructs. Because of the delivery mode in a magazine format, intervention participants might expect to see brands commonly associated and typically seen in other kinds of media. For example, the Dole brand promoting fruit consumption or Nike brand depicting physically active African-American women could contribute to the visual imagery of the magazines. In addition, partnership with organizations trusted in the African-American community could have enhanced source credibility for messages about mammography screening.

Applications of tailoring to patient education and counseling

Tailored health messages have also been used in clinical populations to promote disease management or health promotion. For example, tailored messages have been shown to enhance asthma self-management (Thoonen *et al.* 2002), assist in decision making regarding hormone replacement therapy (McBride *et al.* 2002), encourage colorectal cancer screening in primary care settings, and control blood pressure (Bosworth *et al.* 2005). These studies also find that tailoring is effective in changing outcomes relevant to patient-centered interests, such as greater confidence in decision making and satisfaction with decisions (McBride *et al.* 2002), reducing information needs and increasing patient satisfaction in asthma self-management (Thoonen *et al.* 2002), enhancing readiness for screening (Jerant *et al.* 2007), and increasing self-confidence in disease management (Bosworth *et al.* 2005). These results suggest that the benefits of tailored health communication are not confined to community samples focusing on prevention of disease or illness, or the promotion of health-enhancing behaviors, but can be used to enhance clinical encounters or satisfaction with medical-related decision making. Table 13.3 summarizes a study that focused on increasing women's breast cancer risk and confidence in making decisions about hormone replacement therapy.

Table 13.3 A tailored intervention to aid decision making about hormone replacement therapy (HRT).

Problem focus: Increase women's accuracy of perceived breast cancer risk, confidence in decision making for HRT, and decision satisfaction

Theoretical foundation: None stated

Target population: Women aged 45–54 who were willing to receive materials about HRT

Study design: Two-group randomized trials to either delayed or active intervention

Tailored messages: (1) Decision aid that was tailored on: perceived menopausal status, hysterectomy status, use of HRT in the past, and perceived risk accuracy for breast cancer, and (2) vignettes of women at decision points similar to the recipient

Findings: Tailored decision aid improved the accuracy of breast cancer risk, decision confidence regarding HRT, and decision satisfaction over a nine-month follow-up period

Source: McBride *et al.* (2002)

The McBride *et al.* (2002) study could have capitalized on branding to enhance its effectiveness in several ways. Source credibility could have been enhanced by branding materials with logos from the National Institute of Health (NIH) or Centers for Disease Control and Prevention (CDC), or a similar organization that is trusted for enhancing women's health. Branding may be especially helpful, in this example, because issues surrounding hormone replacement therapy have become confusing and controversial for many women, and credibility of the information source may be questioned. In addition, these kinds of logos could help develop a more long-term relational connection with women. Organizations that are seen as consistently authoritative sources of health information could make longer-term associations with women. The introductory chapter of this volume highlighted the importance of branding for relationship building, and suggested that commitment and trust are crucial components to using the brand to build a relationship. To the extent that women view the NIH or CDC as committed and trustworthy sources of health information, the more likely the brand could be used to build a longer-term relationship as a source of health information.

The rationale underlying the effectiveness of tailored health communication studies, like those reviewed, relates to information processing and motivation. Kreuter *et al.* (1999) suggest that tailoring eliminates unnecessary information, bringing the most important information into relief. The information is seen as more personally relevant and as a result, people are more likely to pay attention, and process the information presented in tailored communications. Information that is processed centrally is more likely to be stored and recalled, thereby becoming more useful for future behavior. This information-processing perspective is consistent with predictions from the elaboration likelihood model (Petty and Cacioppo 1981), which suggests that information processed more actively or centrally is more likely to be stored, recalled and used in the future. Branded messages may be processed more centrally in health communication because they lead to more careful examinations of the message being presented. For example, women might think that the message to carefully consider family cancer history is important and relevant if endorsed by the CDC. In addition, brands are not typically used in health education and health promotion, so brand-associated messages may be more likely to be elaborated upon and therefore recalled at a later date.

Research also supports the idea that information from tailored communication is processed centrally and branded messages may be useful to integrate into tailored communications. Compared with untailored health messages or standard educational materials, tailored health messages are seen as more personally relevant, and are more likely to be read, remembered, saved and discussed with others (Campbell *et al.* 1994; Brug *et al.* 1996, 1998). Because of findings such as this, and the fact that many of the behaviors studied in tailoring studies are linked with cancer prevention and control, a report of the American Society of Preventive Oncology's Behavioral Oncology group identified tailored health interventions as one of four priority intervention areas for cancer prevention and control research development (Miller *et al.* 2004). Capitalizing on brands that are associated with cancer prevention and control, such as the *truth* brand, could take cancer prevention and control activities one step further.

When are tailored messages not effective and can branding bridge this gap?

Despite the rosy picture painted in the tailoring literature, and the recent meta-analysis that points to effectiveness (Noar *et al.* 2007), leading tailoring researchers have suggested that evidence supporting tailoring could be stronger (Kreuter *et al.* 2000). This conclusion is based on the fact that while tailored messages are remembered more than non-tailored communication, there are substantial numbers of participants in tailoring studies who report not remembering or reading the tailored communications they receive during the course of the study (Skinner *et al.* 1994; Bull *et al.* 1999). In addition, in some studies only half of the participants report finding the tailored health communication personally relevant (Brug *et al.* 1996, 1998).

Kreuter *et al.* (1999, 2000) suggest the impact of tailored messages may be dampened for several reasons. First, on a continuum of completely generic messages to perfectly tailored communication, tailored communication falls in the middle of this range. Tailored health messages, especially print-based messages, do not address every possible determinant that is important for behavior. One possibility is that brands, along with the associated ideals, attitudes or emotions they evoke in audience members, could be leveraged to make tailored messages more relevant by invoking a variety of related associations that also tap determinants of behavior. As more tailoring is done via internet and interactive technology, tailoring health messages will become even more sophisticated, and the use of branded messages even more easily executed.

Second, the most commonly used approach for tailoring health messages is referred to as 'behavioral construct tailoring' (Kreuter *et al.* 2000). Public health researchers and practitioners typically rely on standard health behavior change theory constructs to tailor health messages, including stages of change (Prochaska *et al.* 1992), health beliefs (Janz and Becker 1984) and self-efficacy (Bandura 1998). Are these variables really the most important determinants of behavior change? These theoretical approaches do not address important psychosocial and environmental conditions that may be as or more important in enhancing motivation and determining health behavior change. Here brands may be very helpful for tailored interventions because brands are about identity, emotions and values, as discussed in other Chapter 1 in this volume. Few if any health behavior theories include constructs related to identity, emotions or values; brands could therefore help bridge this conceptual gap.

The work of Kreuter and colleagues is a good example of how branding could leverage tailored interventions. As highlighted earlier, Kreuter *et al.*, (2003) make a convincing argument that cultural variables such as religiosity, collectivism, racial pride or perception of time may be equally important factors conditioning the practice of health behaviors than the typical variables studied to date. Many of these variables relate to group identity, values or emotions. Table 13.2 summarizes their study, comparing cultural and behavioral construct tailoring. Brands could have helped strengthen these associations and possibly increased the effects of the intervention.

In our own work, we have begun to examine how couple-level constructs derived from dyad-level theories can be tailored within couples for each couple member, focusing on cancer prevention behaviors and management of chronic disease. The notion of tailoring on couple-based constructs comes from the idea that marriage and other close relationships are important for health (Kiecolt-Glaser and Newton 2001), but are also emotionally and value-laden as well as central to identity for most people. Here again, branding could help strengthen the interpersonally-based constructs we believe may be important determinants for health behavior (Lewis *et al.* 2002, 2006a, 2006b), by evoking greater identification with the health message through values and emotions.

We define couples-based tailoring as any combination of strategies and information intended to reach couple members, based on characteristics that are unique to that couple, related to the outcome of interest, and derived from a couple-based assessment. Some of the dyad-level processes that may be tailored to couples and linked to better health outcomes include communal coping (Lyons *et al.* 1998), dyadic efficacy (Sterba *et al.* 2007), couple communication style (Lewis and Butterfield 2007) and partner accommodation. Whether branded messages could play a role in addressing important interpersonal, social, cultural and environmental determinants of behavior, because of a brand's associated values, emotions and identities, is an important question for future research.

Despite the potential challenges in tailored health communication, including the need to look beyond tailoring to individually-oriented behavioral constructs to capture more of the social context of health behavior, research and practice using tailored health messages is booming. The use of more interactive channels for delivering tailored communications and increasing the diversity of tailored elements in communication will make them more precise and relevant for consumers, and potentially even more effective at changing health behavior. In the previous section, we have highlighted various ways that branding could add value to the tailoring health message enterprise; we now turn to the ways tailoring can add value to branding.

How can tailored health messaging add value to branded health communication?

In the following section we discuss several ways that tailoring can add value to branding, specifically by increasing brand equity. Brand equity is defined as the set of assets linked to a brand that contribute to (or potentially detract from) the value of a product or service (Aaker 1991, 1996). In the present case, the product or service refers to ideas, behaviors, and lifestyles that enhance health promotion or decrease the probability of ideas, behaviors or lifestyles that compromise health.

Tailoring could add value to branded health communications in multiple ways. Tailored health communication could (1) increase positive associations and help develop brand equity during brand implementation; (2) build and maintain brand equity once a brand is established; (3) help to differentiate the message from competitors, thereby making the brand more competitive; and (4) build a deeper relationship with the consumer. Each of these examples center on enhancing brand equity.

As defined earlier, brand equity is the set of brand assets (or liabilities) that are associated with a brand (Aaker 1991). The assets that Aaker (1991) defines as making up brand equity include brand loyalty, brand awareness, perceived quality, brand associations and other proprietary brand assets. In Table 13.4 we define these brand equity assets, describe why they are important based on Aaker's (1991) work, and how tailoring can add value to branding by affecting brand equity.

Table 13.4 How tailored communication can enhance brand equity assets.

Brand equity asset	Definition	Importance	Value added to branding by tailoring
Brand loyalty	The extent to which customers are satisfied, and are committed to the brand	Attracting and retaining customers and building loyalty require active management	Making communication more personally relevant and motivating to each individual, thereby increasing loyalty
Brand awareness	The extent to which a brand is recognized, recalled, and at the top of one's mind (recognition and recall are signals that a brand has presence, substance and stability)	Brand awareness is created through communication repetition and communication relevance	Enhancing awareness more quickly because these messages are centrally processed, decreasing the need for communication repetition, thereby building brand equity more quickly
Perceived quality	Extent to which the brand is perceived of as having value and excellence	Identifying what quality dimensions are important helps define quality for the customer	Addressing the variability in customers' quality perceptions and help deliver credible quality messages to customers
Brand associations	Anything that is mentally linked to a brand (brand position is often associated with the brand, as is the relative price position)	Different customers may hold different associations with a brand; these can affect processing and recall of information, differentiate the brand from a competitor, and create positiveattitudes and feelings	Addressing the variability in customers' associations and help build more positive associations by making associations more personal appealing or relevant
Other proprietary brand assets	The name, symbol and slogan that are indicators of the brand and proprietary to it	Names, symbols and sloganscan become easy to use indicators for the brand and are large assets	Strategically placing slogans and other assets to enhance associations

Table 13.4 illustrates how tailoring can add value to branded health communication by building brand equity in a variety of ways. We develop these examples further by describing how three aspects of tailored health communication – theoretically-based determinants, tailored message libraries, and tailored versus targeted delivery, could enhance various dimensions of brand equity. We use the highly successful *truth* campaign as an example where tailoring could have enhanced brand equity.

Tailored messaging libraries typically incorporate a variety of health messages, pictures, and icons that can be used in a communication based on an individual's responses to some survey assessment. This library concept could offer many branded images and messages rather than one image or message. For example, the *truth*® campaign promoted the positive social image of nonsmoking youth as cool, edgy, hip and rebellious (Evans *et al.* 2005). This presumes that all at-risk youth aspire to this image. This may be the modal social image, but not the only one, and others may be more relevant to at-risk youth. By offering many positive social images, tailored messaging could increase the potential for identification with a branded behavior, and the association that the behavior is 'just like me'. To the extent that competing brands are not tailored, such an association should increase brand loyalty and possibly perceived quality. Tailoring can help branding differentiate the message.

The theoretically-based behavioral determinants typically used in tailored messaging interventions focus on enhancing knowledge, skills and motivation for behavior change. The ability to tie the social image of a brand to theoretically-based behavioral determinants should increase the efficacy of the brand. For example, the *truth*® campaign built a successful brand and social image for nonsmoking youth, but did not attempt to build self-efficacy for refusal skills or address other barriers to behavior change related to smoking. By addressing the unique challenges that each person faces related to the practice of a particular health behavior, tailored messaging should increase the salience and identification with a brand, increase perceived quality, and be more efficacious in its message compared with competing messages. Tailoring could increase brand loyalty and 'adherence' to the branded behavior.

Tailored messaging can go beyond approaches that might build brand equity by targeting communication delivery. Tailored messaging can offer only those messages and images that mean something to the intended recipient. Typically, social marketing campaigns deliver the message to audience segments, based on demographic or psychographic characteristics (Andreasen 1995). Tailoring the delivery of the communication should reduce the clutter (i.e. number of different messages that a person receives) and increase the salience or connection of the message, including images and branded images the recipient receives. The end result would be receiving messages and branded images that pertain most to a particular individual. Tailoring could enhance brand awareness and perceived quality of the brand.

The kinds of behaviors central to health promotion and disease prevention can be complicated, insomuch as they are emotionally, psychologically and contextually embedded in people's lives. Branding these types of behaviors may not be as simple as branding a product such as athletic shoes, where the behavioral outcome is the choice to purchase one pair of shoes over another. Medication adherence among chronically ill patients or nutrition and physical activity patterns among overweight individuals may be more difficult to brand. For these behaviors, it may not be enough to create a positive social image of the desired behavior in order to create lasting behavior change, but it may be necessary for motivating some individuals. In addition, branded images may need to be coupled with specifically tailored information about the importance of the behavior and how to enact the behavior and maintain it over time. In this way, tailoring can help branding tackle more complicated behaviors and enhance the knowledge, skills and motivation needed to change health behavior.

How can we evaluate the value added by tailoring to branding and vice versa?

Above we have made several suggestions regarding the interface of tailoring and branding. There are several ways that these ideas could be evaluated to determine whether tailoring can add value to branded health communication. Below we describe the general questions tailoring and branding research might pose and how these questions could be examined.

To determine if tailoring has added any value to branding or vice versa we would want to answer the question 'What aspects of the branded and tailored message worked and why?' To answer this, research questions based on the rows in Table 13.4 could be applied to a campaign or study that included both branded and tailored health communication. For example, similar to the Kreuter *et al.* (2005) study of both cultural and behavioral construct tailoring, we could implement a controlled study in which one group received branded health communication, one received tailored health communication, one received branded and tailored health communication, and a final group served as a control group. Between-group comparison would reveal whether tailoring could add value to the branded-only approach.

To determine how or why tailoring has added value to the branded health communication we would need to develop measures to probe aspects of brand equity related to the particular behavior or image of the intervention. Such measures have been developed successfully for evaluation of branded campaigns, including the *truth*® campaign (Evans *et al.* 2005). By measuring aspects of brand equity – brand loyalty, brand awareness, perceived quality or other brand associations – we could examine within groups why the tailoring component of an intervention added value to the branded health communication. These measures would help determine if tailoring increased brand loyalty, awareness or quality, and addressed consumers' fundamental values as a result of the intersection between branding and tailoring. Additional questions that could be answered by studies such as this include determining whether branded and tailored communication work better for some groups or some behaviors over others. Finally, determining the cost-effectiveness of branded and tailored communication relative to either approach alone would be an important goal.

The challenge to this sort of research is that it is time-intensive to develop the assessment tools, the databases that house information on individual consumers and the computer algorithms necessary for tailored messaging libraries. There may, however, be ways that public health researchers can capitalize on existing data structures to test some of the questions we pose above. For example, public health researchers could form partnerships with markets that have 'club' programs to track food purchases. A large amount of information is kept on individual consumers when they swipe cards at the point of purchase. Many of the purchases include branded products. Tailored communication, based on information in these kinds of databases, and that seeks to change or enhance purchase of healthy products could be delivered to individuals based on their preferences, past behavior or purchasing behavior. In addition, data-mining techniques could be used with health claim data or medical record information to deliver systematically varied branded and tailored messages to determine in what combination tailoring and branding reduces physician visits, increases adherence to medications or self-management of chronic illness.

Health clubs typically gather information on individual behaviors, preferences, and on physical activity that is a behavior branded extensively by commercial marketers. Public health could potentially brand physical activity successfully as well. Public health researchers could partner with organizations that house individual information on physical activity or leisure activity to examine the added value of tailoring to branded products and services.

Finally, the Noar *et al.* (2007) meta-analysis found 178 articles related to tailoring, but only included 57 studies that focused on print communication and had behavior change as the outcome. By examining some or all of the tailored materials from these 178 studies, it may be possible to determine whether tailored materials become easy to recall, remembered at a later date, motivating, or effective in changing behavioral intention if they are also branded. Formative and process studies that examine these kinds of variables could be done by obtaining these tailored intervention materials, branding them, and then determining if brands would make tailored materials more efficacious.

Conclusion

Public health messages compete for the attention of consumers in a marketplace that is filled with sophisticated messages promoting health-compromising products, behaviors and ideas that are delivered in engaging and motivating ways. Public health messages need to be differentiated from these messages and at the same time match their sophistication and motivational value. It is essential to recognize that public health is competing for the time and attention of consumers. The prevalence of health-compromising versus health-enhancing behaviors suggests that public health is losing the battle for the attention and motivation of the consumer.

In this chapter we have described how tailored health messaging, an effective way of delivering health information could add value to branded health communication, specifically by increasing brand equity. We have also described how branding could add value to tailored health communication. We see this integration as valuable, because technology will make the delivery of branded communication more interactive over time, thereby increasing its breadth and depth. By integrating tailored communication with branded communication, messages could become more personally relevant to consumers, increasing brand awareness, loyalty and quality. The challenge is that tailoring messages requires collecting information on individual consumers and housing this information in data structures that can be linked with health messages. This challenge may require public health researchers and practitioners to partner with organizations and disciplines not typically considered when promoting health. These cross-sectoral and interdisciplinary collaborations may, however, be key to successful branded and tailored campaigns or interventions. Undoubtedly, commercial marketers have already developed such partnerships for the promotion of products that may be health compromising.

Acknowledgements

Preparation of this chapter was supported by a grant from the National Institute of Arthritis and Musculoskeletal Diseases, National Institutes of Health, *Tailored Messaging for Couple Chronic Illness Management* (NIAMS R03 AR054067) and a Professional Development Award to Doug Evans from RTI International.

References

Aaker, D. A. (1991). *Managing brand equity: capitalizing on the value of a brand name*. New York: The Free Press.

Aaker, D. A. (1996). *Building strong brands*. New York: The Free Press.

Andreasen, A. R. (1995). *Marketing social change*. San Francisco, CA: Jossey-Bass.

Bandura, A. (1998). Health promotion from the perspective of social cognitive theory. *Psychology and Health* **13**:623–49.

Bosworth, H. B., Olsen, M. K., Gentry, P., Orr, M., Dudley, T., McCant, F., *et al.* (2005). Nurse administered telephone intervention for blood pressure control: a patient-tailored multifactorial intervention. *Patient Education and Counseling* **57**:5–14.

Brug, J., Steenhuis, I., van Assema, P., Glanz, K., and DeVries, H. (1996). The impact of a computer-tailored nutrition intervention. *Preventive Medicine* **25**:236–42.

Brug, J., Glanz, K., van Assema, P., Kok, G., and Breukelen, G. J. P. V. (1998). The impact of computer-tailored feedback and iterative feedback on fat, fruit, and vegetable intake. *Health Education and Behavior* **25**:517–31.

Bull, F., Jamrozik, K., and Blanksby, B. (1999). Tailored advice on exercise – does it make a difference? *American Journal of Preventive Medicine* **16**:230–9.

Campbell, M.K., Tessaro, I., DeVellis, B., Benedict, S., Kelsey, K., Belton, L., *et al.* (2002). Effects of a tailored health promotion program for female blue-collar workers: health works for women. *Prevention Medicine* **34**:313–23.

Campbell, M. K., DeVellis, B. M., Strecher, V. J., Ammerman, A. S., DeVellis, R. F., and Sandler, R. S. (1994). Improving dietary behavior: the effectiveness of tailored messages in primary settings. *American Journal of Public Health* **84**:783–7.

Campbell, M. K., Demark-Wahnefried, W., Symons, M., Kalsbeek, W., Dodds, J., Cowan, A., *et al.* (1999). Fruit and vegetable consumption and prevention of cancer: the Black Churches United for Better Health project. *American Journal of Public Health* **89**:1390–6.

Evans, D., Wasserman, J., Bertolotti, E., and Martino, S. (2002). Branding behavior: the strategy behind the truth® campaign. *Social Marketing Quarterly* **8**:17–29.

Evans, D., Price, S., and Blahut, S. (2005). Evaluating the truth® brand. *Journal of Health Communication* **10**:181–92.

Fish, L.J. (2006). Capitalizing on the teachable moment: Improving the effectiveness of self-help smoking cessation interventions. Doctoral disssertation submitted to the University of North Carolina at Chapel Hill.

Janz, N. K. and Becker, M. H. (1984). The health belief model: a decade later. *Health Education Quarterly* **11**:1–47.

Jerant, A., Kravitz, R. L., Rooney, M., Amerson, S., Kreuter, M. W., and Franks, P. (2007). Effects of a tailored multimedia computer program on determinants of colorectal cancer screening: a randomized controlled pilot study in physician offices. *Patient Education and Counseling* **66**:67–74.

Kiecolt-Glaser, J. K. and Newton, T. L. (2001). Marriage and health: his and hers. *Psychological Bulletin* **127**:472–503.

Kreuter, M. W., Stretcher, V. J., and Glassman, B. (1999). One size does not fit all: the case for tailoring print materials. *Annals of Behavioral Medicine* **21**:276–83.

Kreuter, M. W., Oswald, D. L., Bull, F. C., and Clark, E. M. (2000). Are tailored health education materials always more effective than non-tailored materials? *Health Education Research* **15**:305–15.

Kreuter, M. W., Lukwago, S. N., Bucholtz, D. C., Clark, E. M., and Sanders-Thompson, V. (2003). Achieving cultural appropriateness in health promotion programs: targeted and tailored approaches. *Health Education and Behavior* **30**:133–46.

Kreuter, M. W., Sugg-Skinner, C., Holt, C. L., Clark, E. M., Haire-Joshu, D., Qiang, F., *et al.* (2005). Cultural tailoring for mammography and fruit and vegetable intake among low-income African-American women in urban public health centers. *Preventive Medicine* **53**:53–62.

Kristal, A. R., Curry, S. J., Shattuck, A. L., Feng, Z., and Li, S. (2000). A randomized trial of a tailored, self-help dietary intervention: the Puget Sound Eating Patterns Study. *Preventive Medicine* **31**:380–9.

Lancaster, T. and Stead, L. F. (2005). Self-help interventions for smoking cessation. Cochrane Database of Systematic Reviews **4**:CD001118.

Lewis, M. A. and Butterfield, R. M. (2007). Social control in marital relationships: effects of one's partner on health behaviors. *Journal of Applied Social Psychology* **37**:298–319.

Lewis, M. A., DeVellis, B., and Sleath, B. (2002). Interpersonal communication and social influence. In K. Glanz, B. K. Rimer and F. M. Lewis (eds.), *Health behavior and health education: theory, research, and practice* (3rd edn). San Francisco, CA: Jossey Bass, pp. 363–402.

Lewis, M. A., Kalinowksi, C. T., Sterba, K. R., Barrett, T. M., and DeVellis, R. F. (2006a). Interpersonal processes and vasculitis management. *Arthritis Care and Research* **55**:670–5.

Lewis, M. A., McBride, C. M., Pollak, K. I., Puleo, E., Butterfield, R. M., and Emmons, K. M. (2006b). Promoting preventive health behavior change among couples: an interdependence and communal coping approach. *Social Science and Medicine* **62**:1369–80.

Lipkus, I. M., Rimer, B. K., Halabi, S., and Stringo, T. S. (2000). Can tailored interventions increase mammography use among HMO women? *American Journal of Preventive Medicine* **18**:1–10.

Lyons, R. F., Mickelson, K. D., Sullivan, M. J. L., and Coyne, J. C. (1998). Coping as a communal process. *Journal of Personal and Social Relationships* **15**:579–605.

Marcus, B., Nigg, C., Riebe, D., and Forsyth, L. (2000). Interactive communication strategies: implications for population-based physical-activity promotion *American Journal of Preventive Medicine* **19**:121–26.

McBride, C. M., Bastian, L. A., Halabi, S., Fish, L., Lipkus, I. M., Bosworth, H. B., *et al.* (2002). A tailored intervention to aid decision-making about hormone replacement therapy. *American Journal of Public Health* **92**:1112–14.

Miller, S. M., Bowen, D. J., Campbell, M. K., Diefenbach, M. A., Gritz, E. R., Jacobsen, P. B., *et al.* (2004). Current research promises and challenges in behavioral oncology: report from the American Society of Preventive Oncology Annual Meeting 2002. *Cancer Epidemiology, Biomarkers and Prevention* **13**:171–80.

National Assessment of Adult Literacy (NAAL). (2007). The health literacy of America's adults: results from the 2003 National Assessment of Adult Literacy. Available at: www.http://nces.ed.gov/naal/index.asp (accessed on June 9 2008).

Noar, S. M., Benac, C. N., and Harris, M. S. (2007). Does tailoring matter? Meta-analytic review of tailored print health behavior change interventions. *Psychological Bulletin* **133**:673–93.

Ogilvy. (2007) Case studies: The National Heart, Lung, and Blood Institute – the Heart Truth campaign. Available at: http://www.ogilvypr.com/case-studies/heart-truth-1.cfm (accessed 3 March 2008).

Petty, R. E. and Cacioppo, J. T. (1981). *Attitudes and persuasion: classic and contemporary approaches.* Dubuque, IA: Brown.

Prochaska, J. O., DiClemente, C. C., and Norcross, J. C. (1992). In search of how people change: applications to addictive behaviors. *American Psychologist* **47**:1102–14.

Prochaska, J. O., DiClemente, C. C., Velicer, W. F., and Rossi, J. S. (1993). Standardized, individualized, interactive, and personalized self-help programs for smoking cessation. *Health Psychology* **12**:399–405.

Rimer, B. K. and Glassman, B. (1999). Is there a use for tailored printed communications in cancer risk communication? *Journal of the National Cancer Institute Monographs* **25**:140–8.

Rimer, B. K. and Kreuter, M. W. (2006). Advancing tailored health communication: a persuasion and message effects perspective. *Journal of Health Communication* **56**:S184–S201.

Rimer, B. K., Conaway, M., Lyna, P., Classman, B., Yarnall, K. S. H., Lipkus, I. M., *et al.* (1999). The impact of tailored interventions on a community health center population. *Patient Education and Counseling* **37**:125–40.

Rimer, B. K., Halabi, S., Skinner, C. S., Kaplan, E. B., Crawford, Y., Samsa, G. P., *et al.* (2001). The short-term impact of tailored mammography decision-making interventions. *Patient Education and Counseling* **43**:269–85.

Skinner, C. S., Stretcher, V. J., and Hospers, H. (1994). Physicians' recommendations for mammography: do tailored messages make a difference? *American Journal of Public Health* **84**:43–9.

Slater, M., and Flora, J. (1991). Health lifestyles: Audience segmentation analysis for public health interventions. *Health Education Quarterly* **18**:221–33.

Squiers, L., Finney Rutten, L., Treiman, K., Bright, M., and Hesse, B. (2005). Cancer patients' information needs across the cancer care continuum: evidence from the Cancer Information Service. *Journal of Health Communication* **10**:15–34.

Squiers, L., Bright, M. A., Finney Rutten, L., Atienza, A., Treiman, K., Moser, R., *et al.* (2006). Awareness of the National Cancer Institute's Cancer Information Service: results from the Health Information National Trends Survey (HINTS). *Journal of Health Communication* **11**(S1):117–33.

Sterba, K. R., DeVellis, R. F., Lewis, M. A., DeVellis, B., Jordon, J. M., Baucom, D. H., *et al.* (2007). Developing and testing a measure of dyadic efficacy for married women with rheumatoid arthritis and their spouses. *Arthritis Care and Research* **57**:294–302.

Strecher, V. J. (1999). Computer-tailored smoking cessation materials: a review and discussion. *Patient Education and Counseling* **36**:107–17.

Stretcher, V. J., Wang, C., Derry, H., Wildenhaus, K., and Johnson, C. (2002). Tailored interventions for multiple risk behaviors. *Health Education Research* **17**:619–26.

Stretcher, V. J., Shiffman, S., and West, R. (2007). Randomized controlled trial of a web-based computer-tailored smoking cessation program as a supplement to nicotine patch therapy. *Addiction* **100**:682–8.

Thoonen, B. P. A., Schermer, T. R. J., Jansen, M., Smeele, I., Jacobs, A. J. E., Grol, R., *et al.* (2002). Asthma education tailored to individual patient needs can optimise partnerships in asthma self-management. *Patient Education and Counseling* **47**:355–60.

14

Challenges and limitations of applying branding in social marketing

Lauren A. McCormack, Megan A. Lewis, and David Driscoll

Summary

- There are some key differences between social marketing and commercial marketing that have implications for branding.
- While branded messages can still be persuasive, they should take a less directional and more informational tone when the clinical or epidemiological evidence is limited or weak.
- All forms of persuasion, including branding, should be handled with care when used in directive health promotion due to the potential risk of breaching the ethical boundaries of public health practice.
- Applying branding in combination with other communication strategies can enhance its effectiveness.

Introduction

Social marketing consists of the application of commercial marketing principles and strategies to promote socially beneficial outcomes (Andreason 1995). Several of the chapters in this volume have explored how social marketing products are often inherently more complex than commercial products. A social marketing product may be intangible, such as a change in attitude or a prospective future benefit associated with giving up something people like, such as smoking (McDermott *et al.* 2005), as opposed to an immediate purchase of a commercial product, such as clothes or soap.

Branding is a marketing technique often used in commercial marketing to help sell a product. As noted in previous chapters, public health brands are the associations that individuals hold for health behaviors, or lifestyles that embody multiple health behaviors. They are communications that elicit a particular set of beneficial associations in the minds of consumers related to health behaviors and lifestyles. Public health brands can be distinguished from commercial brands by their focus on health behaviors or lifestyles that embody multiple health behaviors rather than purchasing behaviors.

When these associations are combined in the mind of the consumer, independent of the perceived benefits of the health behaviors themselves, they form that public health brand's identity. The extent to which the public health brand's identity serves to reduce the costs and augment the benefits of the healthy behaviors in the mind of the consumer relative to the competition is referred to as the brand's equity. Thus, as described in Chapter 2, the objective of branding is to establish and maintain brand equity, and the function of branding is to alter the cost–benefit ratio of the exchange to promote health behaviors.

In this chapter, we begin by reviewing some of the key differences when applying branding in commercial marketing versus social marketing. Within social marketing, a range of different health behaviors can be targeted, and we argue that branding may need to be applied differently depending on the attributes of the specific behavior. For example, one of the key challenges that we foresee is applying social marketing and branding principles when the clinical or epidemiological evidence does not clearly support how the behavior should be changed; this situation is becoming more commonplace. In these cases, the branding process needs to be modified and/or other non-directive approaches to educating the public about their health options should be considered. By non-directive approaches, we mean messages that do not direct people as to what actions they should follow. We discuss these issues and ethical considerations within the context of a continuum of approaches for influencing health behaviors.

Key differences between commercial and social marketing: implications for branding

Elsewhere in this volume, various authors have shown that branding and other commercial marketing principles can be applied to public health behaviors and that more branded public health messages are needed. They have demonstrated through multiple case studies that branding has been successfully applied in a variety of public health domains, to a diverse set of audiences, and in a range of settings. This is possible because some of the goals and objectives of commercial and social marketing are quite similar, and the tools are applied in primarily the same way. In both cases, branding can be used to help establish long-term relationships that extend beyond a single communication episode.

While there are numerous examples of the utility of applying branding techniques in social marketing, we acknowledge that there are some key differences between commercial and social marketing that should be taken into consideration, and that have implications for branding when used in social marketing. We first review some of the key differences (see Table 14.1), some of which have been touched upon in prior chapters, then expand on two of the differences later in the chapter. Through this process, we illustrate possible ways to overcome some of the challenges and limitations, and how to capitalize on opportunities for expanding public health brands in the future.

Table 14.1 Some key differences between commercial and social marketing.

Elements	Commercial marketing	Social marketing
Motives and outcomes	Product sales or service consumption	Health-promoting behavior and social benefit (long-term or at the population-level)
Behavioral complexity; social context	Some are less complicated; others are more complicated	Interrelated and complex; social context can amplify complexity
Availability of supporting evidence for the message	Uses market research about audience response to create the message	Clinical or epidemiological evidence is needed to support the message
Ethical considerations	Ethical considerations present; advertising industry is regulated	Ethical considerations may be greater because persuading people to change health behavior
Financial support	Generally higher – supported by private corporations	Generally lower – supported by government agencies or philanthropic organizations

Motives and outcomes

With commercial marketing, the motive is to increase product sales and/or service consumption. With public health interventions, however, the 'product' is often a change in behavior (Kotler *et al.* 2002) or a call to action – either adoption of a new behavior or suspension of a behavior in which someone is already engaging. The consumer may find the behavior either difficult to adopt or difficult to cease, thereby making it challenging to *sell* the idea to the target audience. For the most part, there is no monetary exchange with the acquisition of public health products (i.e. no 'price'); by contrast, there is frequently a financial component with commercial marketing. There can, however, be other costs when achieving health benefits, including time, effort and psychological costs (Evans and McCormack 2007; Siegal and Lotenberg 2007). The focus of the benefit for public health interventions and social marketing focuses on its health enhancing aspects and the benefit to the society at large and/or over the long term.

Sometimes, the health-enhancing benefits may not be immediate and may take years to experience. In other cases, the benefits may be societal, that is, the benefits are evident at the population level rather than the individual level. Widespread pediatric vaccination for uncommon diseases can have a population-wide protective effect, for example, thus making it unlikely that any child will come in contact with the disease for which they were vaccinated. Having to wait to experience the positive consequences of one's behavior, or not experience them at all, can also be hard to sell and harder to brand. In these cases, not only does the 'promotion' often need to focus on increasing the likelihood that the audience will adopt (or cease) the behavior, but that they will sustain it over time. Creative strategies are needed to help encourage risk-reduction behaviors with a long-term public health benefit (e.g. good nutritional habits) as the rewards may be decades away. Branding might be used to create positive associations and images with the idea of protecting one's community or socially modeling healthy eating to younger generations.

Behavioral complexity and social context

Health behaviors are often interrelated and complex. The social context in which they occur often needs to be factored in when considering how to influence them, and can amplify the complexity. Techniques that target both environmental conditions as well as individuals may be more effective than either alone (Stokols *et al.* 1996). We argue that messages can use the social context to their advantage when branding, as long as they understand it well, including its strengths and limitations. For example, some recent programs to increase levels of physical activity recognize the role played by environment and access to resources. The Active Living by Design Initiative funded by the Robert Wood Johnson Foundation emphasizes innovative approaches to increase physical activity through community design, public policies and communications strategies (http://www.activelivingbydesign.org). The logic behind the initiative is that by providing strategies and support in the community, shorter and longer-term changes can lead to health and lifestyle improvements. The foundation also funds an initiative focused on diabetes self-management (http://www.rwjf.org/applications/solicited/npo).

McCormack *et al.* (2007a) found that people who had a healthcare provider who assisted them in finding physical activity resources were significantly more likely to report sufficient levels of physical activity, controlling for sociodemographic characteristics, self-efficacy, smoking status and body mass index. In these cases, we believe that to be most effective, branded health messages need to be comprehensive enough to address the whole person, their social context, and their environment.

Availability of supporting evidence for the message

Most commercial marketing efforts do not rely on clinical evidence to be able to say that their product is good; however, they may need data supporting the fact that their products are not harmful. This is a major distinguishing factor for public health interventions, which generally require scientific evidence supporting that a certain behavior (e.g. quitting smoking, condom use) has positive health consequences and/or can reduce health risks. As such, commercial marketers may be able to rely more on audience research techniques for crafting their messages (without other input), relative to social marketers.

For the most part, the behaviors that branded public health messages have sought to change thus far have clear-cut evidence supporting their messages. As noted earlier, it is well known that physical activity will enhance health and decrease the probability of multiple other heart-related health conditions (Briss *et al.* 2000; Kahn *et al.* 2002). Given the strength of the supporting evidence, several campaigns have been launched using social marketing principles and branding to encourage increased levels of physical activity. For example, the *VERB, It's What You Do* campaign is a national, multicultural campaign to increase and maintain physical activity among 'tweens' (youth age 9–13) (Wong *et al.* 2004). Intervention materials used in the *VERB* campaign reflect the strong evidence supporting the relationship between physical activity and enhanced health.

Other examples of commonly recommended behaviors previously addressed in public health campaigns include reducing sun exposure (Hill *et al.* 2002), consuming folic acid every day if you may become pregnant (Flores 2007), and not engaging in risky behaviors such as unprotected sex (Wellings 2001) and illicit drug use (Palmgreen *et al.* 2002). In all of these instances, the message is straightforward – clinical or epidemiologic evidence supports the contention that a person can improve their health by adopting or rejecting a specified behavior. For behaviors with strong evidence, we argue that branding can be used as a communication strategy more easily relative to behaviors for which the evidence is less clear. When the evidence is equivocal – which is becoming more commonplace – branding can be more complicated and special considerations, including ethical considerations, are heightened.

Ethical considerations

By definition, interventions that seek to persuade someone to change their behavior have ethical implications (Burdine *et al.* 1987). Ethical considerations may be greater with application of social marketing relative to commercial marketing if their focus is on persuading someone to change something that affects their personal health. First and foremost, the messages and the brand should seek to 'do good' and 'do no harm' and limit the potential for detrimental side effects that might occur. Guttman summarizes some of the key moral obligations and ethical dilemmas relevant to health promotion:

> Ethicists note that moral obligation to do the utmost to better people's health, to avoid doing them any harm, to respect people's autonomy and privacy, to ensure equity and fairness and provide for those who are particularly vulnerable or who have special needs, and to maximize the greatest utility from health promotion efforts, especially when resources are limited.
>
> Guttman (2003: 652)

Balancing all of these factors is not easy and requires careful implementation, especially because there are no standard regulations such as those with the advertising industry.

Financial factors

The final difference between commercial and social marketing that we discuss is that average funding levels are often quite different, although there are some exceptions to this, such as the *VERB* campaign, which at its peak in 2003 received some $60 million in funding (see Chapters 1 and 6). Most public health campaign budgets are limited and implementers need to be cognizant of what they can achieve with limited resources. They often reach out to community-level partners to help them identify and/or connect with the target audience. In-kind contributions can help to offset some of the limits in funding. Given the small size of some public health campaign budgets, it may be even more important to harness the potential power of branding to help differentiate product offerings and build relationships with target audiences (Siegal and Lotenberg 2007).

We have attempted to highlight some of the distinctions between branding when used in commercial as opposed to social marketing applications. These differences include the motives and outcomes sought, the behavioral complexity of the behavior being advocated, the nature of the evidence bases supporting the behavior, potential ethical issues and financial support. Some of these differences have implications for how branding is used, others do not. Branding techniques can still help build relationships in both commercial and public health applications. In the sections that follow, we expand on two of the differences introduced above: the need for supporting clinical evidence and ethical considerations. Public health interventions must be credible, trustworthy and have the public interest as the primary concern. We discuss each issue and how branding needs to be modified accordingly to address these issues, beginning with a continuum of approaches for influencing behaviors.

A continuum of strategies for changing public health behavior: variations based on the available evidence

An overarching goal of *Healthy People 2010* is to help individuals of all ages increase life expectancy and improve their quality of life (US Department of Health and Human Services 2000). One of the ten public health goals is to 'inform, educate, and empower people about health issues' (Rothschild 1999). Application of social marketing principles is an important strategy for influencing public health goals and messages (Kotler *et al.* 2002).

In an effort to describe the evolution of social marketing as a strategy for social change, Fox and Kotler (1980) describe four approaches for changing public health behavior – legal, technological, economic and informational. Legal approaches involve the implementation or passage of policies or laws with the goal of changing behavior. These kinds of approaches can be successful in changing health-related behavior, but are more effective when enforcement of laws takes place along with the implementation of the policy or law as has been shown, for example, in tobacco control (Feighery *et al.* 1991). Technological strategies refer to changes that occur in the environment that affect health or behavioral outcomes. These technologies can include chemical supports (e.g. nicotine patches) or mechanical supports (automatic seatbelts or belt reminder systems in cars) that support behavior change. Economic approaches refer either to monetary penalties attached to an outcome or behavior (e.g. taxes or higher prices on cigarettes) or incentives to induce behavior change. Both approaches have merit with higher cigarette prices being associated with lower purchase rates among youth (Chaploupka 2003) and monetary incentives predicting greater weight loss (Finkelstein *et al.* 2007).

Legal, technological and economic strategies are more passive types of interventions that require lower effort or motivation in terms of use (Stokols *et al.* 1996). They create supportive or non-supportive environmental conditions that affect the probability of a behavior. *Informational* approaches to change refer to strategies that involve presenting 'just the facts' or more persuasive information. Presenting 'the facts' or framing information using persuasive techniques, such as the use of social marketing principles or theoretical constructs to inform intervention components are both effective (Glanz *et al.* 2003). Some evidence shows that information presented more persuasively is more effective at changing behavior than just presenting the facts about a health condition or potential risk (Snyder and Hamilton 2002). Informational techniques are targeted toward individuals or populations through a variety of communication techniques. In public health, more emphasis has been placed on education and law with less application of marketing (Rothschild 1999). Each of these strategies for influencing change can be used independently or in combination depending on the target behavior and audience. Using them in combination may be necessary to influence some behaviors (Siegal and Lotenberg 2007).

When the clinical evidence is equivocal, we argue that non-directive approaches, that is, approaches that provide information or alternatives but do not advocate for a particular choice, are needed for behavior change (Figure 14.1), and that branding should be used judiciously in these cases. In these situations, we are on the informational end of Fox and Kotler's (1980) typology – providing information for decision making and allowing the consumer to determine whether or not to adopt the behavior. The typology reflects a continuum of strategies for changing health behavior ranging from legal to technological to economic to informational. We propose adding two parallel continuums to consider. The first relates to the certainty of the related clinical evidence – it may be unequivocal (which tends to align more with the legal, technological, or even economic behavior change strategies), or equivocal (which aligns with more informational strategies). The second additional continuum is that directive messages align with more legal/technological/economic strategies, and non-directive messages align with more informational strategies.

Health behaviors with limited evidence

As medical science advances, and screening tests, treatments and pharmaceutical agents are developed for which the public health evidence remains uncertain, many public health issues meet the criteria of 'wicked problems' as originally coined by Horst Rittel (Rittell and Weber 1973: 2). This is a growing phenomenon given the state of medical science in certain clinical areas such as genetic testing (Bekker 2003), diagnostic tests for breast

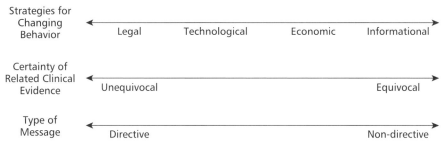

Fig. 14.1 Changing public health behavior: variations based on the degree of evidence. Adapted from Fox and Kotler (1980).

abnormalities (US Department of Health and Human Services 2006) and antidepressants (US Department of Health and Human Services 2007). These are problems for which the solution is complicated by the diversity of stakeholder views and preferences; therefore they are sometimes referred to as 'preference-sensitive decisions'. For these behaviors, we argue that non-directive messages are more appropriate than directive approaches because they do not direct consumers toward a specific path. The goal of non-directive messages is to provide consumers with the available information and educate them about the uncertainty with respect to the clinical evidence. This can include a persuasive element instructing individuals to weigh the advantages and disadvantages of the different options carefully (e.g. treatment *a* versus treatment *b*), then select an option based on their own preferences or situation. Some more in-depth examples may be helpful at this point to illustrate when non-directive messages are appropriate.

Fish consumption

Environmental health offers a multitude of preference-sensitive decisions for which informational or non-directive campaigns are appropriate. Fish can be a rich source of polyunsaturated fatty acids, which have been demonstrated to reduce the risk of cardio-vascular disease and stroke, and may also be critical to the development of the brain *in utero* (Cohen *et al.* 1995; Konig *et al.* 2005). Fish are also a source of environmental contaminants including methylmercury (Burger *et al.* 2007). Methylmercury is a potent neurotoxin that causes developmental delays in young or unborn children even in low doses and has been linked to neurological and cardiovascular degeneration in adults with higher doses (Cohen *et al.* 2005).

Individuals must be aware of personal vulnerability, and make informed decisions regarding what kinds of fish are safe to eat and in what amounts. The number of Americans who die from heart attacks and strokes far exceeds those who die from any other cause (MMWR 2004), and thus risk communications that reduce overall rates of fish consumption would increase the overall US mortality rate (Teutsch and Cohen 2005). The goals of risk communications regarding fish consumption are thus to promote informed decisions to reduce exposure to contaminated fish among vulnerable subpopulations without reducing fish consumption in the general population (USEPA 2004; IOM 2006).

Newborn screening

Newborn screening has had a tremendous positive impact on public health in the last several decades, resulting in reductions in mortality, mental retardation and other serious disabilities (Watson 2006). While some of the benefits are indisputable, other benefits may vary depending on the perspective of the stakeholder, be it the individual, the family or society. This is particularly important, as the number of conditions that may be screened is growing, and systems are not yet in place to communicate adequate information to decision makers about the potential drawbacks of screening, such as false positives and identifying other genetic abnormalities along the way (Bailey *et al.* 2006). Both of these issues raise ethical considerations. In the pro-screening environment in which we live (Schwartz *et al.* 2004), it may be difficult for someone to understand the need for simply informing and educating consumers and not persuading them or mandating a behavior. As genetic testing becomes a more readily available option in the public health arena, the issues of medical uncertainty may become more apparent.

Prostate cancer screening

Finally, the decision to be screened for prostate cancer can be controversial because there is disagreement about the reliability and efficacy of the prostate-specific antigen (PSA) test and the potential harm associated with treatment (impotence and incontinence). Leading medical groups have different recommendations about prostate cancer screening (e.g. the American Cancer Society recommends that asymptomatic men aged 50 and older who have a life expectancy of at least ten years be offered the PSA test annually, while the American College of Preventive Medicine recommends against routine population screening). The US Preventive Services Task Force concluded that it could not recommend either for or against routinely screening men for prostate cancer because there was insufficient evidence to determine whether the benefits outweighed the harms for the screened population. Given this uncertainty, many major medical organizations recommend using an informed decision-making process to make this decision.

With these three different examples, we sought to illustrate the range of issues that may require non-directive communication approaches and how the associated behaviors differ from behaviors with clear-cut evidence such as quitting smoking or enhancing physical activity. To date, branding has been applied primarily, if not exclusively, to behaviors with uncontroversial evidence. Is branding a strategy that can only be used for certain public health behaviors or only when the clinical evidence is strong, or can it be used regardless? Would it be as effective in enhancing appropriate fish consumption, newborn screening, or prostate cancer screening? Or are these examples of situations in which branding is less useful given the complexity of the decision-making situation? What are the considerations and limits when applying branding to these public health issues for which the clinical evidence is not uniform or uncertain? How does one apply branding in these cases?

While there are some issues to consider when branding public health products, we think it is still possible to do so even when the clinical evidence is uncertain or incomplete. When the evidence is limited or weak, as is the case with non-directive health promotion, empowering consumers to make informed decisions is the correct course of action. In these situations, campaigns should provide the necessary information for consumers to make decisions in accordance with their values and preferences.

Informed decision making

Informed decision making (IDM) is an example of a non-directive technique that can be used in conjunction with branding. As described previously, IDM is a communication strategy that requires the decision maker to understand the nature of the disease or condition being addressed as well as the clinical service and its likely consequences. The decision maker must also consider his or her preferences as appropriate; participate in decision making at a personally desirable level; and either make a decision that is consistent with his or her preferences and values or elect to defer a decision to a later time (Briss *et al.* 2004; Mullen *et al.* 2006). For IDM to take place, consumers must often be provided with the skills to allow them to adopt informed behaviors based on the evidence provided. IDM is thus a behavior, but the outcome of that behavior, or the product, cannot be generalized and described in relation to other products. Thus, for prospective IDM promotion programs using social marketing, the key attribute of comparison is not the product, but the process by which that product was selected (i.e. was it an informed process?).

McCormack and colleagues (2007b) developed a set of intervention materials to promote IDM regarding prostate cancer screening for a community-based intervention study. The materials included an educational video with scenarios of men making different PSA screening choices, a ten-minute script for a physician to use in a community-based forum along with a poster to illustrate key talking points, a website, tri-fold brochures, and a shirt-pocket card for men to have with them when they go into the doctor's office. The messages were cast relative to behaviors, with more concrete evidence for contrast (heart disease, stroke and colon cancer) and some branding elements applied for greater impact. Prior research suggested that starting with more intuitive messages, such as those regarding these health issues, might overcome cognitive dissonance with the IDM message and suggest that the PSA test represents a different kind of decision (Driscoll and Harris-Kojetin 2002).

All of the materials were marked with a *You Decide* logo and theme (see Fig. 14. 2). In the physician community presentation forum, the PSA issue was positioned as one that gave men the power, the right and the ability to make their own decision about the test, regardless of what they had done in the past or what other men were doing. The format and contents of the materials were heavily influenced by audience research including three rounds of individual and group interviews with members of the intervention communities.

The PSA materials conveyed that men should carefully consider the risks and benefits of the PSA test, assess their own values and preferences, and make the screening decision that was right for them. After exposure to the intervention, intervention group members were found to be more knowledgeable about the PSA test and prostate cancer relative to

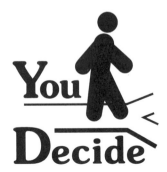

Fig. 14.2 *You Decide* logo used in intervention materials to promote informed decision-making about prostate cancer screening.

control group members according to a ten-item index (McCormack *et al.* 2007b). At six months after exposure to the intervention they were more likely to participate in the PSA decision-making process at their preferred level; however, the difference between the intervention and control group was no longer significant at 12 months post-intervention (McCormack *et al.* 2007c).

Ethical considerations when applying branding in public health marketing

Branding is thought to affect outcomes by building strong positive associations with a behavior or idea primarily through social imagery and modeling of healthful behavioral alternatives (Evans *et al.* 2004). Thus, as opposed to many health communication or social marketing campaigns, where visuals, words and other elements convey the message, the *active* ingredient in branding is the imagery through which the health messages are delivered. Given the potency of social imagery for generating strong emotions, connections and identification with an idea, behavior or product, branding can be an especially powerful form of persuasion (Evans *et al.* 2005). All forms of persuasion, including branding, should be handled with care when used in directive health promotion due to the potential risk of breaching the ethical boundaries of public health practice. In particular, the use of branding may not fully consider the public health principles of individual autonomy and respect for individuals and communities (Public Health Leadership Society 2002).

Directive public health messages are, almost by definition, autonomy-reducing. They take the form of proscriptions (e.g. Don't smoke!) or prescription (e.g. Eat right, exercise more!) messages, telling people what they should or should not do. Although public health messages can be ethically presented or communicated in ways that promote informed decision making, when presented as persuasive communication they become autonomy-reducing. The stronger the persuasive communication is, the more autonomy-reducing the communication potentially becomes.

For branding, this raises some ethical concerns. First, strong evidence is needed to justify the use of branding directive messages. The behavior being advocated should be well supported by evidence, and the benefits of a particular behavior must outweigh the risks or the harms. For example, branding is well justified in smoking prevention, as is the case with the *truth* campaign (Evans *et al.* 2005). The evidence surrounding the harms of smoking is incontrovertible, and branding can successfully counteract the powerful and prevalent messages propagated by the smoking industry in order to encourage people to smoke.

Different types of persuasion tools have been used in health communications and branding practices. As discussed in Guttman (2003), these include exaggeration, omission, use of fear, emotional appeals and personal responsibility. For example, some branded (and non-branded) campaigns try to convince their audience that they should adopt healthier behaviors because they owe it to themselves, their families or society. This may cause people who do not adopt the recommendation to be viewed as 'unwilling, lazy, and weak in character' (Guttman 2003: 661), which could result in stress, anxiety and guilt. While this may not be the goal of the campaign and the branded message, it may nonetheless be the result. Critics have argued that certain tools of persuasion can be viewed as manipulative (Faden 1987), and this will be a growing concern for social marketing and branding.

The issue of moral justification has also been raised in the ethics discussions, that is, weighing the goals of the individual versus the goals of the society and who has the right to make decisions about what is good for the public's health (Andreason 2001; Grier and Bryant 2005).

Addressing some of the ethical considerations when applying marketing and branding techniques might involve ensuring that the message communicates a complete set of information – both the pros, and if relevant, the cons to adopting the behavior. The messages should effectively translate the latest scientific evidence as clearly as possible to the ordinary consumer (Edwards *et al.* 2003) using recent plain language techniques (http://www.plainlanguage.org/). Do the messages use linguistically appropriate terminology that is written at the appropriate health literacy level? While the branding seeks to motivate people, it should be truthful and not misleading in terms of what the positive outcomes will be if the behavior is adopted (Guttman 2003).

One needs to ensure that the messages and the branding process are culturally sensitive and appropriate (Gudykunst and Mody 2002); this issue will continue to grow in importance as our society becomes increasingly more diverse (Nelson *et al.* 2002). Do they take into consideration particular cultural values or traditions of the audience segments that they are targeting? For example, food-related messages aimed at segments of the populations need to factor in that subgroups may have certain staple foods that will not be eliminated from the diet regardless of their nutritional value.

In all situations, but particularly when the message is based on uncertain evidence, branding for may need to be applied with caution. Branding in these cases may not adequately capture the complexity of messages needed to enhance autonomy in decision making, and may undermine respect for individuals and community because all sides of an argument cannot be adequately portrayed. Given its persuasive potency, and by implication its autonomy-reducing potential, and the possibility of undermining respect for individuals and communities, public health practitioners should be aware of ethical considerations and use caution when employing branding.

Conclusions

In recent years, social marketers and public health planners have increased use of commercial marketing principles to persuade their audience to adopt a certain behavior (Andreason 2003; Grier and Bryant 2005). Several of these examples have been described in previous chapters of this volume. Branding has also become an important strategy in social marketing aimed at improving population health, as recently highlighted by Siegal and Lotenberg. They describe that 'Branding and brand management techniques can help ensure that a consistent identity is communicated and delivered to supporters, partners, target audiences, thereby enabling public health marketers to build strong relationships with all these groups' (Siegal and Lotenberg 2007: 228).

In this chapter, we have argued that branding sometimes needs to be applied differently in social marketing relative to commercial marketing, and that there are a few key instances when this becomes even more critical. The first is when the clinical evidence is uncertain. While branded messages can still be persuasive, they should take a less directional and more informational tone when the clinical or epidemiological evidence is limited. The second key issue relates to ethical considerations, which we have said must be carefully factored in when applying commercial marketing principles and branding to health behaviors.

Creative solutions may be helpful in achieving these goals. For example, using branding in combination with other communication strategies is one possible approach. A specific example is leveraging the existing healthcare and health insurance systems to help achieve more widespread healthy behaviors. While there are certain elements of the US health insurance system that present challenges when using branding for public health products, there are also potential opportunities on which to capitalize. Health messages are more effective if the messenger is viewed as a credible source of information (McGuire 2001), and health education campaigns commonly use partnerships to enhance their programs (Lefebvre 2006). Many large health insurers, university healthcare systems and employers could take advantage of this because they are well-known entities with solid reputations, particularly when they partner with other reputable organizations with supporting guidelines (e.g. federal or state governments, medical societies or associations). The various partners could work in tandem to send consistent information to consumers using individual and/or joint brands. Presumably, this would increase the likelihood that consumers would become aware of the messages and they could build on each other. Jointly-branded messages, for example, may go a long way towards promoting behavior change by building awareness, increasing loyalty and reinforcing the message. This process helps to redefine the public health product by conveying its widespread support and building relationships across key organizations that influence people's healthcare behaviors. Bringing more and different partners and collaborators together has been specifically identified as a way that branding can contribute to social marketing (McDivitt 2003).

Partnerships, especially with private sector partners, are also likely to bring additional financial resources to underfunded public health programs. This could simultaneously address a potential concern about spending resources on branding and developing relationships with one's market when social marketing campaigns generally do not have the resources to address basic activities (McDivitt 2003). It is important that all parties involved be honest and upfront about their goals and objectives (Lefebvre 2006).

References

Andreasen, A. (1995). *Marketing social change*. San Francisco, CA: Jossey-Bass.

Andreason, A. (2001). *Ethics in social marketing*. Washington, DC: Georgetown University Press.

Andreason, A. (2003). The life trajectory of social marketing. *Marketing Theory* 3:293–303.

Bailey, D., Beskow, L., Davis, A., and Skinner, D. (2006). Changing perspectives on the benefits of newborn screening. *Mental Retardation and Developmental Disabilities Research Reviews* **12**:270–9.

Bekker, H. (2003). Genetic testing: facilitating informed choices. *Encyclopedia of the Human Genome*.

Briss, P. A., Zaza, S., Pappaioanou, M., *et al.* (2000). Developing an evidence-based guide to community preventive services – methods. The Task Force on Community Preventive Services. *American Journal of Preventive Medicine* **18**(S1):35–43.

Briss, P., Rimer, B., Reilley, B., *et al.* (2004). Promoting informed decisions about cancer screening in communities and healthcare systems. *American Journal of Preventive Medicine* **26**:67–80.

Burdine, J. N., McLeroy, K. B., and Gottlieb, N. H. (1987). Ethical dilemmas in health promotion: an introduction. *Health Education Quarterly* **14**:7–9.

Burger, J., Gochfelf, M., Jeitner, C., Burke, S., Stamm, T. (2007). Metal levels in flathead sole (*Hippoglossoides elassodon*) and great sculpin (*Myoxocephalus polyacanthocephalus*) from Adak Island, Alaska: potential risk to predators and fishermen. *Chemosphere* **103**:62–9.

Chaloupka, F. J. (2003) Contextual factors and youth tobacco use: policy linkages. *Addiction* **98**(S1):147–50.

Cohen, J. T., Bellinger, D. C., Connor, W. E., Kris-Etherton, P. M., Lawrence, R. S., Savitz, D. A., *et al.* (2005). A quantitative risk–benefit analysis of changes in population fish consumption. *American Journal of Preventive Medicine* **29**:325–34.

Cohen, J. T., Bellinger, D. C., and Shaywitz, B. A. (2005). A quantitative analysis of prenatal methyl mercury exposure and cognitive development. *American Journal of Preventive Medicine* **29**:353–65.

Driscoll, D. and Harris-Kojetin, L. (2002). *Final patient messages for prostate-specific antigen (PSA) screening for prostate cancer. Medicare screening messages project*. Research Triangle Park, NC: RTI International.

Edwards, A., Unigwe, S., Elwy, G., Hood, K (2003). Effects of communicating individual risks in screening programs: Cochrane Systematic Review. *British Medical Journal* **327**:703–9.

Evans, D. and McCormack, L. (forthcoming). Applying social marketing in health care: communicating evidence to change consumer behavior. *Medical Decision Making*.

Evans, D., S. Price, and S. Blahut (2005). Evaluating the truth® brand. *Journal of Health Communication* **10**:181–92.

Evans, W. D., Price, S., Blahut, S., Hersey, J., Niederdeppe, J., and Ray, S. (2004). Social imagery, tobacco independence, and the truth® campaign. *Journal of Health Communication* **9**:425–41.

Faden, R. R. (1987). Ethical issues in government sponsored public health campaigns. *Health Education Quarterly* **14**:227–37.

Feighery, E., Altman, D. G., and Shaffer, G. (1991). The effects of combining education and enforcement to reduce tobacco sales to minors. A study of four northern California communities. *Journal of the American Medical Association* **266**:3168–71.

Flores, A. L., Prue, C. E., and Daniel, K. L. (2007). Broadcasting behavior change: a comparison of the effectiveness of paid and unpaid media to increase folic acid awareness, knowledge, and consumption among Hispanic women of childbearing age. *Health Promotion Practice* **8**:145–53.

Fox, K. F. A. and Kotler, P. (1980). The marketing of social causes: the first 10 years. *Journal of Marketing* **44**:24–33.

Glanz, K., Rimer, B. K., and Lewis, F. M. (eds.). (2003). *Health behavior and health education: theory, research, and practice*. San Francisco, CA: Jossey-Bass.

Grier, S., and Bryant, C. (2005). Social marketing in public health. *Annual Review of Public Health* **26**:319–39.

Gudykunst, W. B. and Mody, B. (2002). *Handbook of international and intercultural communication* (2nd edn). Thousand Oaks, CA: Sage.

Guttman, N. (2003). Ethics in health communication interventions. In T. Thompson *et al.* (eds.) *Handbook in health communication*. Mahwah, NJ: Lawrence Erlbaum Associates.

Hill, D., Marks, R., and Borland, R. (2002). Changes in sun-related attitudes and behaviors, and reduced sunburn prevalence in a population at high risk of melanoma. In R. Hornik (ed.) *Public health communication: evidence for behavior change*. Mahwah, NJ: Lawrence Erlbaum Associates.

Institute of Medicine (IOM). (2006). Seafood choices: balancing benefits and risks. Available at: http://www.nap.edu/catalog/11762.html (accessed 19 October 2007).

Kahn, E. B., Ramsey, L. T., Brownson, R. C., Heath, G. W., Howze, E. H., Powell, K. E., *et al.*, and the Task Force on Community Preventive Services. (2002). The effectiveness of interventions to increase physical activity: a systematic review. *American Journal of Preventive Medicine* **22**(4S):73–105.

König, A., Bouzan, C., Cohen, J. T., Connor, W. E., Kris-Etherton, P. M., Gray, G. M., *et al.* (2005). A quantitative analysis of fish consumption and coronary heart disease mortality. *American Journal of Preventive Medicine*, **29**:335–46.

Kotler, P., Roberto, N., and Lee, N. (2002). *Social marketing: Improving the quality of life* (2nd edn). Thousand Oaks, CA: Sage.

Lefebvre, C. (2006). Partnerships for social marketing programs: an example from the Bone Health Campaign. *Social Marketing Quarterly* **12**:41–54.

McCormack, L., Williams-Piehota, P., Burton, J., O'Toole, M., Bann, C., Karns, S., *et al.* (2007a). Physical activity levels among those in diabetes self-management demonstration programs. [under review].

McCormack, L., Treiman, K., Bann, C., Williams-Piehota, P., Driscoll, D., Poehlman, J., *et al.* (2007b). Decision making about PSA screening: effects of a community-based intervention. [under review].

McCormack, L., Bann, C., Williams-Piehota, P., Driscoll, D., Soloe, C., Poehlman, J., *et al.* (2007c). Communication message strategies for increasing knowledge about prostate cancer screening. [under review].

McDermott, L., Stead, M., and Hastings, G. (2005). What is and what is not social marketing: the challenge of reviewing the evidence. *Journal of Marketing Management* **21**:545–53.

McDivitt, J. (2003). Is there a role for branding in social marketing? *Social Marketing Quarterly* **9**:11–17.

McGuire, W. J. (2001). Input and output variables currently promising for constructing persuasive communications. In R. Rice and C. Atkin, C. (eds). *Public communication campaigns* (3rd edn).

MMWR Weekly. (2007) Prevalence of Heart Disease – United States 2005. *MMWR Weekly* **56**(6):113–18.

Mullen, P. D., Allen, J. D., Glanz, K., *et al.* (2006). Measures used in studies of informed decision making about cancer screening: a systematic review. *Annals of Behavioral Medicine* **32**:188–201.

Nelson, D., Woodward, J., Brownson, R., Remington, P., and Parventa, C. (2002). Future directions. In D. Nelson, *et al.* (eds.), *Communicating public health information effectively: a guide for practitioners*. City, State: American Public Health Association.

Palmgreen, P., Donahew, L., Lorch, E., Hoyle, R., and Stephenson, M. (2002). Television campaigns and sensation seeking targeting time series approach. In R. Hornik (ed.) *Public health communication: evidence for behavior change*. Mahwah, NJ: Lawrence Erlbaum Associates.

Public Health Leadership Society. (2002). Principles of the ethical practice of public health, Version 2.2. Available at: http://www.apha.org/programs/education/progeduethicalguidelines.htm.

Rittell, H. W. J. and Webber, M. M. (1973). Dilemmas in a general theory of planning. *Policy Sciences* **4**:155–69.

Rothschild, M. L. (1999). Carrots, sticks and promises: a conceptual framework for the behavior management of public health and social issues. *Journal of Marketing* **63**:24–37.

Siegal, M., and Lotenberg, L. (2007). *Marketing public health: Strategies to promote social change*. Sudbury: Jones and Barlett Publishers.

Stokols, D., Allen, J., and Bellingham, R. L. (1996). The social ecology of health promotion: implications for research and practice. *American Journal of Health Promotion* **10**:247–51.

Schwartz, L. M., Woloshin, S., Fowler, F. J., Jr., and Welch, H. G. 2004 Enthusiasm for cancer screening in the United States. *Journal of the American Medical Association* **291**:71–8.

Teutsch, S. M. and Cohen, J. T. (2005). Health trade-offs from policies to alter fish consumption. *American Journal of Preventive Medicine* 29:324.

US Department of Health and Human Services. (2000). *Healthy People 2010. Volume 1: Understanding and improving health* (2nd edn). Washington, DC: US Government Printing Office.

US Department of Health and Human Services, Agency for Healthcare Research and Quality. (2006). Effectiveness of noninvasive diagnostic tests for breast abnormalities. Available at: http://effectivehealthcare.ahrq.org/reports/topic.cfm?topic=2&sid=32&rType=4&sType=2#2 (accessed 10 December 2007).

US Department of Health and Human Services, Agency for Healthcare Research and Quality. (2007). Choosing antidepressants for adults. Available at: http://effectivehealthcare.ahrq.org/reports/topic.cfm?topic=8&sid=39&rType=9 (accessed 10 December 2007).

US Environmental Protection Agency (EPA). (2004). *What you need to know about mercury in fish and shellfish*. Available at: http://www.epa.gov/waterscience/fishadvice/advice.html (accessed 19 October 2007).

Watson, M. (2006). Current status of newborn screening: decision making about the conditions to include in screening programs. *Mental Retardation and Developmental Disabilities Research Reviews* 12:230–5.

Wellings, K. (2001). Evaluating AIDS public education in Europe. In R. Hornik (ed.) *Public health communication: evidence for behavior change*. Mahwah, NJ: Lawrence Erlbaum Associates.

Wong, F., Huhman, M., Heitzler, C., Asbury, L., Bretthauer-Mueller, R., McCarthy, S., *et al.* (2004). VERB(tm) – a social marketing campaign to increase physical activity among youth. *Preventing Chronic Disease* 1. Available at: http://www.cdc.gov/pcd/issues/2004/jul/04_0043.htm (accessed 19 October 2007).

15

Future directions for public health branding

W. Douglas Evans and Gerard Hastings

Summary

◆ Public health branding has existed for as long as social marketing, but has only recently been effectively harnessed and applied.

◆ Lessons from successful branding efforts in HIV, tobacco control and nutrition/physical activity can be used in other health domains.

◆ Promising new domains for public health branding include healthcare (prescribers and consumers) and children's media use, among other health risk behaviors.

◆ More branded messages, use of new media and technologies, and research in this area are needed.

Introduction

Brands have been a part of social marketing from its early days. Public service campaigns in the 1960s and 1970s, such as Smokey and Bear and McGruff the Crime Dog, are examples of branded characters used in fire and crime prevention campaigns. But the *strategic* use of brands and branding in public health, based on behavioral theory, to change specific knowledge, attitudes and health behaviors is a relatively new approach. As discussed throughout this volume, brands and branding have only recently joined the public health lexicon.

The strategic use of brands to promote healthy behaviors and prevent risk behaviors has significant promise in public health because, very often, multiple behaviors need to be changed and maintained in order to have lasting health outcome benefits. Brands have potential to embody multiple behaviors and behavior change messages. As many health behaviors are complex, health behavior change is often more difficult than affecting consumer choice, thus making the development of improved branding strategies a critical objective for public health in order to prevent and control morbidity and mortality. This chapter focuses on how we can develop more and better public health brands in the future.

Our competitive position

As an integral part of social marketing, brands and brand managers inherit both the challenges and opportunities of the field. In particular, public health brands live with a familiar elephant in the room: bigger and stronger competition. Compared with commercial marketers, we have smaller budgets, less time and space to promote our brands, and operate in an environment surrounded by intense promotion of competing messages and behavioral alternatives.

The competition can be direct or indirect. Oppositional brands, such as *truth* and other tobacco countermarketing campigns, face commercial brands head on. But their direct competition, such as the tobacco industry, has longstanding, well-funded promotional campaigns, sophisticated pricing and placement strategies, and widely recognized products. Other public health brands, such as community-based and culturally-specific efforts, and many efforts in developing world contexts, face numerous forms of indirect competition. This may be in terms of accessibility of channels, social influences, and cultural norms that act as barriers to the behavior change promoted by the public health brand, such as *loveLife* or *Suami SIAGA*, as Evans and Haider discuss in Chapter 11.

The problem is one of exposure, and of winning market share conceived as reaching and occupying space in the minds and lives of audiences, and taking space away from the competition. Ultimately, the problem is our ability (or inability) to create conditions in the larger social and media environment that foster behavior change mediated by public health brand equity.

In this volume, we have reviewed public health brands using several different promotion strategies, including oppositional marketing, use of various cultural settings, different channels and message strategies, but each of these approaches suffers from the same malady. As Gordon *et al.* point out in Chapter 4, the competition – direct or indirect – has built-in advantages that public health cannot easily overcome.

Nevertheless, our competitive disadvantage offers several choices to social marketers and opportunities for innovation. We have advantages and opportunities in public health that can to some extent offset our disadvantages in resources and total audience exposure. Given that commercial marketers will always have bigger budgets and be on the air virtually 24/7, and public health never will, we face several fundamental questions:

- What branding strategies can public health use to beat the competition?
- How can brands be used strategically to magnify the effects of social marketing messages?
- How can we create more effective, more audience-centered brands?
- How can we take advantage of social trends (e.g. green movement, distrust of authority) that favor us over the competition?
- How can we strategically utilize technology to our advantage?

In the following, we focus on the future of public health branding and offer some initial suggestions to answer these strategic questions. We illustrate new domains into which branding can expand, new questions to address and methods to use in branding studies, and conclude by outlining an agenda for the development of branding as a strategic component of social marketing in the future.

New domains

Areas of opportunity

As we have seen in this volume, public health brands work by building positive relationships with the audience in order to increase the value of promoted behaviors and encourage exchange in the form of health behavior adoption. One way social marketers do this is by addressing the competition. The *truth* and *VERB* campaigns developed behavioral alternatives and creative branded messaging to overcome two different kinds of competition: tobacco industry marketing and brand promotion on the one hand, and a broader social and media environment promoting physical inactivity on the other. They succeeded by offering more appealing, healthful behaviors for the audience *to do* instead of simply targeting the unhealthy behavior itself. Campaign advertisements provided behavioral alternatives to smoking (rebelling against industry manipulation, and expressing independent thinking) and to physical inactivity (making sports and exercise fun and thrilling), thereby outdoing the competition's message that its products, or alternative behaviors, were socially desirable. As noted in Chapter 1, public health branding has also had similar successes in nutrition and HIV/AIDS.

We have also seen that public health brands can address multiple levels in the social ecology, and have been used to influence 'upstream' factors as well as 'downstream' individual behavior. Social marketing in tobacco control has been used to promote policy change and legislation, leading to changes in social norms and the acceptability of smoking (Evans *et al.* 2006). As discussed in Chapter 12 of this volume, public health organizations use branding strategies to create a reputation that promotes social mobilization and influences public debate and opinion. Social marketers have a strategic choice to make in terms of which level(s) of the social ecology to address, given limited resources and competition for public attention.

New domains for public health branding should be chosen with an eye to which topics and levels of social ecology appear susceptible to strategies demonstrated successful by earlier brands. That is, topics of major social impact for which there are also readily 'brand-able' healthful behavioral alternatives, and for which there is a clear opportunity for brand promotion, should be our target. In the following, we suggest two examples that appear to meet these broad criteria and discuss the opportunity to build new brands.

Children's media use

Children's media use in the developed world is at record high levels. In the USA, data from the Kaiser Family Foundation show that 8–18-year-olds in 2004 reported an average of 7.5 hours of daily electronic media (e.g. TV, internet, music) exposure (including multitasking with more than one media source) in just over 5.75 hours of media use (Roberts and Foehr 2008). In other words, some form of media use occupies the vast majority of these children and adolescents' free time. Greater media use has also been associated with negative health outcomes, such as poor nutritional habits, physical inactivity and obesity (Robinson 1999). Recent research has suggested that the *content* of media may be associated with these negative health effects, but more research is needed in this area (Fitzgibbon *et al.* 2007).

Given the ubiquity of media use, its influence on children's lives, and health implications, it appears to be an excellent candidate for a future branded campaign targeting parents of children and adolescents, and possibly a campaign aimed at children themselves. The goals of such a campaign could be based on lessons learned from previous campaigns in tobacco use and physical activity, including modifying norms about media use, promoting parent involvement, promoting 'smart' media use as socially desirable behavior, and branding interpersonal social engagement as cool (maybe: 'virtual dating isn't even fooling around' – get it?)

A campaign called *The TV Boss* has been developed in the USA (www.thetvboss.org). This campaign can be considered an example of 'direct influence' efforts to raise parents' knowledge and build their skills to control children's television and media use. *The TV Boss* campaign is a good example of the use of branding to reduce media use and limit children's exposure to specific content. Using the major elements of public health brands outlined by Evans *et al.* (forthcoming), it seeks to develop a relationship with the target audience by depicting parents in the same situation that audience members would likely find themselves (e.g. needing to protect kids from the many negative television characters out there). The campaign models parents' concerns and shows them being strong and taking control by blocking negative content. The campaign adds value for audience members by providing them with tools and information, all built around positive norms (parental involvement and control) that tap into parents' needs with respect to their children (especially adolescents).

However, future efforts to limit children's media use and should draw on a broader set of lessons learned from branded campaigns. These include the importance of knowing the audience and targeting messages appropriately; using creative marketing and promotional strategies such as branding healthy lifestyle choices; using multiple channels to increase exposure; and addressing multiple points on the chain of influence leading to individual behavior – upstream policy and structural factors as well as community, interpersonal and individual factors.

There are several potentially fruitful avenues for future messages and campaigns. For pre-adolescent children, parents are a powerful social influence and have substantial opportunities to limit media use and marketing exposure. Social marketers should conduct formative research with parents to understand the home and family media environment, and their role in regulating children's media use. Similar research, though not aimed at designing a social marketing campaign, was conducted by Jordan *et al.* (2006) and could serve as a starting point.

Based on results of this and related research, a campaign targeting possibly two distinct groups – parents of pre-school (aged 2–5) and elementary school (aged 6–11) children – could be developed. Using lessons drawn from recent successful social marketing campaigns (e.g. aspiration to a healthy lifestyle that is portrayed as socially desirable), messages would be crafted specifically for each group with the aim of increasing knowledge of what constitutes appropriate media use (e.g. no more than two hours of screen time per day); improving awareness of the health risks of excessive media use and the potential risks of marketing exposure; and modifying parent attitudes and practices regarding children's media use. The overarching goal would be to change the social norm about media use from one of permissiveness to one of parental involvement and management of the home and family media environment.

For adolescents (aged 12–17), and potentially also a secondary audience of young adults (aged 18–24), separate formative research should be conducted on their knowledge, attitudes, beliefs and practices related to media use and how they use their time with media as compared with other pursuits, including television, music and new media. The goal of this campaign would be to *brand* limited media use as socially desirable, as the new, hip and cool way to live. Media use would not be demonized, but it would be situated in the context of a larger, socially desirable lifestyle in which television, the internet and devices are part of a wider array of pursuits (e.g. living a physically active, outgoing, socially engaged lifestyle). Messages would be aimed at changing social norms about media use (e.g. consciousness of limitations of multi-tasking, value of interpersonal interaction in balance with human–media interaction). Advertising to promote the brand would use social modeling (e.g. portrayals of hip, edgy, cool kids as using media in moderation, or balancing media use and multi-tasking with popularity among peers and direct (not online) social interaction as desired goals. For example: 'Media use – it's cool but don't let it rule (your life)'.

A number of innovative strategies that are currently in development may be useful for social marketing in future messages and campaigns:

- *Improved audience segmentation.* Market research data (like commercial marketers) could be used to identify better behavioral predictors and message strategies.
- *Tailoring.* Refined predictors could be used to develop tailored messages for very specific groups, such as adolescents that visit certain websites.
- *Co-branding with trusted brands.* Like commercial marketers, social marketers can link their branded messages to other trusted brands (e.g. co-branding a nutrition social marketing message for parents of pre-school children with the Sesame Workshop).
- *Use of technology.* Internet, handheld devices and other media frequently used by young people could be used to compete with industry using 'viral marketing' and potentially lower advertising costs.
- *Social networking.* Social marketing messages could be placed in media used by children and adolescents to network, thus taking advantage of potential social diffusion effects (e.g. through MySpace, Facebook, iPods).

While no panacea, these approaches would continue the so-far successful trends in social marketing demonstrated in tobacco control, diet and physical activity, and HIV/AIDS prevention. Specifically, they use the proven techniques of commercial marketing to compete for a larger share of children's time, attention and behavior away from the television, computer or handheld device screen.

Branding for healthcare providers and consumers

While relatively little work has been done to apply social marketing in healthcare, there is tremendous potential as the field addresses topics and utilizes behavior change strategies that are directly applicable to healthcare. Pharmaceutical companies have been very successful in developing branded direct-to-consumer and provider-oriented marketing strategies (Steinman *et al.* 2006). Indeed, many of the specific strategies used in healthcare to change consumer behavior have been proven effective in health promotion fields such as tobacco control, as well as by the 'competition', as in the effective tactics used by pharmaceutical companies in marketing drugs both to physicians and consumers, and making prescription drugs a normal part of people's lifestyles (e.g. erectile dysfunction medications).

In particular, there is evidence from five trials in different healthcare settings that using outreach visits in combination with a social marketing approach can be effective, especially when targeted at high prescribers of particular medications (Soumerari and Avorn 1990). While in-person visits are effective, they are also quite expensive. Multiple interventions have been demonstrated to be effective taking into account these evidence-based principles that do not involve in-office visits. The use of multiple types of interventions seems to be very valuable (Soumerari and Avorn 1990).

Potentially significant barriers to changing prescribing behavior may occur at a variety of social ecological levels, including structural (e.g. financial disincentives), organizational (e.g. inappropriate skill mix, lack of facilities or equipment), peer group (e.g. local standards of care not in line with desired practice), individual (e.g. knowledge, skills, information overload within busy consultations leading to acts of omission or error) and patient expectations, such as those inspired by direct-to-consumer pharmaceutical advertising (Grimshaw *et al.* 2002). These barriers may be overcome by employing approaches modeled on public health branding, such as those employed in by tobacco countermarketing and other oppositional marketing.

While there are relatively few examples of brands developed for social marketing programs in healthcare, there are lessons available from the success of pharmaceutical marketing to practitioners and consumers. As noted, pharmaceutical companies have developed and implemented effective strategies for changing practitioner behavior. These methods offer practical lessons and opportunities for social marketers seeking to change practitioner and consumer behavior. For example, Pfizer employed strategies such as using physician speakers to promote off-label use of gabapentin through continuing medical education events, advisory boards and consultant meetings at which physicians would participate in informal information-gathering that amounted to 'exploratory research' for Pfizer. These effective industry marketing tactics suggest that competing approaches utilizing the same underlying strategies – delivery of highly credible information from trusted sources – can inform prescriber and consumer knowledge and practices.

The following guidelines appear to underlie effective pharmaceutical marketing and may be useful in developing brands to influence physician and consumer behavior related to drug prescription and consumption:

- define specific behavioral alternatives (i.e. do *what* instead of prescribe or consume Cialis or Viagra?);
- identify a value proposition for the alternative behavior (i.e. why is it better than the exchange realized by prescribing or consuming Viagra?);
- use market research;
- establish credibility;
- target 'high-potential' physicians;
- involve 'opinion leaders';
- ensure two-sided communication;
- promote enactment of behavioral alternatives (i.e. how does the audience get engaged?);
- use repetition and reinforcement.

In summary, there is a solid basis to believe that branding can be an effective tool to change providers' and consumers' drug prescription and use behaviors, just as it has been in health promotion and disease prevention. The relevance of oppositional marketing suggests an opportunity to use proven strategies from tobacco control and physical activity. The evidence on social marketing suggests that its underlying principles of behavior change can be used to influence healthcare provider behavior and consumer decision making through multiple message strategies and channels. Moreover, the healthcare treatment setting in the physician's office offers an additional channel to reinforce brand promotion through mass media. As a trusted source, providers' reinforcement of branded health messages about prescription drugs or other healthcare treatment topics, could add value beyond the effects of mass communication.

New research

Research priorities

The branding review by Evans *et al.* (forthcoming) suggests that, like other public health strategies, there is reasonably good evaluation and research on public health brands. However, there are relatively few experimental or quasi-experimental studies, or studies using sophisticated branding measures or analyses of the effects of branding associations or attributes on behavior, such as have been used in advertising research (Aaker 1996; Keller 1998).

There is some question in the field of social marketing whether randomized experiments are feasible or even desirable, but overall there is a need for more rigorous study designs and there are good examples of experimental branding studies in the published literature (Evans *et al.* 2007). If our commercial counterparts use such methods, and they do (but rarely publish, for proprietary reasons), then we would be wise to use equally sophisticated methods. Moreover, the limited resources available for public health marketing suggest there is a heightened need to know which branding strategies work. A solid evidence base on branding effectiveness will raise the stature of the overall strategy in the scientific community. New research can build upon recent work in public health brand measurement to improve the effectiveness of future branding efforts.

Future research questions

Previous research on public health branding efficacy and effectiveness has shown that brand equity serves as mediator (i.e. a mechanism of behavior change) and that it can prevent health-risk behaviors and encourage adoption of alternative behaviors over time (Evans *et al.* 2005, 2007). Yet there are many questions surrounding how public health brands work, for whom, in what contexts, and for what content and behaviors? The following are some of the major questions future research should address:

◆ To what extent, and under what conditions, do brand equity effects increase as a function of exposure? In other words, to what extent is there a dose–response relationship for the exposure–brand equity relationship as demonstrated for exposure–behavior in response to social marketing campaigns?

◆ How does the relationship between public health brands and their audiences change over time? That is, how do audiences' perceptions change based on factors such as messages and social and other media influences?

◆ How well do public health brands survive fluctuating media buys and periods of low or no audience exposure?

◆ What effects do changes in social norms (e.g. nutrition fads) and other moderators such as the media and marketing environment (e.g. new technologies) have on brand equity and its mediating effects?

◆ How can social marketers improve the effectiveness of brands in maintaining adopted health behavior over time?

To answer these questions, more efficacy research (i.e. experiments in which messages are delivered and reactions measured under controlled conditions) is needed to examine specific questions about how branding works to change behavior. With ongoing internet panel studies now widespread (e.g. Knowledge Networks, Harris Interactive, and numerous market research panels in the USA and Europe), there are relatively low-cost opportunities to design experiments and expose study participants to messages and test reactions over time. Efficacy research is increasingly being used to help understand the mechanisms of behavior change and improve social marketing messages and branding (Evans *et al.* 2008). As many social marketing campaigns are implemented under conditions that make controlled experiments difficult, efficacy studies have advantages when the goal is to understand message reactions and identify underlying behavioral mechanisms.

Effectiveness research on the implementation of social marketing in healthcare would naturally follow efficacy studies. Examples from tobacco control, nutrition and physical activity, and HIV/AIDS suggest that this would entail evaluations of campaigns that utilize audience segmentation and targeted messaging, aimed at specific audiences. This suggests an opportunity to build a broad research agenda on social marketing and public health branding.

There are a number of potentially effective targeted and tailored message strategies that would naturally be subject of the proposed research agenda, including:

- target messages based on sociodemographic factors, cultural beliefs or values, psychosocial determinants or geographic location;
- personalize risk data – use stories, narratives, and anecdotes;
- use graphics and other pictorial materials to clarify messages;
- be sensitive to local norms, such as culture, speech and dress;
- use a variety of approaches, such as written, oral and electronic;
- use clear, non-technical 'plain' language appropriate to the target audience.

Conclusions

Branding is especially important in public health precisely because of challenges we face compared with the competition – lower budgets, limited exposure, time-limited campaigns, etc. The quality and effectiveness of public health brands may be even more important than in the commercial sector precisely because of these limitations. We have less margin for error because our resources are fewer. While a commercial marketer can sometimes count on sheer exposure to drive home a message through repetition and multiple channels, public health messages reach audiences less frequently and therefore must be more effective to cut through the media clutter and have a behavioral effect.

Social marketers need to 'think brand' more than ever before. Too many campaigns and promotional efforts are done without a strategic branding approach or even the building blocks of branding, such as competitive analysis or clear behavioral objectives. Branding has been around for as long as social marketing has existed, but has neither been well understood nor used strategically until recent years. This may in part be due to (1) a lack of sufficient communication and cross-fertilization between the fields of marketing and public health, and (2) the lack of training of public health professionals in marketing principles. The fields of marketing and public health need to work together more closely, and schools of public health need to embrace health marketing and focus attention on relevant training in collaboration with schools of business and marketing.

Finally, research and evaluation is needed not only to build better public brands, but also to build an evidence base and the credibility of this approach with the public health community. One challenge we face is lack of knowledge about how brands work, and how to make them work better to affect upstream social environments and organizations, and individual behaviors downstream. We can address this by engaging more researchers in branding research to answer questions such as those raised earlier.

Another challenge is the lack of appreciation in the health sciences research community for the potential of branding to impact public health. As we have seen throughout this volume, branding can make a tremendous difference at a population level in terms of reduced morbidity, mortality and healthcare costs. If used strategically, it can change our society for the better. But in order to do that, social marketers need to build the evidence base and support among their natural constituencies, including researchers. In turn, increased funding, visibility and credibility for social marketing can pave the way for real and lasting strategies to effect social change.

References

Aaker, D. (1996). *Building strong brands.* New York, NY: Simon & Schuster Inc.

Evans, W.D., Davis, K.C., Zhang, Y. (2008). Social marketing research with new media: Case Study of the Parents Speak Up National Campaign Evaluation. *Cases in Public Health Communication and Marketing* **2**:1–18.

Evans W.D., Blistein, J. Hersey, J., Renaud, J., Yaroch, A. (forthcoming). Systematic review of public health branding. *Journal of Health Communication.*

Evans, W. D., Necheles, J., Longjohn, M., and Christoffel, K. (2007). The 5-4-3-2-1 Go! intervention: social marketing strategies for nutrition. *Journal of Nutrition Education and Behavior* **39**(S1):S55–S59.

Evans, W. D., Powers, A., Hersey, J., and Renaud, J. (2006). The influence of social environment and social image on adolescent smoking. *Health Psychology* **25**:26–33.

Evans, W. D., Ulasevich, A., Stillman, F., and Viswanath, V. (2006). 'The ASSIST newspaper tracking system. In F. Stillman and W. Trochim (eds) *Evaluation of Project ASSIST: a blueprint for state-level tobacco control.* Bethesda, MD: National Cancer Institute Press. pp. 185–211.

Fitzgibbon, M., Gans, K., Evans, W. D., Viswanath, V., Johnson-Taylor, W., Krebs-Smith, S., *et al.* (2007). Communicating healthy eating: lessons learned and future directions. *Journal of Nutrition Education and Behavior* **39**(S1):S63–S71.

Grimshaw, J. M., Eccles, M. P., Walker, A. E., and Thomas, R. E. (2002). Changing physicians' behavior: what works and thoughts on getting more things to work. *Journal of Continuing Education in Health Professions* **22**:237–43.

Jordan, A., Hersey, J., McDivitt, J., and Heitzler, C. (2006) Reducing children's television-viewing time: a qualitative study of parents and their children. *Pediatrics* **118**:1303–10.

Keller, K. L. (1998). Branding perspectives on social marketing. *Advances in Consumer Research* **25**:299–302.

Roberts, D. F. and Foehr, U. G. (2008). Young people's electronic media exposure. *Future of children: media technology in the lives of children and youth.* Princeton, NJ: Princeton University Press.

Robinson, T. N. (1999). Reducing children's television viewing to prevent obesity: a randomized controlled trial. *Journal of the American Medical Association* **282**:1561–7.

Soumerai, S. B. and Avorn, J. (1990). Principles of educational outreach 'academic detailing' to improve clinical decision making. *Journal of the American Medical Association* **263**:549–56.

Steinman, M., Bero, L., Chren, M., and Lord Field, C.S. (2006). The promotion of Gabapentin: An analysis of internal industry documents. *Annals of Internal Medicine* **145**:284–93.

Index